"I have always admired Dr. Agatston's contributions in the areas of healthy nutrition and heart attack prevention. He and I share a concern about the obesity epidemic and a passion for helping people achieve better health. Dr. Agatston's approach to healthy eating is flexible and friendly—it really fits into a busy, active life, like mine! Being a former world-class athlete and fitness advocate, I know the building blocks to a healthy life."

— **Dara Torres,** 12-time Olympic medalist, 5-time Olympian, mother, *New York Times* best-selling author, and fitness entrepreneur

"Dr. Agatston has worked for decades to help our communities improve their health, in South Beach and beyond. His diet not only helps people lose weight, but also helps prevent disease and leads to better health overall. I know firsthand how this diet can help you feel better and give you the energy to live your life and pursue your goals."

— **Philip Levine,** Former Mayor of Miami Beach

"Dr. Agatston is a man with a Midas touch, a pioneer in preventive cardiology and medicine. His breakthrough work on identifying early deposition of atherosclerosis has revolutionized how we prevent heart disease. In this fascinating book, Dr. Agatston takes us on a whirlwind tour exploring the complicated mechanisms and consequences of our dietary choices. Our current diet and related obesity are the leading cause for risk of heart disease. What do we do about it? Dr. Agatston, a leading preventive cardiology clinician and scientist, gives us the prescription for how we can detect the early signs of disease years sooner, and how we can change our health outcomes by changing our diets. I strongly recommend his book to all seeking the latest science of weight loss in an easy-to-follow plan that will help people like me achieve a healthy weight, enjoy better health, and ultimately reduce the risk of the number one killer disease in the U.S.: heart disease."

— **Khurram Nasir, M.D., M.P.H., M.Sc.,** Chief, Division of Cardiovascular Prevention and Wellness, Houston Methodist, and Adjunct Associate Professor of Medicine, Yale University

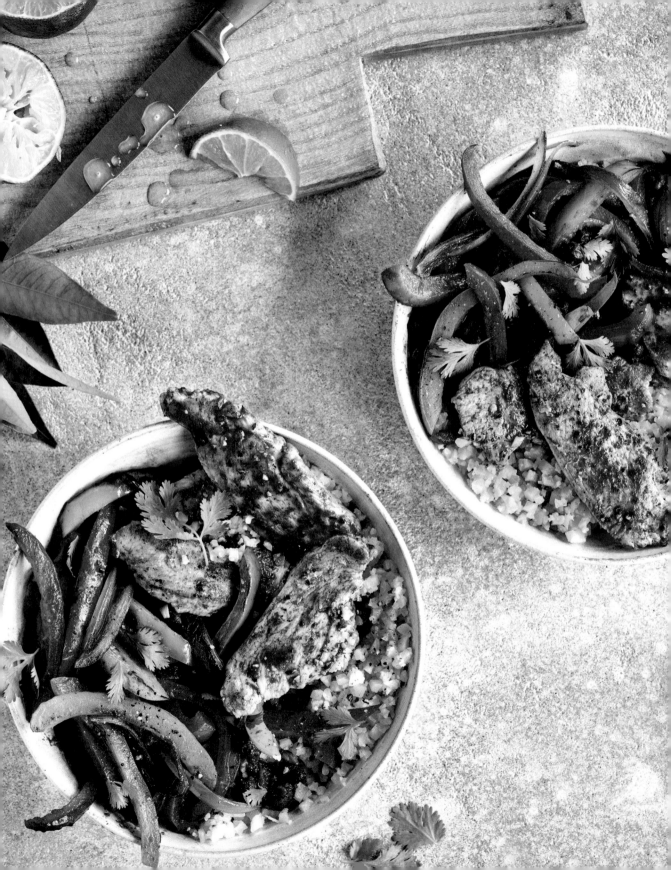

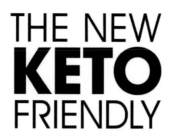

THE NEW
KETO
FRIENDLY

SOUTH
BEACH
DIET

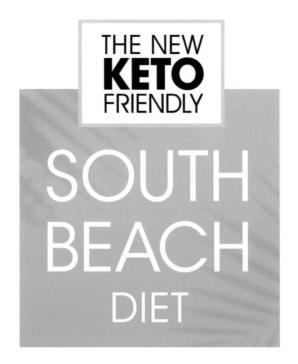

THE NEW KETO FRIENDLY

SOUTH BEACH DIET

Rev Your Metabolism and Improve Your Health
with the Latest Science of Weight Loss

ARTHUR AGATSTON, M.D.

with Judi Woolger, M.D.

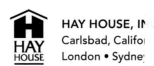

HAY HOUSE, INC
Carlsbad, Califor
London • Sydney

Published in the United States by: Hay House, Inc.: www.hayhouse.com® • **Published in Australia by:** Hay House Australia Pty. Ltd.: www.hayhouse.com.au • **Published in the United Kingdom by:** Hay House UK, Ltd.: www.hayhouse.co.uk • **Published in India by:** Hay House Publishers India: www.hayhouse.co.in

Indexer: J S Editorial, LLC
Cover design: Julie Davison and Chris MacDonald
Interior design: Julie Davison
Interior photos: Photos on pages 193, 196, 216, 217, and 245 used under license from Shutterstock.com

Cataloging-in-Publication Data is on file at the Library of Congress

Hardcover ISBN: 978-1-4019-5917-3
E-book ISBN: 978-1-4019-5918-0
Audiobook ISBN: 978-1-4019-59371

10 9 8 7 6 5 4 3 2 1
1st edition, December 2019

Printed in the United States of America

SUSTAINABLE FORESTRY INITIATIVE
Certified Chain of Custody
Promoting Sustainable Forestry
www.sfiprogram.org
SFI-01268
SFI label applies to the text stock

My wife and invaluable partner

in this project and I dedicate this book

to our new granddaughter, Ellie.

CONTENTS

INTRODUCTION

Dear Reader:

Almost 20 years ago, *The South Beach Diet* helped revolutionize the nutrition world with a plan that focused on good carbs, good fats, and healthy proteins. It helped people "lose belly fat first" while improving their health and encouraging habits to prevent diabetes and heart attacks. The science behind the diet was solid, and its principles have stood the test of time. But nutrition and medical science have continued to progress rapidly. In our clinical practice, my colleagues and I have integrated new information into our diet strategy with great success.

While we have learned a great deal, there are still many nutrition myths that persist in the popular culture and even in much of the medical community. The list of those myths is pretty long, but let me tease you with a few advances that you'll learn about in this book:

- Insulin resistance is the core nutritional problem in America and the world today, and it starts many years before it is usually diagnosed.

- For many of us, addiction to sugar appears to be a major factor in the development of insulin resistance.

- Sugar, particularly its fructose component, is akin to a slow-acting poison in the quantities we are consuming today.

- The dangerous consequences of our excess sugar and refined carbohydrate diets begin years before our blood sugars become abnormal, a stage I have come to call "pre-prediabetes."

- During this period of pre-prediabetes, you are likely already developing a fatty liver and arteriosclerosis in your arteries, but you don't know it because the symptoms have not yet appeared.

- Animal and plant saturated fats do not have adverse effects on your cholesterol levels, nor do they increase your risk of heart attack or stroke.

- Dairy fat is healthy fat.

- Omega-6 vegetable oils, in the quantities consumed by Americans, are not healthy fats, even when not hydrogenated.

- Omega-3 fish oils are important for good health (and we will make sure you learn how to reap their benefits).

- In America, protein consumption decreases with age, contributing to loss of muscle and bone mass. This in turn leads to physical limitations associated with aging. This can be prevented by maintaining a healthy protein intake along with regular exercise.

- Intermittent fasting can be a useful tool to break sugar addiction, jump-start your diet when you transgress or hit a plateau, and maintain a healthy lifestyle long term.

- Low-sodium (salt) diets are unhealthy for some people and it is important to know how your own body responds to salt.

- Fruits and vegetables should not be lumped together in nutrition recommendations. Many fruits are high in fructose and can be diet busters.

- Full ketosis can be an effective way to lose weight and reverse diabetes, but this strategy should be initiated under a doctor's supervision. A keto-friendly approach is effective, sustainable, and preferable for most people.

This book—the updated, "keto-friendly" South Beach Diet—is based on the same core South Beach Diet principles, enhanced with the latest nutrition advances. While some of the science is complicated, the plan itself is simple.

I'm excited to share this book with you because this new approach gives you the benefits of a keto diet in a lifestyle-friendly way. With its flexibility and highly satisfying foods, the Keto-Friendly South Beach Diet is easy to start and easy to stick with over time. You will lose weight, get healthier, and feel better, and these principles will become an easy-to-maintain lifestyle.

I wish you the best of luck on your journey to good health.

Arthur Agatston, M.D.

PART I

UNDERSTANDING THE KETO-FRIENDLY SOUTH BEACH DIET

CHAPTER 1

THE STORY OF THE SOUTH BEACH DIET

What if I told you that there's a good chance you're addicted to sugar? And I don't mean that you just can't resist a nice slice of chocolate cake when it's put in front of you. I mean truly, physiologically addicted to the point where you're sneaking snacks behind your family's back? At least, that was the case with me. And it led me to gain weight while supposedly on my own diet! And sugar addiction was only half the story.

This revelation about sugar addiction started me on a journey that led to some surprising discoveries and "aha" moments that helped connect the dots on important new advances in the science of weight loss. I incorporated these into my own diet, and then that of my patients. The result was a new diet plan that focuses on more efficient fat burning in an easier-to-stick-to plan, among other things—all summarized here in *The New Keto-Friendly*

South Beach Diet. But first, the story of the series of events that led me here.

THE SOUTH BEACH DIET

You may know me as the doctor who created *The South Beach Diet*, a book published back in 2003 during the era of the low-carb Atkins and the low-fat Ornish diets. But the South Beach Diet was different. It wasn't simply low carb, and it definitely wasn't low fat. It was a diet focused on healthy carbs and healthy fats. It encouraged normal-sized portions of meat, lots of vegetables, and good fats from foods such as fish, olive oil, and nuts.

The original South Beach Diet was divided into three phases. The first phase required giving up sugar, bread, pasta, potatoes, baked goods, alcohol, and fruit—all foods that quickly break down into simple sugars and cause surges in blood sugar (glucose) and insulin. This initial phase was the diet's most critical. It was designed to control your insulin levels, get rid of your sugar and carbohydrate cravings, and to burn fat. It was, even then, what we now call very keto friendly. And it worked.

On Phase 1 people lost weight quickly and their belly fat was the first to go. In the more lenient Phase 2 that started two weeks after Phase 1, you gradually and selectively added low-glycemic whole grains and whole fruits into your diet and you stayed on Phase 2 until you reached your weight-loss goal. Phase 3 was the maintenance phase.

> # Many of our South Beach Dieters wanted to stay on Phase 1 for longer than the prescribed two weeks.

Because I had experienced the same cravings as many of my patients, I became the first official South Beach Dieter. I had great success, but I observed something important early on: many of our South Beach Dieters wanted to stay on Phase 1 for longer than the prescribed two weeks. We initially thought this was driven primarily by a desire to continue the faster Phase 1 weight loss, but these lovers of Phase 1 reported that it wasn't really just about quicker weight loss. They reported that when they cut out carbohydrates, they felt wonderful. They noticed that many of their health issues, such as brain fog, migraine headaches, irritable bowel symptoms, arthritic pains, and skin conditions

like acne and psoriasis, went away. This was a welcome and unexpected surprise. For many, Phase 2 ultimately seemed like a path back to their old dietary habits, with the weight and chronic health issues returning.

CONFESSIONS OF AN OVERWEIGHT "DIET" DOCTOR

Over the next few years, I realized that I had a very similar experience. When I was on Phase 1 of the South Beach Diet, I would lose my cravings and feel fantastic, but once I moved on to Phase 2 and added back whole grains and fruits, I would eventually "cheat"—on my own diet. In times of stress, during the holidays, or when traveling, I would inevitably consume the wrong carbs—usually something with sugar— and suddenly things would spin out of control. When I allowed myself a chocolate chip cookie (I was already an admitted chocoholic), I didn't stop at just one or two, but kept going until there weren't any left.

It wasn't just grains. I also found cantaloupe to be a "diet buster" for me. Even though I had written extensively about insulin resistance and swings in blood sugar, I thought this behavior was due to a lack of discipline. My cravings were under control after two weeks on Phase 1, so why couldn't I eat a half of a cookie? I got pretty frustrated at my poor self-control, along with the return of my belly!

Then, in the summer of 2018, a series of events changed my life and the trajectory of the South Beach Diet. It started with an incident that was, frankly, not uncommon. While on vacation with my wife and two sons, I enjoyed a typical healthy dinner of salmon and roasted broccoli. But dessert was not so healthy. After dinner, my older son warmed up a blueberry pie from our favorite local farm stand. I dug right in and was wolfing it down when I heard my wife say, "Arthur, slow down." My younger son added, "Come on, Dad." I heeded their kind interventions, said okay, and paused to catch my breath.

But after dinner, once the coast was clear, I surreptitiously returned to the kitchen and finished the whole pie. Not just what was left on my plate, but what was left of the *entire pie*. And all the while, I was telling myself that blueberries were, after all, good for me. Brilliant!

MY "AHA" MOMENT

Then things changed. Over summer vacations, I have always enjoyed catching up on my reading, including medical literature and books that I did not have time to absorb during the year. One topic I focused on that summer was developments in neuroscience, which were moving especially fast thanks to the advances in functional magnetic resonance imaging, or functional MRI. With this advanced imaging technology, it was possible to see (in real time) areas in the brain lighting up in response to certain thoughts and activities, such as practicing mindfulness or learning a new physical skill like juggling.

It was just around the time of my blueberry pie incident that I read *The Hacking of the American Mind,* by a famous sugar researcher and low-sugar advocate, Dr. Robert H. Lustig. His book explained the causes of addiction in general and sugar addiction in particular. I

learned that research using functional MRI had demonstrated that addiction to sugar was real. When individuals like me were exposed to a favorite sugar-laden food, such as blueberry pie, the same area of the brain lit up and the same metabolic pathways were stimulated as when people who are addicted to alcohol or tobacco are smoking or drinking. Sugar addiction, I realized, was very real and a big contributor to obesity, diabetes, and probably the majority of the chronic conditions associated with the Standard American Diet, what we refer to as SAD.

In my work creating the original South Beach Diet, I was focused on how eating too many refined carbohydrates and sugars raised insulin levels, causing cravings and wreaking havoc on our metabolism. Now, I realized that insulin resistance and sugar addiction combined to create a powerful force: a double whammy that results in feeling out of control and overeating while, ironically, leaving you feeling hungry despite your oversized meals and snacks.

As I continued digging deeper into the importance of sugar addiction, it also became clear that my own addiction had started in my teens and early twenties, when I was super slim with absolutely normal blood sugars. I found new studies demonstrating that the great majority of overweight teenagers and young adults (many like me who were thin), already had metabolic problems that were not being detected on routine blood testing. The real cause of their problems was being missed. This heightened my alarm about the dangers of sugar addiction and the negative effects of elevated insulin—effects that most often go undetected for years, even decades.

I also recognized that my personal failures on Phase 2 of the South Beach Diet and my sneaky late-night trips to the kitchen were unmistakable signs that I was dealing with both insulin resistance and a true sugar addiction. I realized that even though my cravings had subsided after two weeks on Phase I, my addiction hadn't. I was unable to stop eating after a small slice of pie. It wasn't a lack of discipline or willpower. It wasn't my fault. If your experience is similar, it's not your fault either.

This may seem like bad news, but it's actually quite empowering. When you understand that the reason you keep falling off the diet wagon has nothing to do with a character flaw, it becomes much easier to change your behavior. You are not weak or undisciplined. You are most likely insulin resistant and addicted to sugar. The good news is that with our current knowledge, these challenges can be conquered.

PATIENT STORY

Anna W.: No More Sugar Addiction

Our patient Anna W., a 60-year-old accountant, was frustrated by her high blood pressure, anxiety, and depression. In addition to being overweight, she had excess fat in her liver (known as "fatty liver"). While Anna was changing in an exam room, our nurse came into my office with her chart and said, *"Oh my gosh. This poor woman is sobbing and hysterical."* Sure enough, Anna was sobbing. She told us she couldn't function at work. She sat at her desk, eating constantly. She had given up smoking 20 years before but had substituted eating as her new addiction. She was eating anything sweet she could find. She was stressed about work and caring for her 90-year-old mother and 16-year-old daughter. She wasn't sleeping. Her weight on that day was 204 pounds.

After two hours of conversation, she calmed down and agreed that something needed to change. After speaking with Anna, the nutritionist called me and said she had never counseled anyone so attached to sugar and so afraid to let go of it. Nonetheless, Anna acquiesced to our plan.

The first days were difficult; Anna needed constant emotional support. But, after a week, something happened that she did not expect; she actually felt better. She could think clearly and have a conversation without crying. She missed sugar, but it was no longer a deep craving. Several months later, Anna weighed in at 158 pounds. Now she walks every weekend and tries to fit in some weekday exercise. She got a promotion at work. Yes, Anna still has stressors, but she is coping much better. With no crying, no chronic anxiety, and less fear, her blood pressure is down and her head is clear.

THE NEW KETO-FRIENDLY
SOUTH BEACH DIET IS BORN

For the record, when I was surreptitiously shoving forkfuls of blueberry pie into my mouth, I knew very well that I was getting a much larger dose of sugar than I would get from eating a handful of blueberries. I was simply in denial and trying to justify my behavior. This makes sense to me now, since denial is a characteristic of addiction. But what I learned that summer elevated my concern about the danger of sugar addiction in addition to the impact of high-glycemic carbohydrates on our health. This convinced me that it was time to share my new insights in an updated South Beach Diet.

But back to my experience in the summer of 2018. I set August 1 as my "D-Day" to return to the fat burning and keto-friendly Phase 1 of the South Beach Diet . . . forever if necessary, not just for two weeks. I also added full-fat dairy to the diet, based on a mountain of new medical studies. I was excited to jump into Phase 1 again because, with my new knowledge, I was convinced that what had always sabotaged my good intentions was hormonally driven. Now that I better understood what was happening, I felt I could overcome it; and I have.

I quickly lost my cravings, as I always had on Phase 1. With great optimism, I continued on Phase 1 beyond the originally prescribed two weeks and was feeling great. My first big challenge came during an early fall trip to visit my cousin Susie, in State College, Pennsylvania, for a Penn State football game. This had become an annual adventure, and in rushing to get there, I forgot that Susie (who is a fabulous baker) traditionally greeted us with freshly baked brownies. On past visits, I would make a

disclaimer that, while I shouldn't be eating such high-sugar and -starch goodies, in deference to her efforts I would have just one. In no time, I would be on my way to finishing the whole plate. But this time, I was feeling so great on my extended Phase 1 (already having lost much of my belly fat), that I didn't want to take a chance of sliding backward. Also, I did not experience my usual cravings. So I declined her offer and, in my mind at least, quite rudely passed on the brownie component of my cousin's hospitality.

From that time on, I have faced parties, weddings, Thanksgiving, and the Christmas season without much difficulty and with amazingly few transgressions. I have happily found that I could have a bite of key lime pie at South Beach's Joe's Stone Crab without inhaling the whole thing. The keto-friendly extended Phase 1 was working. Even better, I realized that once I was on Phase 1 for a month, it felt easy. It was this experience and a series of "aha" moments that led me to create *The New Keto-Friendly South Beach Diet.*

BENEFITS BEYOND WEIGHT LOSS

It is important to convey that it isn't just freedom from sugar addiction and insulin-induced cravings that keeps me on track. I just feel so much better mentally and physically that I can't imagine regressing.

One initially unexpected reward I received on the new diet came when I reached the well-described stage of fat adaptation, which happens when you minimize sugars and refined carbohydrates for a period of weeks to months. The original South Beach Diet Phase 1 was not long enough to reach this point, but the new Keto-Friendly South Beach Diet is. Weight loss is a major benefit of fat adaptation, but the positives of this stage extend beyond your waist circumference. When I returned to Miami Beach after my summer vacation, I also returned to my boxing training, which I had done regularly for about five years. I train with former highly ranked professional boxer Juan Arroyo. Juan trains me vigorously for one hour, three days a week.

My first training after about six weeks on Phase 1 came at 7 A.M. on a Tuesday morning. I normally got pretty tired after a few rounds in the south Florida heat and would sit out a round or two before continuing to train. But on this hot and humid morning, I went the full hour without taking a round off. I was amazed by my endurance. I was now efficiently burning fat, and it felt great.

Since starting my new approach, I've maintained a 15- to 20-pound weight loss—almost all from my belly—with surprising ease. I feel better than ever, both mentally and physically, and after more than a year I'm confident that I will succeed in the long term, for three major reasons:

- First, I feel so good that I never want to go back. I'm more alert and energetic, and my concentration has improved. My sleep apnea has totally resolved, and I sleep well throughout the night. Feeling great is the best motivator.

- Second, I've lost my sugar addiction and completely reversed my insulin resistance. Now, I'm able to enjoy a chocolate brownie (or a slice of blueberry pie) without inhaling the entire plate.

- Third, I've found that eating this way is easy to do and easy to stick with. The food satisfies me, and the plan is simple, friendly, and flexible so it works in everyday life.

My wife has also benefitted from this new keto-friendly way of life, but in different ways. While I lost my carbohydrate cravings and sugar addiction (and my belly), my wife experienced amazing improvement in migraine headaches and joint pain, symptoms she had been dealing with for a long time. She is so happy to be free of them that she will never turn back.

WHY DIET RECOMMENDATIONS KEEP CHANGING

Now, before we jump into the nitty gritty of *The New Keto-Friendly South Beach Diet*, I want to address the fact that, over the years, diet advice has often been confusing and sometimes conflicting. I know you've probably thought at some point during your weight loss or health-seeking journey: "Can't anyone make up their minds?!" Low fat one day, high fat the next. Carbs are good for you and then they're not. Everyone advised eating low-fat or fat-free dairy, and now you're telling me to eat full-fat dairy? First, Phase 1 lasted two weeks; now it goes on for a month or longer.

It's understandable if you feel like the scientific and medical communities keep throwing you curveballs, but there are good reasons for this. The accelerating march of technology, and the integration of new information that goes along with it, allow us to more precisely understand our complicated human body. With advanced diagnostic techniques such as the functional MRI and much more sophisticated and effective cholesterol screening, we're able to reach more reliable conclusions and recommend more reliable therapies to help you stay healthy.

A major objective of this book is to help you navigate through the evolving science in health and nutrition.

As new and improved technologies are introduced, our knowledge base will only continue to grow. This new knowledge will most certainly create confusion as well. A major objective of this book is to help you navigate through the evolving science in health and nutrition so you can benefit from these technological advances and improve your own health.

I'm excited to share the revelations from my personal journey of discovery, and the experiences that we have had in our clinical practice, to help you get past any confusion.

This is not to suggest that we have all the answers. We will continue to learn and many more discoveries will be made in the future. But the good news is that we have the tools and technology to dramatically improve your health right now.

So, if you are obese, overweight, or even at a normal weight but tend to gain weight in your belly—or if you are simply not feeling the vitality you would like—this book can help. Try it for a month and see how you feel. Watch your belly melt away along with your cravings. Feel your energy levels soar. I'm confident that if you follow our guidelines, you'll find this lifestyle easier than you expect, and you will reap the same benefits that my patients, my wife, and I have. I expect that you, too, will feel better than ever and won't want to turn back.

CHAPTER 2

WHAT IS KETO FRIENDLY?

The Keto-Friendly South Beach Diet is not just low carb. It's definitely not low fat. And it's not a strict ketogenic diet.

This new approach includes the best of the original South Beach Diet (good carbs and good fats) as well as some of the best practices of the keto diet, including low carb/high "full" fat—especially dairy—and a longer initial phase to reverse sugar addiction and become "fat adapted." *And* it incorporates additional science-backed recommendations that promote fat burning and numerous health benefits such as weight loss, increased energy, mental clarity, and the resolution of insulin resistance. Unlike strict ketogenic diets, this plan does not require that you stay in ketosis—or even be in ketosis—to reap these benefits.

The keto-friendly approach offers the fat burning benefits of keto but it's easier to start, and easier to sustain as a lifestyle. The plan outlined in this book is the culmination of years of evolving science and years of applying these new concepts and discoveries in my own practice. Our patients have experienced remarkable results as they have adopted these lifestyle changes.

PUTTING KETO FRIENDLY INTO PRACTICE

Once I returned to Miami Beach after my summer of 2018 enlightenment, I continued to feel better and better on my prolonged Phase 1 eating plan. This is what pioneers in the keto diet, Drs. Stephen Phinney, Jeff Volek, and Tim Noakes recognized as "keto adaptation," but is also referred to as "fat adaptation" and it occurs on a keto-*friendly* diet as well as a keto diet.

One of the first manifestations of this phenomenon was my enhanced boxing endurance, which extended to my tennis game as well. In addition, my cravings for sweets and refined carbs seemed to disappear. When I returned to my office and socialized with friends and colleagues, I felt like the caricature of the ex-smoker who is so excited after quitting that they go around pulling cigarettes out of people's mouths. Our dietitians and my physician colleagues all bought in, and we began putting our patients on this new prolonged Phase 1 (keto-friendly) plan. I must have told my blueberry pie story a hundred times, but I never tired of relating my experience. I felt so great, I had to spread the word.

We were, and continue to be, very excited by the results our patients and friends have experienced: bellies melting away, joint and abdominal pains resolving, reports of better mental and physical prowess. Our patients tell us that when they stay on this keto-friendly diet, their appetite is greatly reduced and cravings virtually disappear. We tweaked our approach to tailor it to individual patients depending on their needs and preferences. We found intermittent fasting, popularized by Dr. Jason Fung, to be a valuable additional strategy for many of them. New research on the role of protein, especially as we age, led to further adjustments in our recommendations as well.

Along with my enthusiastic team, I continued to aggressively delve into the rapidly growing scientific literature in the nutrition and low-carb field. The discovery of what I call pre-prediabetes, via an insulin secretion test, opened up a whole new world of earlier diagnosis of insulin resistance. The insulin secretion test gave us a better tool for determining who is at risk for diabetes and chronic disease. This in turn allowed us to identify an entirely new population of patients who could most benefit from this keto-friendly diet. It also allowed us to more precisely monitor our patients' progress. We have learned a great deal from this new approach.

WHAT YOU WILL EAT

The Keto-Friendly South Beach Diet allows a higher level of carbohydrates than strict keto, but it is still solidly low carb and fat burning. It recommends higher amounts of healthy fats, including full-fat dairy, than the original South Beach Diet. It also includes more protein than strict keto diets, which is especially important as you get older, and is one of the keys to feeling satisfied after a meal. On a strict keto diet, carbohydrates are typically restricted to fewer than 5 percent of total calories, with fat providing around 75 percent and protein accounting for the remaining 20 percent. But on Phase 1 of the Keto-Friendly South Beach Diet plan, you'll get around 10 to 20 percent of your calories from carbohydrates, 55 to 65 percent from fat, and 25 to 30 percent from protein, although this is only a guide. On this plan, you will ultimately learn what works best for you.

PATIENT STORY

Alan K.: Lost His Cravings and 30 Pounds

Alan K., 72 years old, had been an acquaintance for many years. When he first came to see us, he weighed 240 pounds. We suggested he change his diet, but he was reluctant to commit. He couldn't cook, which made a modification in eating habits even more intimidating. He was very down on himself and lacked faith in his ability to succeed on a diet, which made it very hard for him to get started. In his first year as our patient, he hit a high of 315 pounds. Alan was depressed and was experiencing severe fatigue as well as profuse sweating. He was clearly insulin resistant. He also suffered with constipation and ate a bowl of fiber cereal every night in an attempt to relieve the problem. His digestive difficulties continued and he was always hungry. He tried to diet, but it didn't work.

Alan began cancelling appointments because he was embarrassed about his perceived lack of discipline. We finally convinced him to come in and talk about it because his weight gain was severely jeopardizing his health. We learned that instead of following our recommendations, he was inadvertently sabotaging his attempts at healthy dieting by following advice he remembered hearing and reading "somewhere." He was eating a high-carb cereal every night. He was hungry all the time. He was also eating a frozen "vegetable pasta" dish, thinking it was mainly vegetables rather than a white-flour pasta with a few veggies mixed in.

He blamed himself for his inability to sustain a diet, but finally agreed to follow our keto-friendly plan. He was clearly sugar addicted. We told him his hunger was not his fault; his hormones were telling him to eat! With almost daily support from our staff and the understanding that his problem was hormonal, not a lack of discipline, things turned around. He began sticking to this new way of eating. His appetite was greatly reduced and he no longer felt cravings. After four months, he had lost 30 pounds. Today, his sweating issue is almost gone and his digestive symptoms have resolved. His blood pressure medications have been reduced considerably. Alan feels better than he has in years, better health-wise and better about himself.

SATIETY AND SATISFACTION

On this keto-friendly diet, you will eat lots of satisfying foods such as whole-milk yogurt, cheeses, and butter. In fact, incorporating full-fat dairy foods into your meal plan is a key to keeping you full and satisfied. You will also eat plenty of quality proteins, including a variety of meat, poultry, and seafood—another difference between keto-friendly and a strict keto diet. You won't just eat grilled chicken breast with steamed broccoli; you'll eat chicken thighs with a side of buttered snap peas, or steak with Gorgonzola cream sauce and Parmesan roasted brussels sprouts. You won't only eat hard-boiled eggs (although they are great); you'll also eat chive and prosciutto egg cups with a creamy latte. Using simple, great-tasting substitutions (replacing white flour with almond flour, or using a natural, no-sugar sweetener such as erythritol, for example), you'll even eat indulgent foods like cheesy garlic breadsticks and delicious chocolate brownies. Overall, the diet laid out for you in this book is truly friendly, in that we encourage a wider variety of foods than strict keto diets allow in order to give you the advantage of all the nutrients they contain and because we know you do not have to be in ketosis in order for it to work. With the addition of more fats and the healthy balance of vegetables and proteins, this updated South Beach Diet is satiating, satisfying, and nutritious.

> ## This diet was designed to include satisfying foods that cut cravings, fill you up, and make it easier to stick to over time.

This diet was designed to include satisfying foods that cut cravings, fill you up, and make it easier to stick to over time. We've found that this approach is easy to sustain and it works. In fact, by putting your body into fat-burning mode, it can help you to boost your metabolism and burn from around 100 to 500 more calories per day (at the same calorie consumption level) compared to high-carb, low-fat diets. But the diet's benefits are not limited to weight loss. I know firsthand it can also help improve your sleep, reduce inflammation and joint pain, increase your energy, and enhance your mental acuity while preventing diabetes and chronic disease.

ONE SIZE DOES NOT FIT ALL

It's a cliché but true: in the area of nutrition, one meal plan does not fit all. Though we give guidance in this book and in the daily meal plans, we know people have different food preferences and needs based on individual tastes, backgrounds, and medical histories. Is there diabetes in the family? Is there heart disease in the family? Have you gradually gained belly fat over the years, suggesting that you're insulin resistant? Does your weight yo-yo easily, also a sign of insulin resistance?

We prescribe simple principles that can be successfully followed with a wide variety of food choices to accommodate your needs and preferences. From carnivore to vegan, you will do well if you follow the guidelines set out in this book. Meat lover or vegetarian, keeping sugar to a minimum is rule number one!

In order to make good food choices and transform your diet into a healthy lifestyle whether you're traveling, cooking at home, or dining out, it is important to understand as much of the science behind the plan as possible. This awareness will help keep you on track no matter where you find yourself—be it a friend's birthday party, a fast food establishment, or stuck in an airport. Almost any diet that prescribes exactly what to eat at each meal can result in short-term weight loss, but it's not a lifestyle solution. When you understand the diet's principles, it can be more easily personalized to fit into your everyday life. So, while we provide you with meal plans and menu recommendations, we also explain the "why" behind the plan.

You will hear me say this many times, but it's something that I believe: in order to lose weight and improve your health, you need a plan that works for the long term in real life. This is where keto *friendly* comes in.

FAT BURNING IN KETO VERSUS KETO FRIENDLY

To fulfill our body's constant requirement for energy—whether at rest, sleeping, or exercising—we are always burning a combination of carbohydrates and fat. As we lower our carbohydrate intake, we burn more fat and less glucose from carbs. In general, the lower our carb intake, the more fat we burn. When daily carbohydrate intake goes really low (20 grams or less), and we are burning mainly fat, our livers have difficulty burning all of the fat for immediate energy and some is transformed into ketones. Ketones are molecules that enter the blood stream and can be burned for fuel primarily by brain and muscle tissues.

Investigation is continuing on the effect of ketones on brain function, inflammation, and other areas. A ketogenic diet has, for example, been of proven benefit for children with seizure disorders but we do not yet know if there are any further therapeutic benefits of reaching and sustaining ketosis. What is clear at this time is that carbohydrate intake in the range recommended in the Keto-Friendly South Beach Diet also makes you into a fat-burning machine, with the associated health benefits. One advantage

we do see with patients reaching ketosis is the ability to monitor compliance with low carbohydrate intake. This provides valuable feedback for the doctor and the patient.

The benefit of measuring ketone levels has been elegantly demonstrated by the Virta group in Indiana. Led by Drs. Sarah Hallberg, Stephen Phinney, and Jeff Volek, the group has reported excellent success at reversing even long-standing diabetes by regularly measuring ketone levels while patients were on a "well-formulated" keto diet. Their patients were carefully monitored by physicians and specially trained health care coaches.

Strict ketogenic diets, especially in patients on medications for high blood pressure or high blood sugars, should be done under the supervision of a physician who has familiarity with low carb and keto diets. We use strict keto diets for certain patients who have type 2 diabetes that may be difficult to reverse, as well as for others who are at high risk for diabetes and who do not mind the close monitoring and the blood sticks which are frequent during initiation of the ketogenic diet. But I have found with the majority of my patients that our keto-friendly, more flexible approach works just as well and is easier to adopt and sustain over time.

THE KETO-FRIENDLY APPROACH

The diet in this book falls into the category of a less strict, "keto-friendly" low-carb diet. The plan allows roughly between 20 and 50 grams of net carbs per day to start, increasing to as much as 75 to 100 grams after fat adaptation and loss of belly fat and insulin resistance. This diet does not require you to monitor ketone levels.

As you will learn, when you lower the insulin levels in your bloodstream, the resulting hormonal effect on the cells in your body allows you to essentially "unlock" your fat stores, and your belly fat melts away without being in full ketosis. This has been demonstrated in many low-carbohydrate clinical trials. In one major study, people with insulin resistance who followed a similar low-carb diet burned up to 478 more calories per day than those on a higher-carb diet—eating the same number of daily calories.

> When you lower the insulin levels in your bloodstream, the resulting hormonal effect on the cells in your body allows you to essentially "unlock" your fat stores, and your belly fat melts away.

In our practice, we have reversed diabetes and prediabetes with the original South Beach Diet, but over the past year, with the longer keto-friendly Phase 1 and our understanding of sugar addiction, our patients have found it easier to adopt this way of eating as a lifestyle. When our patients begin to experience the extra benefits of fat adaptation, as I did, there is no turning back.

KEEPING IT FRIENDLY

Some people absolutely do not want to give up their occasional glass of wine, their dish of blueberries with yogurt in the morning, or other favorites. Some of these choices could slow their rate of weight loss, but the occasional deviation will not hinder significant weight loss and improved blood chemistries over time. However, some choices can turn into what we call "diet busters," meaning they lead to more frequent lapses and can stop weight loss. In our experience, overdoing it with nuts, too much high-sugar fruit, too much dairy, and the hidden sugar in packaged foods are the most common diet busters. What reaches the threshold of a diet buster varies between individuals. When they occur early in your diet before fat adaptation, these occasional indulgences are more likely to take you off track. Later on, these occasional treats will not impact your success. We believe that for a diet to turn into a lifestyle, it needs to be something you can live with. That said, this plan does depend on your particular metabolism, your degree of insulin resistance, and your overall compliance.

A majority of Americans suffer from some degree of insulin resistance, but most can reverse this without measuring their ketones. I did.

IT RUNS IN THE FAMILY

The story of a recent typical patient illustrates the importance of looking beneath the surface of your family history. A 51-year-old gentleman came to see me because a screening test revealed calcium in his coronary arteries, a sign of early arteriosclerosis. The question was "why the coronary arteriosclerosis?" If we know the cause, we can better prevent its progression to a heart attack. He had the screening because his father had just died of a heart attack. Our patient reported his father had had a previous heart attack at age 55 and had undergone heart bypass in his mid-70s but was "not diabetic." When I asked if his father was overweight, the answer was "not really," which was an important clue.

What did he mean by "not really?" "What about a belly?" I asked. "Yeah, my dad had a bit of a belly as he got older." That meant his dad almost certainly had prediabetes or diabetes, even if undiagnosed, and it probably led to his father's coronary artery disease and ultimately to his death. It also meant that my patient was at risk too, and that insulin resistance was likely the cause of his coronary calcium. He did turn out to have evidence of insulin resistance at a stage when the keto-friendly lifestyle regimen could prevent its progression, and consequently the progression of his coronary arteriosclerosis as well. Prediabetes and even diabetes often went undiagnosed and still does. The fact that diabetes and certainly prediabetes were not diagnosed in a parent does not mean they didn't have it.

12 RULES FOR KETO-FRIENDLY EATING

So, depending on your weight, your medical history, your family history, and your own preferences, a more or less strict low-carb approach may be appropriate.

I have done very well with the Keto-Friendly South Beach Diet. It truly is a plan I can do for life. I don't have to count carbs or anything else daily, but I *do* make the right food choices and pay close attention to food labels. I review ingredients, being careful to look for things such as hidden added sugars. For me, minimizing sugar has made the difference. So, we definitely recommend limiting carbs when you get started on this plan. But you shouldn't be overburdened by counting if you follow the Foods to Enjoy List.

ARE YOU INSULIN RESISTANT?

- Have you gained weight regularly in adulthood?

- Do you carry your excess weight in your belly?

- Do you easily yo-yo when you diet?

- Do you experience cravings soon after meals?

- Do you have a family history of type 2 diabetes?

- Do you eat lots of bread, pasta, pastries, sugary snacks and drinks?

If you said yes to most of these questions, chances are you may be insulin resistant. Check with your doctor.

Once you lose your excess fat, especially from your belly, you can be more relaxed with your food choices. But if you are addicted to sugar, you need to be extremely careful. Then, even small indiscretions can become a slippery slope. You know who you are. When you have lost your cravings, have become fat adapted, and are feeling the many benefits of our approach, these occasional indulgences are more easily handled and much less likely to sabotage your diet.

All this comes back to the maxim "one size does not fit all." The key is to follow the principles laid out in this book. Once you understand the principles, you can make appropriate adjustments as you go until you find the right balance for you, one you can sustain long term as a healthy way of life. Let the 12 Rules for Keto-Friendly Eating be your guide; each of these rules will be explained in upcoming chapters. And remember: this diet is keto friendly, so shoot for following these rules most of the time, for the long term.

Don't be too hard on yourself when you don't strictly comply. You are already eating a much better diet and you cannot always reach the high bar. Just regroup and get back on track.

12 RULES FOR KETO-FRIENDLY EATING

1. Minimize sugars.

2. Strictly avoid refined carbohydrates.

3. Limit snacking.

4. Favor fewer, larger meals over frequent small meals.

5. Maximize the healthiest fats.

6. Consume full-fat dairy.

7. Limit omega-6 vegetable oils.

8. Eat a variety of non-starchy vegetables.

9. Enjoy a wide variety of meats, poultry, and seafood.

10. Eat primarily whole foods.

11. Eat slowly.

12. Be flexible.

CHAPTER 3

THE SCIENCE BEHIND THE DIET

It's All about Insulin

When I am fated to sit in an airport because I arrive compulsively early or because my plane is delayed, I find myself inadvertently conducting population research. I try not to stare, but over the years I have observed a growing number of Americans (and non-Americans) with large bellies. These protruding middles are a sure sign that they have fat in their livers and around their internal organs, also known as visceral fat. While some heavy people carry most of their excess weight in their hips and thighs, known as "pears," most overweight individuals carry their excess weight in their bellies, often while maintaining thin arms and thin legs; these people are known as "apples." My concern has always been not just about the obvious obesity epidemic but also that so many of my fellow travelers were clearly prediabetic or diabetic and didn't know it.

PRE-PREDIABETES

Many people with protruding bellies do not think of themselves as obese or even overweight, and most have no idea that their organs are already deteriorating. Without a change in diet and lifestyle, their health outlook is bleak. Although they have plenty of calories stored as fat in their bellies, these people still make beelines to the food court and return with so much to eat and drink, you'd think they were starving. Indeed, that is how they feel and now we know why.

Today, I am even more concerned about the obesity epidemic because I am convinced that all of those with bellies, even if they don't meet the current criteria for diabetes or prediabetes, are what I call "pre-prediabetics." I use that term to describe people who, although their blood sugars are still normal, are already suffering from the disease process that will eventually lead to diabetes and its associated chronic illnesses—unless they take proper action. It is likely they already have excess fat in their livers and arteriosclerosis in their arteries, and they may also be suffering from "brain fog," headaches, joint pain, dizziness, chronic fatigue, depression, anxiety, skin problems, and many other maladies. A particularly disturbing fact is that we're now seeing these early signs of trouble in teenagers, and even in elementary school–age children.

INSULIN RESISTANCE

What these pre-prediabetics and often their doctors don't appreciate is that all their varied signs and symptoms are from a *single and treatable cause*—insulin resistance. Insulin resistance is a decrease in the sensitivity of the liver, muscle, fat, and other organs to the important actions of the hormone insulin. Insulin resistance ultimately leads to progressive failure of insulin production in the pancreas. This is called "beta cell failure" since it is the beta cells of the pancreas that manufacture insulin.

While insulin resistance and beta cell failure are the two mechanisms that eventually lead to type 2 diabetes (formerly known as adult onset diabetes), their ill effects begin to impact your health about 20 years before your blood sugar is abnormal and a diagnosis of type 2 diabetes is made. Simply said, if you are chronically elevating your insulin levels by eating too many refined carbs and sugars, there's a good chance you are already insulin resistant.

To understand how the Keto-Friendly South Beach Diet can help, it's important to learn the basics of how insulin works.

WHAT EVERYBODY NEEDS TO KNOW ABOUT INSULIN

Insulin is an essential hormone you have no doubt heard of, but you may think it's not relevant unless you have diabetes. The big headline here is that *everyone* should be concerned about insulin, because the majority of Americans have an insulin problem whether they know it or not.

> Everyone should be concerned about insulin, because the majority of Americans have an insulin problem whether they know it or not.

When insulin is functioning normally, it efficiently regulates our body's use of energy which is supplied by the food we eat. Insulin is secreted into the bloodstream during and shortly after eating a meal to lower your glucose (also known as blood sugar) by moving it from your bloodstream into your tissues. Once in your tissues, the glucose is burned for immediate energy or stored as glycogen for later use. Many of you have heard of and may have experienced "hypoglycemia" (low blood sugar) when your insulin levels overshoot after a meal and lower your blood sugar to the point where you become weak, dizzy, and extremely hungry. Fat also enters your tissues with the help of insulin after a meal and, like glucose, is either burned for energy or stored for later use. Fat, however, does not raise your insulin levels nearly as much as sugar or refined carbohydrates.

Other hormones are involved but insulin is the major player for directing how we distribute, burn, and store the energy we consume as food and drink. When we eat more food than is required for our immediate energy needs, insulin signals our cells to store the extra energy for later use, when food may not be available. Our cells store fat in the form of triglycerides, and glucose in the form of glycogen. Strings of attached glucose molecules are called "starch" when found in plant foods such as potatoes, rice, and wheat, and are called "glycogen" when stored in humans and other mammals. When we need energy but are not eating, such as during periods between meals or when we sleep, it becomes necessary to access our fuel reserves of fat (triglycerides) and carbohydrates (glycogen).

GENERATING & STORING ENERGY

So, when insulin levels fall after a meal, it signals our tissues to break down our glycogen stores into glucose and our triglyceride stores into free fatty acids. Both glucose and free fatty acids are directly burned inside our cells' mitochondria, which are our body's energy generators. The mitochondria produce ATP (adenosine triphosphate) molecules from the burned glucose and free fatty acids. The ATP is directly transformed into energy in all the cells of our body, keeping our organs alive and functioning. This is how our body's energy requirements are satisfied between meals, when we are sleeping, or during longer periods without food, such as fasting or famine. Protein throughout our body can also act as a fuel reserve, especially when our glycogen stores are depleted, and our fat reserves have dropped from extended fasting or famine. But protein intake, like fat, has minimum effect on insulin levels and does not cause insulin resistance.

Insulin promotes energy storage in several ways. It stimulates enzymes that turn excess carbohydrates in our diet into glycogen for storage, but when the glycogen stores in our muscles and livers are full, insulin stimulates other enzymes in our liver to turn the remaining carbohydrates into fatty acids and then into triglycerides for storage in liver cells. This is important because carbohydrates in their storage form of glycogen can only hold enough energy reserves to last for a few days.

A NOTE FOR ATHLETES

If you happen to be a marathon runner, you know that your glycogen stores become depleted about 3 hours into a marathon. After you burn through your glycogen stores, you switch to burning fat, but unless you are "fat adapted" this is not done efficiently and you become exhausted. This phenomenon is called "hitting the wall," and is why long-distance runners have traditionally carb loaded with pasta and other starches before a race. They are loading up their glycogen stores in the hopes of delaying hitting the wall.

Today, more and more endurance athletes are eating low-carb keto or keto-friendly diets in order to become fat adapted, as I was when I returned to my boxing after six weeks of low-carb eating. These fat-adapted athletes do not hit the wall and are winning endurance events because their fat stores last throughout the race and into recovery. In fact, under normal circumstances, fat stores can hold enough energy reserves to sustain an individual for weeks with calorie-free fluid replacement alone.

WHEN INSULIN GOES INTO OVERDRIVE

Insulin levels go up during and immediately after a meal to facilitate the movement of glucose from our bloodstream into our tissues. When insulin rises, it also signals our brain that we are full and can stop eating. Then after our meal, insulin levels normally fall. But there are times when insulin levels are sustained at high levels even after meals. These persistent high levels cause our tissues to become resistant to insulin's action, a condition we already described as insulin resistance. The tissues send signals to the pancreas to produce even more insulin to overcome the insulin resistance.

When higher insulin levels do overcome the tissues' insulin resistance, it causes an exaggerated fall in blood sugar known as "reactive hypoglycemia." This stimulates more hunger for sugar and starches, which are quickly absorbed when eaten, correcting the low blood sugar. You feel temporarily better, but the sugar and starch cause a further rise in insulin, leading to a vicious cycle of big swings in blood sugar. This eventually results in constantly elevated insulin levels that put us in a continuous fat-storage mode. Even after meals, our insulin resistant brains tell us, "You are still hungry. Keep eating.

Store more fat." It's hard to imagine, but when you're insulin resistant, even though your body has enough stored fuel to survive for weeks without eating, you feel like you are starving because your high insulin levels prevent you from accessing your ample fat reserves.

> Even after meals, our insulin resistant brains tell us, "You are still hungry. Keep eating. Store more fat."

WHY WE'RE SO HUNGRY

During earlier times, when feast was inevitably followed by famine, insulin resistance and the resultant fat storage was an important survival mechanism. In summer and fall months, when food was plentiful, humans would eat more, develop insulin resistance, and go into a fat-storage mode that helped them survive the inevitable winter famine. The problem in the United States today is that we experience a constant state of feast that is never followed by famine. Too many of us remain in our insulin resistant fat-storage mode indefinitely, always hungry despite an abundance of fuel.

Our sustained high insulin levels block the enzymes that would release glucose from glycogen and free fatty acids from triglycerides, to be burned for energy and keep us satiated. This is why insulin resistant individuals are hungry all day; their insulin levels never fall other than transiently after meals, resulting in reactive hypoglycemia that causes even more hunger, exacerbating weight gain and continued insulin resistance. In this fat storage mode, we consume a lot more calories. But simply limiting calories will not work to satisfy your hunger and keep weight off for the long term if you are making the wrong food choices. So, calories count, but counting calories won't work unless you learn to choose foods wisely.

The diet and principles laid out in this book will get you off the insulin/blood sugar roller coaster by lowering your insulin levels so that you can unlock your body's own fuel stores for needed energy.

WHAT WE CAN LEARN FROM THE GRIZZLY BEAR

One of the best illustrations to help you understand the critical role of insulin in humans is a year in the life of the grizzly bear. The grizzly bear must store enough fuel, in the form of fat, during late summer and fall to supply it with energy throughout its winter hibernation. The bears accomplish this by increasing their daily intake from a few thousand calories to about 20,000 calories, which packs on about three pounds per day.

Is this radical change in behavior a conscious decision handed down via parental instructions? I don't think so. Neither is it due to supersized meals served at a local restaurant. It is, instead, hormonally driven. Scientists have been studying bear hibernation to learn more about human hormones, and their ranks do not include "bear psychologists" trying to figure out what stresses are making the grizzlies gain so much weight every summer and fall.

We do know that nature helps the grizzly bears achieve their weight gain with an annual sustained increase in their insulin levels, causing them to become insulin resistant. Continuous high insulin levels in the bears, as in humans, block the release of stored fat, so the grizzly must eat more to supply its current needs. Exaggerated insulin secretion after a feeding causes reactive hypoglycemia just as it does in humans, to generate cravings.

Normally during and after meals, higher insulin levels signal the bear to stop eating. But this hormonal reflex is not helpful if you are trying to gain hundreds of pounds in preparation for a long hibernation. The survival solution for bears before their winter sleep, and for humans before a winter famine, is persistently high insulin levels. This period of continuously high insulin overstimulates the bear's insulin brain receptors, which become much less responsive to the "stop eating" signals. This is brain insulin resistance. The grizzlies continue consuming excess calories, storing fat for the winter. This period is called "hyperphagia," a time of excessive eating due to excessive appetite. It is not from lack of stored energy, which is already substantial, and certainly not from lack of grizzly discipline. The bears are in fat-storage mode—a mode in which more and more Americans find themselves.

The next way nature aids the grizzly is through the ripening of fruit with its sweet sugar content. As the voracious grizzlies thoroughly deplete the region's trees of their sweet berries, the bear's insulin levels rise even more. This causes bigger swings in blood sugar, making the bears even more ravenous. These insulin resistant bears will climb trees to steal honey from beehives, undeterred by stinging bees. If you live in bear country, you know this is not a good time to leave out garbage or to keep seeds in bird feeders; the bears will find them. They have become addicted to sugar. After a weight gain of hundreds of pounds accompanied by an increase in blood pressure, the bears are ready for their well-earned winter slumber in their cozy dens.

When the bears begin their hibernation, their fruit and food consumption abruptly comes to a halt. They are beginning a fast, so their insulin levels fall. This drop in insulin unlocks their fat stores by allowing the previously blocked enzymes to function. The stored triglycerides are released as free fatty acids and glycogen stores become glucose. This provides the energy needs for the bear's still functioning brain, heart, kidneys, lungs, and other organs. The bears must also burn enough fuel to keep their warm-blooded bodies from freezing. This is achieved by a signal from the falling insulin level to "brown fat," located under the skin, to burn enough fuel to increase the bear's metabolism and maintain its core temperature.

Insulin resistant, overweight men and women who greatly reduce their carb intake have a drop in insulin levels similar to hibernating grizzlies. Like the bears, these overweight individuals can also increase their metabolism by burning brown fat.

IT'S ABOUT INSULIN, NOT BLOOD SUGAR

Recent studies indicate that about two-thirds of Americans, and much of the world, are suffering from insulin resistance. So how has this problem become epidemic? I believe an important reason is that our focus has been on the wrong target—blood glucose, commonly known as blood sugar—rather than the real culprit, insulin. The reason for this is a simple accident in the evolution of medical technology.

> Insulin resistant, overweight men and women who greatly reduce their carb intake have a drop in insulin levels similar to hibernating grizzlies.

Doctors were able to measure blood glucose in clinical practice about 80 years before technology made it practical to measure blood insulin levels. For decades, our focus has been on a consequence of diabetes, high blood sugars, not on its cause, insulin resistance. Because our focus was on blood sugar rather than insulin, lowering blood sugar became the goal for the treatment of type 2 diabetics and pre-diabetics. Unfortunately, when type 2 diabetics are treated with insulin, or with medications that stimulate more insulin production from the pancreas, the complications of diabetes only get worse. The goal for treating type 2 diabetes, pre-diabetes, and pre-prediabetes should be to lower insulin levels and to reverse insulin resistance. The only time to use insulin in type 2 diabetics is at a stage when the pancreatic insulin producing beta cells are nearly completely dysfunctional and cannot produce insulin.

FAT & SICK

When high insulin levels are sustained over a long period of time, we get fat and sick. We see this today in epidemic numbers. The ravages of inappropriately high insulin levels begin many years before blood sugars become elevated. Blood sugars are not sustained at high levels until the beta cells of the pancreas begin to fail and cannot produce enough insulin to overcome the insulin resistance of the organs. By only measuring blood sugar, with no analysis of insulin responsiveness, the early signs of insulin resistance and its damage to our organs go unrecognized until blood sugars are abnormal.

Even with the ability to measure insulin levels, we routinely measure them in the fasting state. This does not reflect the inappropriately high insulin response occurring after meals, evident early in insulin resistance. These persistently high insulin levels cause the depositing of excess fat in our organs and blood vessels for many years before our doctors may become aware. The first awareness may come with an abnormal liver function test or even a heart attack. In order to truly understand whether or not you are insulin resistant, despite a normal blood sugar, your insulin must be measured fasting and then at intervals after a meal or ingestion of a glucose drink.

PATIENT STORY

Danielle C.: Reversing Prediabetes through Diet

Our patient Danielle C., 50 years old, came to see us after her previous doctor told her she was prediabetic—which she was. She was scared and wanted help. Danielle had digestive issues and low-level depression. She had asked her former doctor about the keto diet, but not knowing much about it, he discouraged her from doing it and didn't offer any real alternative. Our team told her just the opposite about her diet; that a low-carb, keto-friendly diet was exactly what she needed to address her insulin resistance and that our plan would be easy and flexible. After a year and a half, Danielle has made this lower-carb plan a lifestyle, finding it easy to stick with. She lost the 10 to 15 pounds she needed to lose, her mood has lifted, and her digestive issues have resolved. Her testing for prediabetes and insulin resistance are normal. Most importantly, Danielle reports she is feeling great.

A SHORT HISTORY OF INSULIN

In type 1 diabetes (formerly known as juvenile diabetes), the problem is not too much insulin, as in insulin resistance and type 2 diabetes, but not *enough* insulin. Type 1 diabetes was first diagnosed in antiquity because its presentation was so dramatic. Children and young adults would suddenly become emaciated, rapidly losing weight despite eating and drinking voraciously. They would then go into a coma and die. These type 1 diabetics had suffered damage to their insulin-producing pancreatic beta cells, possibly due to a viral or some other infection. With little or no insulin production, they could not move energy—in the form of glucose, fats, and proteins—from their bloodstream into their tissues. It all went out through their kidneys into their urine. This meant that despite consuming plenty of food, these type 1 diabetics essentially starved to death from malnutrition. It was appreciated early on that there was a lot of sugar in these patients' urine, but it was not until the late 1800s that it was learned that the problem started in the pancreas.

In the early 1920s, Dr. Frederick Banting was able to isolate insulin from a beef pancreas and inject it into a young woman who was wasting away. As the injected insulin moved the excessive blood sugar into her cells and organs, the patient underwent a miraculous trans-formation, gaining weight and energy. It appeared that the cure for diabetes had arrived. An immediate issue became the danger of using too much insulin and dropping the blood sugar too low (hypoglycemia), putting the patient back at high risk for death.

Hypoglycemia could only be prevented if a patient's blood sugar could be easily, accu-rately, and frequently measured to make appropriate adjustments to insulin dosages. This was accomplished by the development of just such a blood test, and with that new tool, doctors started testing for high blood sugars in patients without known diabetes. They found many patients with high blood sugar, but these patients were usually adults and did not look like they were starving like the juveniles. Quite the opposite, they tended to be overweight and died of heart attacks and strokes, not of malnutrition and coma.

Doctors recognized the difference and labeled this syndrome "adult onset diabetes." But they thought the high blood sugar was still a problem of insufficient insulin, which they could not measure. So they focused on the blood sugar and treated adult onset diabetes in the same way they treated juvenile diabetes, with insulin injections and later with oral drugs that stimulated the pancreatic beta cells to produce more insulin. This approach did not prevent heart attacks and strokes in these patients; in fact, it increased them. It was not until the discovery in the 1960s of a new method for measuring protein hormones called the "immunoassay" that doctors were able to measure insulin. That is when we finally learned that the issue in type 2 diabetes was not too *little* insulin, but too *much*—the opposite of what had been believed.

THE LIFESAVING TEST YOU NEED TO KNOW ABOUT

The realization that the insulin resistance/ diabetes process begins 20 years before blood sugars become abnormal has clarified much of what my colleagues and I observe daily in our practice. In the past, patients would come to me with evidence of coronary arteriosclerosis manifested by a high coronary calcium score (more on this test later) and limited knowledge of their family medical history. They may have had an elevated blood pressure or high triglycerides, but their blood sugars and hemoglobin A1Cs (a test reflecting their average blood sugar over the past 3 months) were normal. I would check for the uncommon genetic disorder that might cause coronary artery disease, but more often than not, these tests were normal too. But then I learned about a test that measured the insulin secretion response to glucose. By measuring this response, I now had a tool to explain my patients' coronary arteriosclerosis and I had a strategy to stop its progression.

My epiphany about the importance of measuring insulin secretion in nondiabetics and non-prediabetics started after I read Dr. David Ludwig's breakthrough study published in *The British Medical Journal* in November 2018. He observed young, overweight but not diabetic Framingham State University students and faculty members who were randomly placed on a high, medium, or low-carbohydrate diet. What was new was that Dr. Ludwig classified these patients as high, medium, or low insulin secretors based on their insulin response to the standard oral glucose drink.

The study showed that the high-insulin secretors assigned to the low-carb diet burned, on average, 478 more calories per day compared to baseline. In other words, their insulin dropped and their metabolism went up dramatically. The metabolism of the high-insulin secretors on the high-carb, low-fat diet went in the opposite direction: it slowed.

After this study, we started routinely measuring insulin secretion after a glucose drink—the same drink used in the standard oral glucose tolerance test (OGTT). In the general population, the OGTT has been replaced by the hemoglobin A1C test because it provides similar information and requires just one blood draw instead of five. The big difference is that we measure the insulin response instead of just the glucose response, using it as an oral insulin tolerance test (OITT). We first used the test to predict who would respond best to our keto-friendly meal plan, and it worked.

THE KRAFT TEST

I learned from a lecture by prevention guru Ivor Cummings that an innovative pathologist, Dr. Joseph R. Kraft, had developed this test and used it on 15,000 patients in the 1970s. This was a time when insulin level testing first became available for research but was not yet available for clinical practice. Kraft's work was largely ignored by the diabetes and nutrition establishment, something that has happened to many pioneers and innovators, and that is why I hadn't heard about him or his work.

He wrote a book published in 2008, *Diabetes Epidemic & You*, summarizing his vast experience. Dr. Kraft, who died a few years ago at age 96, had already found that insulin resistance (as documented by his insulin secretion test) starts many years before the oral glucose tolerance test becomes abnormal. He argued, as others have recently, that the disease process should be labeled "type 2 diabetes" when his "Kraft insulin test" first becomes abnormal. He concluded that waiting for an elevated glucose test was too late in the process.

Dr. Ralph DeFronzo, one of the foremost researchers in this field, has demonstrated in clinical trials that the early stages of what are termed "diabetic microvascular diseases" of the kidneys, eyes, and nerves can begin by the time a diagnosis of prediabetes or diabetes is made. He also has shown that severe insulin resistance as well as pancreatic beta cell dysfunction can occur at a time when the OGTT and hemoglobin A1C are classified as normal.

Dr. Kraft, with his OITT secretion, established how changing patterns of insulin secretion progress from a normal pattern (when there is no insulin resistance) to predictable changes in the patterns as insulin resistance progresses and is ultimately accompanied by beta cell dysfunction. This opens up a whole new world of diagnosing and quantifying insulin resistance during the pre-prediabetes phase.

Now, with the simple test developed by Dr. Kraft in the 1970s, we are identifying these patients and treating them when deterioration to their organs can be stopped or even reversed. Since the doctors in our practice have been performing the Kraft oral insulin tolerance test, we have identified many patients who have coronary artery calcium, high blood pressure, fatty livers, and other signs of preclinical disease with normal blood sugars and hemoglobin A1Cs—but abnormal Kraft OITT patterns. With the Keto-Friendly South Beach Diet, we have observed improvement in their blood pressure and liver function tests, along with the melting away of their excess visceral fat. We have also observed prompt decreases in their triglycerides.

THE DIABESITY PANDEMIC

Diabetes and obesity are now pandemics. The global prevalence of diabetes was calculated at 425 million people in 2017, and the number is projected to increase to 629 million people by 2045, a nearly 50 percent increase. So far, the actual increase in diabetes prevalence has greatly exceeded even the dire predictions both in the United States and abroad. This means that this pandemic is on course to overwhelm our healthcare systems. I hope to convince you that with current technology, we can inexpensively diagnose and treat this condition during its early insulin resistance stage, many years before its ravages present themselves clinically.

In the meantime, you can take simple, powerful steps by making changes in your diet that can have you looking and feeling better both inside and out.

CHAPTER 4

THE STANDARD AMERICAN DIET

What We Know Now

I grew up before the obesity/diabetes epidemic and, as many of you from my generation may recall, we had very few overweight kids in school. There were exactly two in my elementary school grade of more than a hundred students. These children, who came from overweight families, were not diabetic and did not develop diabetes as adults. There was likely an inherited trait that caused their fat to be stored safely under their skin as subcutaneous fat, not as visceral fat positioned dangerously in their liver and around their organs.

Among my classmates, friends, and their families, obesity was rare. This was not for lack of available food; the age of the supermarket had arrived. There was plenty to eat, and I can still recall my mother's words: "Arthur, clean your plate. Kids are starving in China." Dessert was happily provided if I finished my vegetables. But we were not given snacks after dinner and had just one midafternoon snack after school.

None of us were ever told to stop eating because we would gain too much weight. Kids were not overweight, and neither were their parents, yet we never heard of anyone counting calories. How did so many people maintain stable weights without consciously watching what they ate or counting calories?

WEIGHT SET POINTS

The answer was simply that we had built-in "weight set points" that were hormonally regulated. Body weight is regulated, just like a body's temperature set point is at 98.6. When you lose weight, your metabolism will slow down and your appetite will increase. This prompts you to eat more, so you regain the weight and return to your set point.

On the opposite end, when you gain weight, your metabolism revs up and your hunger diminishes, so you lose weight. Your body sends these messages to your brain through the action of leptin and other hormones, the most important being insulin. It was these hormones, not calories, that told us when we were full and when we were hungry.

For example, insulin levels normally rise during pregnancy and drop after the newborn is weaned. This is so mothers eat enough to store energy for themselves, their growing fetus, and their newborn. It is also hormones that prevent starving young women with little fat stores from becoming pregnant; they would not have the fuel reserve to feed themselves and their baby.

It is this natural, hormonally driven weight set point that kept the weight of Americans so stable without paying attention to calories; that is, until the 1980s.

DESTROYING OUR WEIGHT SET POINTS

If we have hormonally guarded set points, then how did we get so fat? It could not have come simply from eating too much and moving too little, our sedentary lives, screen time, and "supersizing"—because our set point hormones would have kicked in to reverse the weight gain as they always had. Our set points could only have changed with a shift in our hormonal balance. And that is what happened. The major hormone that went out of balance was— yes, *insulin*. It was elevated insulin levels that caused us to store more fat and burn less. But what knocked our hormones out of balance?

LOW FAT MADE US FAT

Several important events coincided to rapidly change the hormonal balance of Americans and launch the "diabesity" epidemic that continues to this day. Our mixed-up hormones have created a population that generally feels lousy and in whom we are even seeing, for the very first time, a shortened life expectancy.

Based on earlier flawed studies and the medical association recommendations stemming from them, in 1980 the Dietary Guidelines for Americans were updated to encourage a significant reduction in fat intake. It is at that time that our obesity rates abruptly began to increase. Why? These recommendations were made under the false assumption that fat was causing heart attacks, diabetes, and obesity. Sugar was considered a source of calories, just like any other food, except devoid of vitamins and minerals. That is what I learned in medical school in the 1970s during our very limited nutrition education.

I vividly recall a trip home around that time when my Uncle Abby, a math professor, was visiting. As he observed my selection of a sugar-loaded doughnut in place of lunch (yes, my sugar addiction was already showing), he suggested that a more balanced meal might be healthier, and that he didn't think all that sugar was a good idea. As a smart medical student, I thought I knew better, replying that, "Other than causing cavities, there's no problem with sugar." It was calories like any other food's calories. Math professor one, smart medical student zero.

We've come a long way in understanding how what we eat impacts our health. As a preventive cardiologist, and a member of the nutrition committee of the American College of Cardiology, I make nutrition a core piece of my practice and encourage nutrition education whenever I can.

Another recommendation was to substitute unsaturated, partially hydrogenated trans-fat vegetable oils in margarines, salad dressings, and cooking oils for traditional saturated fat–based products. Nobody knew anything about trans fats or had any idea how vegetable oil products were manufactured. They were certainly not natural and not from vegetables.

THE NATIONAL GUIDELINES

Did Americans follow these recommendations? Definitely. Our total fat, saturated fat, milk, dairy, and red meat consumption went down as a percentage of our caloric intake while our consumption of grains, fruits, vegetables, and vegetable oils went up—but we still got fatter and sicker, with a growing incidence of diabetes.

At first, these recommendations seemed to make sense. But, among other things, the refined grains and fruit juices we were eating were full of rapidly absorbed carbohydrates and sugar, and these had a major impact on our insulin levels. The national guidelines turned out to be the largest population health experiment in history, and it went badly. We are still experiencing its unintended consequences and so is our health care system. How did these nutrition changes throw us out of hormonal balance?

> The national guidelines turned out to be the largest population health experiment in history, and it went badly.

OUR HORMONE BALANCE DESTROYED

When fat was reduced in grocery products, the resulting food often tasted like cardboard. Many remember the unofficial rule that anything that tastes like cardboard must be good for us. This posed a challenge for the food industry; after eliminating the fat, what could be substituted to bring back the taste? Sugar was low fat and it tasted good, and given the conventional wisdom—that a calorie is a calorie and calories were fungible—there was no problem with using sugar to replace the fat and improve the taste of food, right? Wrong. This is when bad carbs and sugar began to increase dramatically in our diets, and adversely affect our health.

THE SUGAR EXPLOSION

Beginning with the introduction of the sugar plantation in the 1500s, successive technological advances, particularly in the mid-1880s, made refined sugar less expensive to cultivate and process and thus more accessible. Faster and cheaper forms of transportation during the industrial revolution also contributed to a fairly brisk increase in sugar consumption throughout the first two thirds of the 20th century, with a pause during World War II. But the American experience with sugar changed dramatically owing to another technological advance in the 1970s, with the introduction of high-fructose corn syrup (HFCS).

High-fructose corn syrup is made up of two "simple sugars," glucose and fructose, which are the same as the simple sugars found in cane sugar (table sugar). This new form was initially cheaper than cane sugar and was easier to incorporate into packaged goods in which most of the fat had been removed to satisfy the new "get the fat out" national recommendations. High-fructose corn syrup largely solved the low-fat taste problem.

The new low-fat recommendation coupled with the availability of HFCS created a double whammy, resulting in a huge spike in our per capita sugar consumption. This exponential increase in sugar consumption accelerated insulin resistance, upsetting our hormonal balance and consequently our weight set points. This in turn caused a hefty increase in our waist circumferences and greatly contributed to our epidemic of sugar addiction, obesity, insulin resistance, diabetes, and the resulting complications.

HOW SUGAR UPSETS OUR HORMONES

Let's look at an illustration of how a change in sugar intake upsets our normal hormonal responses. In a study performed by renowned Harvard researcher Dr. David Ludwig and his colleagues, one group of kids was given a drink of a sugary cola before they entered a fast food restaurant; they were then instructed to order and eat whatever they wanted. A second group of kids was sent into the same restaurant, with the same instructions to order and eat whatever they wanted, but without the soft drink beforehand. The soft drink group ate more, because the hormones telling their brains "You are full, stop eating" were blocked by the sugary soft drink, and the hunger hormone usually suppressed by eating or drinking was not.

In a normal adolescent, a natural increase in insulin causes extra calorie intake at the time of their growth spurt. But what if the normal adolescent rise in insulin is exacerbated by soft drinks and other sources of sugars along with refined carbohydrates such as cookies and other baked goods? Their hormones get out of control, keeping them in a fat-storage mode. This is how we have produced an epidemic of overweight, obese, and insulin-resistant teenagers.

HFCS OR CANE SUGAR?

HFCS, found in many soft drinks and packaged foods, has often been demonized as the main source of our obesity and diabetes problem, and for good reason. Knowing this, many food manufacturers have substituted cane sugar. This may make the product label look better, but it has not helped our waistlines. Both HFCS and regular cane sugar are made up of glucose and fructose in nearly the same proportions. The problem with the HFCS was that it was added to a high percentage of our processed, packaged foods, such as white bread, often leaving us unaware of our total sugar intake. And, even if we knew about the added sugar, we thought fat was the enemy. Unlike the days when we added one or two sugar cubes to our coffee, or sprinkled our cereal with a teaspoon of sugar, we were now unaware of how much sugar we were consuming.

THE DANGERS OF GRAZING

As we have discussed, our increased sugar intake causes increased insulin levels and increased hunger. We experience big swings in our blood sugar, making us hungry every few hours. For the last few decades, these hunger episodes were satisfied with frequent snacks, or what is now called "grazing." Supersizing our meals was the fast food industry's answer to our increased hunger. Studies show that adults and kids today are eating many more times per day than they did back in the 1970s. These frequent feedings cause repeated bumps in our insulin levels that keep our fat locked in our bellies and keep us hungry throughout the day and night. Thus, our total calorie intake has increased because we are walking around hungry all the time and because our disrupted hormones have too many of us in a fat-storage mode. It is important to understand that our snacking and supersizing are a result of our disrupted hormonal setpoints, not their cause.

THE PERILS OF PROCESSED FOODS

Processed foods hit the mainstream market around 1965, when convenience was a new priority for most Americans. People were excited to have an alternative to standing over a stove for hours cooking for themselves and their families. Processed foods were supposed to save time and make life easier and more enjoyable. What do we mean by processed foods? Technically, "processing" can include anything that changes food from its original form, which can include anything from cooking to preserving. So of course, not all "processed" foods are "bad."

> It is important to understand that our snacking and supersizing are a result of our disrupted hormonal setpoints, not their cause.

But can food processing go too far? It can and it did. One of the first things many food manufacturers do to create certain processed foods is to remove or disrupt the fiber structure of the carbohydrates. In addition to being lower in fiber, many processed foods are lower in omega-3 fatty acids and micronutrients, including vitamins and minerals, while being higher in omega-6 fatty acids, salt, additives, emulsifiers, and sugar.

But that's not all. Processed foods are one of the biggest sources of sugar in our diet.

Sugar doesn't just make food taste good; it also increases its shelf life. Manufacturers make use of both of these attributes when they add sugar to extend the life of some processed or shelf-stable foods that they make in bulk, saving both time and money.

I have to admit that I particularly fell for the "zero fat, zero cholesterol" label of one of the most popular processed goodies of the 1980s and 1990s. I never thought about the 9 grams of sugar in a single cookie. After all, it wasn't fat. But beyond the sugar and starch content of these non-fat/reduced-fat foods, their refined ingredients also sped up the absorption of glucose, causing a spike in insulin.

INCRETINS: A KEY TO FEELING FULL

To best comprehend the effect of food processing on your diet and your health, it is important to understand the functions of two small intestinal hormones that are not well known to the public or to most physicians. They are called incretins, hormones secreted from inside the intestinal wall by K cells in the upper section of the small intestine or L cells located farther down. These cells are responsible for secreting two hormones—GIP (a hormone that raises insulin), and GLP-1 (a hormone that signals your brain that you are full). You can guess which of these is a problem if it's over-secreting.

GLP-1

When you eat whole foods, the glucose from starch is absorbed more slowly because it is surrounded by fiber (as in steel-cut oats) or is part of a dense whole food that incorporates protein (such as quinoa). Such foods move farther down the small intestine before their fiber or protein is stripped away by intestinal enzymes, thereby exposing their glucose to L cells, rather than the K cells in the upper section of the intestine. These L cells secrete a hormone into the bloodstream called GLP-1 (glucagon-like peptide 1). GLP-1 then travels to the brain and signals that we are satiated and should stop eating. Traditional whole foods with their structure intact pass gradually through the small intestine and the K cells and the L cells, creating a good balance between GIP and GLP-1.

GIP

This balance is upset in favor of GIP when we stray from the whole vegetables, fruits, and grains we were designed to eat. When we eat refined carbohydrates and sugar, the food is absorbed quickly at the upper end of the small intestine, where there is a high concentration of K cells. When these K cells are stimulated by glucose from starch and sugar, the hormone GIP (glucose-dependent insulinotropic polypeptide) is secreted into the bloodstream. GIP then travels to the pancreas, where it stimulates pancreatic beta cells to secrete insulin. This insulin secretion increases blood insulin levels by several times over the level produced by the direct effect of glucose alone. This exaggerated insulin rise is called the "incretin effect."

The relative amounts of the "bad incretin" GIP from the upper intestine to the "good incretin" GLP-1 from farther down explains a lot about higher insulin levels after eating refined carbohydrates and sugar.

Let's review some basics: Whole foods with their plant structure intact are digested gradually in the small intestine. They stimulate the release of the proper ratio of GIP to GLP-1, as we've discussed. Carbohydrates from grains, fruits, or vegetables that have had their fibrous skeletons disrupted with processing are virtually "pre-digested" by the manufacturing process and are absorbed predominantly in the upper small intestine, thereby producing excess GIP and consequently excess insulin.

INSTANT VERSUS STEEL-CUT OATMEAL

An example of the difference between processed and minimally processed carbohydrates is instant oatmeal compared with steel-cut oatmeal. While the fiber remains in the instant oatmeal, it is no longer surrounding the starch core. Without the need to first digest the fiber before reaching the starchy middle, the fiber no longer works to slow digestion. Thus, the starch is exposed to enzymes in the upper small intestine rather than farther down. These enzymes quickly break it down into its glucose components, which are rapidly absorbed through the intestinal wall, releasing the bad incretin, GIP.

If, as with slow-cooked steel-cut oatmeal, the fiber surrounding the starch remains intact, enzymes in your digestive system have difficulty accessing the starch and glucose release is slower. Less GIP is released and, as the oatmeal travels farther down the intestine, more appetite-suppressing GLP-1 is secreted.

The difference between instant and steel-cut oatmeal is not just theoretical. Dr. David Ludwig's group did an elegant study in teenage boys in which all the teens were given a breakfast and lunch of the same food, except that one group was given instant oatmeal for both meals and the other group was served steel-cut oatmeal. The total amount of fiber in instant oatmeal is nearly the same as in whole-grain, steel-cut oatmeal, but, as you have just learned, processing has broken down its fibrous skeleton and it is not surrounding and protecting its starch core from intestinal enzymes. The two groups were then allowed to eat anything they wanted for the rest of the day from a range of foods provided to them. The steel-cut oatmeal group consumed about 500 fewer calories than the instant oatmeal group thanks to less GIP and more GLP-1 secretion.

> The difference between instant and steel-cut oatmeal is not just theoretical.

This experiment beautifully demonstrated that even with the same nutrients, digestion can vary enormously depending on the degree of processing. On a practical level, this means you cannot judge the quality of the food by just counting total carbs and total fiber. That information does not tell you where the glucose is being absorbed. You have to ask yourself whether the structure of the carbohydrate is intact, as it is in a whole food.

This principle applies mainly to carbohydrates, starches, and sugars in grains, fruits, and vegetables. The digestion of processed fats and proteins alone is not influenced. Protein can slow digestion when present with a carbohydrate, such as in pasta made with eggs. In contrast to carbs, the processing of protein or fats has minimal effect on the incretins.

AMERICANS NEED CONVENIENT, HEALTHY PROCESSED FOODS

You may be thinking at this point that I'm asking you to avoid processed foods altogether. But that's not the case. The purpose of this book is to help change the way America (and the world for that matter) eats. I am well aware that most of us are not returning to the family farm or taking daily trips to the farmer's market and spending a lot of time on food preparation. Although eating fresh, whole food is optimal and many of us are very interested in and are cooking at home with fresh ingredients, we can't always access all fresh ingredients or carve out time to prepare meals made from scratch. I have always said that to conquer our epidemic of obesity, we have to make healthy food more convenient and convenient food healthier. Studies have shown that healthy prepared foods can help us lose weight.

To illustrate these points, let me convey the experience of another low-carb guru, Dr. Eric C. Westman, director of the Duke Lifestyle Medicine Clinic. Dr. Westman treats many overweight patients who do not cook their own meals and who routinely frequent fast-food restaurants. For very practical reasons, to optimize compliance, Dr. Westman often advises his patients that when they go to these restaurants, they should get the hamburger but with a salad and no fries, and take off the bun. He has had great success with his approach, tailored to his particular overweight population.

An example of healthy processed foods is flash-frozen vegetables. Flash freezing is a process that preserves freshness and nutrients. There is also no significant loss of nutrients when fish or poultry are frozen. So remember, let's not let "perfect be the enemy of the good." We don't have to be perfect to lose weight and reverse insulin resistance. Consuming healthy, convenient foods can mean the difference between success and failure.

Most so-called "vegetable oils" do not actually come from vegetables, but are derived primarily from seeds or legumes by complex and artificial means.

PROCESSING, VEGETABLE OILS & TRANS FATS

One exception to the rule that the processing of fats is innocuous is when it comes to vegetable oils. Dietary guidelines, first published in the late 1970s and updated periodically thereafter, encouraged a relatively new type of oil to replace the frowned-upon saturated fats found in butter, lard, and tropical oils. The spectacular growth of vegetable oils over the past 50 years turned out to be another unintended experiment with the health of Americans. These replacement oils—omega-6 vegetable oils, otherwise known as trans fats—were initially partially hydrogenated. Now they are processed by newer, more complicated methods.

Most so-called "vegetable oils" do not actually come from vegetables, but are instead derived primarily from seeds or legumes by complex and artificial means. Seed oils were first extracted through manufacturing technology invented in the mid-1800s, in order to make use of the large volume of cottonseeds that were waste products from cotton cultivation. Cottonseed oil was cheaper than whale oil and successfully supplanted it to lubricate the machinery of the industrial revolution. But when John David Rockefeller struck oil and made petroleum less expensive than cottonseed oil, cottonseeds once again became waste products. That was until James Boyce, while working on methods of extracting usable oil from cottonseeds for soap, developed the process of industrial hydrogenation. This made seed oils stable at room temperature. When used as shortening, these partially hydrogenated oils gave foods a longer shelf life. Thus, partially hydrogenated vegetable shortening was born.

This discovery led to the first commercial vegetable shortening, introduced in 1911 as "Crisco" (crystalized cottonseed oil). These partially hydrogenated oils, today better known as "trans fats," had a long shelf life because bacteria could not digest their hydrogenated bonds. The likelihood that the hydrogenation would change how they were digested by humans was not a consideration—they tasted good and did not quickly spoil. Vegetable oils and hydrogenated vegetable oils became the most common oils in our food supply, and by the 1980s supplanted saturated fats such as coconut oils and palm oils in commercial fast food chains and largely replaced butter in our homes. Once ingested, they became incorporated into our tissues, and even made it into breast milk.

In 1980, these vegetable oils were included in dietary guidelines because they were considered "polyunsaturated fats," which had been shown to lower total cholesterol. It was assumed that by lowering cholesterol, vegetable oils would lower heart attack rates. They didn't. It turned out that these partially hydrogenated trans fats *increased* our bad LDL cholesterol and lowered the good HDL.

This uncontrolled nutrition experiment with large volumes of a new oil might have been expected to produce unintended consequences and it did. We now know that it turned out as badly as the low-fat experiment. Consumption of trans fats increases your risk for heart attacks, diabetes, obesity, and other chronic diseases. Trans fats, after first being officially classified as "not generally recognized as safe" by the U.S. Food and Drug Administration, were banned as of 2018.

NON-HYDROGENATED VEGETABLE OILS

While there is no longer controversy regarding trans fats (they are bad), once partially hydrogenated vegetable oils came into disrepute, and oils from saturated fats were still considered unhealthy, the question became, what oils could be substituted? The commercial answer has been to go back to the drawing board and use processed non-hydrogenated vegetable oils—another experiment with our health.

While there is still debate regarding non-hydrogenated vegetable oils, some facts are certain. Vegetable oils are omega-6 oils, essential in small amounts as normally present in nuts and seeds. Their consumption in large quantities of artificially extracted oils is unique to modern times. As the use of vegetable oils has increased, so have our rates of heart attacks, diabetes, and the other chronic diseases of the West. We also know that increased levels of omega-6 measured in our tissues correlate with heart disease.

Of further concern is that omega-6 oils are inherently unstable and easily oxidized, which is why they were hydrogenated for commercial use in the first place. When they are used in commercial frying and baking, they are susceptible to oxidation and turning into dangerous compounds. This does not mean that non-hydrogenated vegetable oils have contributed to chronic disease, but they have not yet been proven safe. I would not volunteer for another experiment with my health, and suggest you decline as well, especially when we have so many safe alternatives. Avoid consuming more than minimal amounts of omega-6 vegetable oils, if any at all.

CHECK YOUR OMEGA-3 INDEX

The other problem with our intake of omega-6 vegetable oils is that it drives down the levels of anti-inflammatory omega-3 in our cell membranes. The higher your omega-6, the lower your omega-3—even if you are consuming a good amount of fish.

You have heard mixed messages regarding the benefits of eating fish and/or taking omega-3 fish oil supplements. This is another area of confusion that has been largely resolved with advances in technology. To understand the benefits of anti-inflammatory fish oil, and the dangers of pro-inflammatory omega-6 vegetable oils, you have to look at the amounts of omega-3 and omega-6 that are actually getting into the membranes of all the cells in your body. Cell membranes are made up of saturated and monounsaturated fats. Omega-3 and omega-6 together make up a relatively small percentage of cell membrane fats, usually around 10 percent. But since the introduction of omega-6 oils, the relative amounts have changed drastically.

FOUR SOURCES OF CONFUSION

Confusion over omega-3 supplementation has occurred for four major reasons. First, in many clinical trials, the dose of the omega-3 supplement often was inadequate to significantly increase omega-3 cell membrane levels. Second, omega-3 supplements as well as oil from fish are absorbed at different rates in different individuals. Third, the amount of actual fish oil in over-the-counter fish-oil supplements is frequently not as advertised. And fourth, even with taking a good amount of fish oil via supplements, if omega-6 rich vegetable oils are also consumed, the amount of omega-3 getting into your cell membranes is suppressed.

Fortunately, all of these limitations can now be overcome—again by advances in technology. In recent years, reliable measurements of the omega-3 and the omega-6 levels in our red blood cell membranes (which reflects the amounts in all of our cell membranes) can be easily and accurately measured in clinical practice as well as in clinical trials. We can also measure the ratio of omega-6 to omega-3. This ratio is important because it tells us if a low omega-3 level is indeed due to too much omega-6 vegetable oil in our diets. Before the rapid rise of omega-6 vegetable oils, our average cell membrane ratio of omega-6 to omega-3 was between 1 to 1 and 4 to 1. In recent decades, this ratio has jumped dramatically, often to well over 10 to 1. Such levels are unprecedented in human history. We messed with Mother Nature—to our detriment.

There are excellent alternatives for vegetable oils in the form of olive oil, avocado oil, coconut oil, lard, and butter—options we have consumed for millennia. Don't be part of another nutrition experiment.

We know now that past national recommendations concerning oils and fats were based on incomplete science. The march of science and technology has put another piece of the health care puzzle in place.

EXCESSIVE SUGAR IS POISON

The unprecedented amount of sugar we are ingesting today is killing us. It doesn't kill as fast as an infection or a quick-acting poison might. Rather, sugar's danger is most akin to smoking. Smoking kills slowly, diminishing our health along the way—causing cancer, emphysema, heart disease, bad skin, and so much more. Smokers endure a long stage of subclinical or preclinical disease when their organs are suffering, but without special testing, they are unaware. Often when smokers quit, symptoms disappear that they had not recognized were related to

smoking. Also, the more cigarettes you smoke, the higher the risk of health problems.

This is analogous to the many ill effects of consuming too much sugar. In its preclinical stage, it can cause liver damage (fatty liver), pancreatic damage, vascular damage, high blood pressure, anxiety, depression, low testosterone, erectile dysfunction, kidney damage, skin problems, and countless other disorders. Once recognized, these disorders are almost always treated as separate conditions, and too often with drugs rather than diet and lifestyle modifications. They are all from the same cause: too much sugar and refined carbohydrates causing insulin resistance and pancreatic beta cell dysfunction. And sugar, like smoking, can be addictive.

The effects of sugar can be diagnosed early, when reversal of the process is most easily achieved. We were warned about the evils of too much sugar back in 1972 by John Yudkin, an English physiologist, in his landmark book *Pure, White and Deadly*. Unfortunately, the nutrition establishment ignored his wisdom. In truth, until recently, there was a lot we didn't know about the metabolism of the fructose component of cane sugar and high-fructose corn syrup. What we have now learned explains much about America's, and the world's, road to obesity, diabetes, and chronic disease.

NEW VIEWS ON FRUCTOSE

Back when we developed the original South Beach Diet, we talked a lot about the glycemic index, a measure of how much a standard quantity of a carbohydrate raises your blood sugar. While this is a useful concept, it has limitations, and its characterization of fructose turned out to be misleading though we couldn't have known it at the time. We often remarked that starches such as white potatoes or white bread had a higher glycemic index than table sugar and were therefore just as bad or worse to consume. We were wrong.

What have we learned since? Sugar is a disaccharide, meaning it is made of two simple sugar molecules, in this case, one glucose and one fructose, bound together. After ingestion, these molecules are quickly separated by enzymes in the upper small intestine. While glucose from your meal directly increases blood glucose and insulin and is used by all the cells in your body, nearly all of the fructose goes from the small intestine directly to your liver for its metabolism. It hardly appears in your bloodstream and does not directly raise your blood sugar or your insulin levels. This explains why table sugar or even HFCS does not have as high a glycemic index as white bread or white potatoes whose starch components are 100 percent glucose molecules.

So what's so bad about fructose? Let us count the ways.

THE DANGER OF FRUCTOSE

If you ingest a tablespoon of sugar, the glucose component is distributed to your entire body through your bloodstream. Of the approximately 20 percent that ends up in your liver, most is stored as glycogen (chains of glucose molecules), some is burned in your mitochondria (your cells' and your entire body's energy generator) for immediate energy needs, and a small amount is turned into fat by a process called "de novo lipogenesis" (DNL) meaning "new fat formation." This fat is packaged as triglycerides (the storage form of fat) along with cholesterol into particles called VLDL (very-low-density lipoprotein). This VLDL delivers its cargo to the rest of the body as needed.

Fructose is more dangerous than glucose because first, almost all fructose goes from the intestine directly to the liver. Second, it cannot be stored as glycogen. That means that it must either be burned by mitochondria for immediate energy or be turned into fat by DNL. Because the amount of fructose entering the liver is triple the amount of glucose and none is diverted for storage as glycogen, if eaten in large quantities it overwhelms the mitochondria's capacity to burn it all and is turned into fat. In the days of having a sugar cube in your coffee or a cookie for dessert or a snack, the mitochondria could burn most of the relatively small quantity of fructose entering the liver. But today, with the huge increase in sugar consumption, we are diverting most of it to the formation of fat. This causes a lot of health problems.

FRUCTOSE CAUSES LIVER INSULIN RESISTANCE

One result of fructose metabolism in the liver is that some of the excess fat it produces blocks the action of insulin on liver cells, causing liver insulin resistance. This in turn allows less glucose to enter the liver. With less glucose coming in from the bloodstream, the liver starts manufacturing glucose itself, further raising the levels of blood sugar and further stimulating insulin secretion from the pancreas. This is how fructose indirectly raises blood sugar and insulin levels and worsens insulin resistance.

The liver tries to get rid of the large volume of fat produced by excessive fructose by stuffing it into VLDL particles, whose job it is to carry triglycerides and cholesterol out of the liver to the organs where it is needed. But the VLDL does not function normally, because it is deformed by being overloaded with fat. It delivers some of its excess fat (in the form of triglycerides) to fat cells around the liver and other internal organs, which you have learned is visceral fat. What we can't easily see from the outside is the excess fat that gets delivered into abdominal organs including the liver, pancreas, and skeletal muscle. But if you see the typical protruding belly, you can be sure there is excess fat in the liver, pancreas, and muscle. The extra fat carried by the VLDL into the blood stream is reflected on routine blood tests as elevated triglycerides.

The overstuffed, deformed VLDL particles are not efficiently cleared from the blood stream by their usual receptors because they don't fit well. They gradually break down into smaller than normal LDL particles, which are also not efficiently cleared from the blood. While hanging around in the bloodstream longer than usual, they go through changes that make them more likely to penetrate into the walls of arteries and build up arteriosclerotic plaques. This is how too much sugar and refined carbohydrates get transformed into the fat that leads to heart attacks and strokes.

Some of the additional fat produced by fructose that cannot be stuffed into the VLDL pours into liver cells, producing a fatty liver. Without a change in diet, the fat can disrupt the structure of the liver cells, leading to inflammation and hepatitis. Eventually the inflammation may progress to scarring, known as cirrhosis of the liver.

The consequences of nonalcoholic liver disease (from too much fructose) have overtaken alcohol in the United States and around the world as the number one cause of cirrhosis of the liver, liver failure, and the need for liver transplant. Once liver glycogen stores are full, continued intake of glucose from refined high-glycemic carbohydrates also is turned into fat, further contributing to fatty liver.

HIGH INSULIN LEVELS CAUSE HIGH BLOOD PRESSURE

High insulin levels also increase salt retention by the kidneys, which in turn causes fluid retention and high blood pressure. This is a major cause of our epidemic of high blood pressure. We traditionally called high blood pressure "essential hypertension," meaning we didn't know the cause. But now that we can measure insulin levels and their effect on salt retention in the kidneys, it appears that the high insulin levels associated with insulin resistance are a major cause of what was called essential hypertension. The good news is that it can be resolved with diet alone, without the need for medications in many cases.

OBESITY IN TEENS

This whole process, beginning with excess DNL and the depositing of fat in the liver, occurs early in the development of insulin resistance. Dr. Robert Lustig and his research group at the University of California, San Francisco, have been leaders in educating the medical community and the public on the particular dangers of excess fructose. As a pediatric endocrinologist, he has been on the front lines of addressing our obesity epidemic in teens, pre-teens, and even toddlers. In a groundbreaking clinical trial started in 2016, his group showed that overweight teenagers already have excess liver fat production (DNL) associated with fatty liver, visceral fat, and high triglycerides.

In a very well-controlled trial, Dr. Lustig eliminated fructose-laden sugars—but not starches—in meals delivered to a group of overweight teens. After just 10 days, they dramatically decreased their DNL. This means that without the high volume of fructose, their livers promptly stopped manufacturing, and actually started burning, their excess fat. This was all documented as a sharp drop in blood triglycerides (from less VLDL), less liver fat, and improved liver function. Thus, the whole process can be rapidly reversed, and the teenagers can lose weight and cure their insulin resistance, obesity, and all their related problems. Just from eliminating fructose-laden sugars.

> We used to think that frequent meals helped stabilize blood sugar and insulin levels. We now know they do the opposite.

It is critical to understand that the blood sugar levels in these teenagers were *normal* and were likely to remain so for many years. This is because their young, healthy pancreases were able to secrete enough insulin to overcome their insulin resistance and keep their blood sugars from becoming elevated. Remember, it was Dr. Lustig who also raised the alarm regarding the dangers of sugar addiction in adults and teenagers. Addiction to video games, smartphones, and now "vaping" all share the same pathway in the brain.

FRUCTOSE AND AGING

As we age, however, if we don't greatly reduce our sugar intake, insulin resistance worsens and pancreatic beta cell function gradually deteriorates. We get fatter and sicker under the burden of preclinical disease including fatty liver, inflammation of joints and other tissues, and arteriosclerotic arteries.

Throughout the United States and much of the rest of the world, fructose is being consumed in record amounts. And, as you have learned, when fructose overwhelms the liver's ability to burn it for energy, it turns into fat, resulting in insulin resistance, high blood sugar, high blood pressure, high triglycerides, low HDL, small LDL particles, inflammation, and visceral belly fat. Thus, fructose alone can account for all the elements of metabolic syndrome and prediabetes. And it does this before we even appreciate what is making our bellies grow and causing us to feel so lousy.

FOOD TIMING, SNACKING, MIXED MEALS & FASTING

As we have emphasized, persistent high levels of insulin are the major reason Americans are fat and sick. So, what do we do about this? Perhaps the easiest and most rational approach for lowering insulin levels is simply not to eat. This logic has led to the recent popularity of fasting. While we do not recommend prolonged fasting (defined as more than 24 hours) without the close medical supervision of a physician with special expertise in this area, the strategy of limiting snacking and meals can be effective.

We used to think that frequent meals helped stabilize blood sugar and insulin levels. We now know they do the opposite, and the reason is GIP. Every time you consume carbohydrates, your blood glucose rises and, accordingly, so does your insulin level. But with the additional pancreatic beta cell stimulation by GIP, your insulin secretion is amplified and the sum of the successive insulin responses from many small meals or snacks is significantly higher than the response from one large meal containing the same foods.

Frequent bumps in insulin throughout the day also have the effect of locking in your stored fat, preventing it from being released to satisfy your energy needs. So not snacking and even skipping a meal keeps your insulin levels low and encourages the release of fat stores from your liver and visceral belly fat. That said, if you're feeling hungry or need to put off a meal, instead have a snack free of sugar and refined carbohydrate that will have a minimal effect on your insulin levels.

Another unappreciated effect of incretins is what happens when processed carbs are consumed with fat in a mixed meal. While fat alone has a minimal effect on insulin secretion, when it is mixed with refined carbs, there is a large surge in GIP secretion and consequently in insulin secretion. One other finding from the world of incretin research is that a carb load *after* your meal raises GIP and insulin less than when consumed as an hors d'oeuvre *before* your meal. Maybe dessert is served after the main course for a good reason.

RESOLVING PARADOXES

Whether we believed in the saturated fat, cholesterol hypothesis reflected in national nutritional guidelines or the more recent low-carb, insulin hypothesis, there have always appeared to be exceptions that contributed to further confusion. By applying what we have learned about the evils of sugar, refined carbohydrates, the role of incretin hormones, and keeping our focus on insulin, we can resolve these apparent paradoxes.

When it comes to the fat/cholesterol/heart theory, there has always been reason for confusion. Why were high-fat, high-protein, and low-carb societies—including the Eskimos, the Maasai tribe of Africa, the Mongols, the Sioux Indians, and colonial Americans—free of obesity and chronic disease despite their high meat and protein and saturated fat diets? In the field of nutrition, there has always been discussion of "the French paradox": If the French are consuming so much saturated fat in their cheeses, creams, sauces, pastries, and foie gras, why do so few of them suffer heart attacks?

Foie gras is produced by stuffing geese with starch-rich corn, which turns into fat in their livers after their glycogen stores are full and their mitochondria can't burn the huge volume of glucose. This results in a very fatty liver, exactly what starch and sugar do in humans.

But eating these fatty livers did not make the French fat or diabetic; eating the corn directly would have.

The French diet is traditionally low in processed carbs and sugar. They never adopted high-fructose corn syrup. The French also never embraced artificially manufactured omega-6 vegetable oils. We now know that their high saturated fat intake, while increasing total cholesterol and total LDL, does so by increasing large LDL, not the dangerous small LDL that penetrates into our arterial wall causing arteriosclerosis. Other populations that have had a traditionally high intake of dairy and meat, the Mongols in northern Asia and the Maasai of Africa, have been both bigger and stronger than their grain-eating neighbors.

THE ASIAN PARADOX

What about the so-called Asian paradox? This refers to societies with traditional diets that were high in carbohydrates and low in fat and had virtually no obesity or heart disease. How could this be, with rice as their staple? The famously long-lived Okinawans ate high-carb diets, with sweet potatoes being an essential source of their sustenance. But Asian societies were all very low in sugar consumption. Their rice and sweet potatoes were not highly processed, so the fiber was left intact, leading to a good balance of the incretin hormones GIP and GLP1. They traditionally had one or two meals a day, and they were not interrupting their labor with frequent snacks. This meant that in their traditional diets, the Asians, like the French, did not produce high levels of insulin and remained thin and free of inflammatory and chronic disease.

Unfortunately, but interestingly, all that is now changing. Kids and adults from Okinawa to Paris to Beijing to Mumbai have now been exposed to American fast food with sugar, omega-6 vegetable oils, and refined carbs as well as convenient snacks. With these changes in diet, the rates of insulin resistance, diabetes and the resulting chronic diseases are approaching those of the West.

While traditional high-carb societies did not experience the obesity or the diabetes of the United States today, neither were they as big and strong as traditional high-fat, high-protein, low-carb populations. Among the best examples of the latter are the American Plains Indians, whose lives revolved around the buffalo. These Native Americans have been documented to have been the tallest people of their time. They were taller than the American colonialists, whose relatively high-fat, high-dairy, and high-protein diet in turn had them two inches taller than the British Redcoats, who consumed a higher-carbohydrate diet with abundant corn as their staple. The societies whose nourishment were closest to the hunter-gatherer diet were bigger and stronger, with fewer cavities and fewer nutrient deficiencies, than the grain-dependent agriculturists.

Another fascinating population, this one in Ecuador, is quite instructive. They were written up in *The New England Journal of Medicine* as the "Little Women of Loja." They are very short in stature because they are missing growth hormone receptors. They are also quite overweight. But, their fat is subcutaneous (under the skin), not visceral belly fat. They run very normal blood sugars and have perfectly normal Kraft insulin tests. With excellent insulin sensitivity, they are very long lived and appear to be free of heart disease, diabetes, cancer, Alzheimer's, and other chronic diseases suffered by insulin resistant Westerners.

SUMMING UP THE CHANGES

Western societies have been advancing at an ever more rapid pace. Technology is changing and impacting our patterns of living so fast that we no longer have time to adjust. From my childhood with almost no overweight kids in my class to where we are today is but one illustration. We have already reached a pretty grim point when it comes to our health. Even with all the advances in medical science, we as a society seem to be getting mentally and physically sicker.

But there is cause for optimism. If we can use our new technologies to identify those who are at risk before they are sick, and apply simple diet and lifestyle solutions, we can begin to reverse the current epidemic of preventable chronic disease. In the next chapter, we will outline some of the many areas where a low-carb/keto-friendly diet can prevent many of the diseases thought to be inevitably associated with aging.

PATIENT STORY

Marie N.: Losing Weight by Ditching Refined Carbs

Marie N., age 55, came to our office for an annual exam. She had gained weight after menopause and was about 30 pounds overweight, but was also lucky enough to have a zero on her calcium score. She appeared to be more of a "pear" than an "apple" in shape, but her calcium scan revealed she had excess visceral fat. Her fasting blood sugar was borderline and her hemoglobin A1C was at the upper limits of normal. Her Kraft insulin secretion test demonstrated that she was insulin resistant. She fit the typical pattern of insulin resistance increasing with age, especially after menopause. This explained her postmenopausal weight gain. A review of her eating pattern revealed a typical Standard American Diet. Marie typically ate bacon and eggs in the morning, rounded out with toast or a muffin. Business meetings always included bagels, pastries, or muffins. Lots of business lunches began with a cocktail and bread basket and ended with dessert. Dinners at home were much the same. Worst of all, Marie had four children who would be following in her footsteps.

She was shocked into action. One month later, Marie was back for her first follow-up visit. She had lost 12 pounds. Her mood had improved and she felt more clear-headed with more energy. She reported that her cravings had resolved within the first three days of following the diet. After her office visit, she went out to lunch with friends and turned down the freshly baked bread and gourmet pizza appetizer that she was offered. She commented that, "It is a lot easier to stick with a plan when you feel so much better following it."

CHAPTER 5

THE HEALTH BENEFITS OF A KETO-FRIENDLY LIFESTYLE

Now that you've learned much of the science behind the Keto-Friendly South Beach Diet, let's review how this translates into better health. What are the tangible benefits you can expect when you normalize your insulin levels? There are many. Besides the most outwardly visible benefit—weight loss and clearer skin—the diet can help protect your heart, boost your mood, improve your cognitive function, and increase your energy and endurance. You may also sleep better and notice that you can hang with your kids or grandkids longer.

Even if your primary motivation for picking up the book is weight loss, it's the other benefits that will likely keep you on the diet for the long term. It has been for me and for so many of our patients.

Since my "D-Day" for starting this diet, I've lost between 15 and 20 pounds of fat. I did this within a few months and have kept it off. The reason is because of the extension of the very keto friendly Phase 1. I resolved my sugar cravings so that, even with an occasional refined carb indulgence, I have not been led down the slippery slope back to sugar addiction and belly fat.

But my unbridled enthusiasm and the reason I am confident I will not falter is because I just feel so much better and surprisingly younger. I start and get through my day with more energy, my athletic endurance has increased, and my recovery time after vigorous exercise is faster. My sleep is excellent and I'm looking forward to aging in a healthy way so I can maintain a level of energy that will allow me to keep up with my first grandchild (who was delivered as this book was being written!). And I am frankly obsessed with sharing my new insights, not just with my patients, family, and friends, but with *you*.

THE DAILY WEIGH-IN

One new habit that has helped with my success is weighing myself daily, which provides constant feedback. Daily weigh-ins have been recently shown to aide with weight loss. We recommend this strategy to our patients, who have also found it to be very helpful. One note of caution though: most jumps or drops of weight from day to day are due to fluid gains or losses, not rapid changes in body fat. You will recognize these patterns with experience. Plane flights provide an example of fluid retention that you may recognize by foot and ankle swelling after a long trip. It may be harder to put your shoes back on at the end of a flight because of this fluid retention.

When eating out, there is often excess salt in restaurant fare, which may also cause fluid retention and a jump of several pounds. You will learn not to worry, as the fluid retention and the few extra pounds will resolve over a few days. Similarly, a day of heavy exercise with a lot of sweating can result in a loss of several pounds on the scale the next morning. This is not fat loss and will again normalize over a few days. What is important is to recognize the trends over many days or a couple of weeks

that will reflect changes in body fat. Also, be aware of how your clothes fit and if your belt needs tightening or loosening. You can learn a lot from these daily indicators, and they will help keep you on track.

MEDICAL SCIENCE IS MOVING FAST; CHANGES IN HEALTH CARE DELIVERY ARE NOT

I am frustrated with the slowness of our health care system to incorporate advances in medical science into improved healthcare delivery to our patients. A leading and very perceptive cardiologist, Dr. Sylvan L. Weinberg, wrote a book back in 2000 entitled, *The Golden Age of Medical Science and the Dark Age of Healthcare Delivery*. Boy, was he prescient. Everything Dr. Weinberg described is even more applicable to health care today. That is why I feel it is so important to help you adopt a healthy diet and lifestyle now, so you can take advantage of "the golden age of medical science" and avoid developing the illnesses that leave you exposed to the problems with today's systems of health care delivery.

I am optimistic because of the scientific progress that has advanced our knowledge and the development of a growing low-carbohydrate community that truly "gets it." This community includes physicians, research Ph.D.s, nurses, and nutritionists, as well as some engineers and journalists. I am seeing encouraging progress in getting the word out about the real causes of our diabesity epidemic and how to reverse it. Many are finding success in their local practices and clinics. I am anxious to add my voice and my experience to the cause with this book. Our current ability to identify heart disease years before it causes a heart attack, and to recognize insulin resistance before it causes damage, combine to give us the tools we need to inexpensively prevent so many chronic diseases that are becoming a growing human and economic threat to America and the world.

PROTECT YOUR HEART WITH A KETO-FRIENDLY DIET

Heart disease kills 610,000 Americans every year, making it the leading cause of death in both men and women. Approximately 735,000 Americans have a heart attack every year, while some 133,000 suffer from a stroke. For the great majority, these potentially fatal events will be the first warning that they have cardiovascular disease. Because of better medications for cholesterol and high blood pressure, along with improved procedures, medications, and treatments immediately following a heart attack, death rates from heart disease have been gradually declining—except for younger adults. Adults 45 years old and younger are not included in this trend toward declining death rates from heart disease; the numbers for this younger demographic have plateaued and may now be on the increase. This means that the high-sugar, high-carb, fast food lifestyle of the generations who grew up in the 1980s and 1990s is trumping all our new medications, procedures, and improved hospital care. Not a good sign!

And now for the first time ever, life expectancy in the United States appears to be declining. Just as important is the number of our senior citizens suffering from Alzheimer's and other chronic diseases, making the last years of their lives unnecessarily miserable.

Heart disease started growing in prevalence a few years after World War I and since the 1940s has persisted in being our number one killer, peaking in the 1960s. Because of this, from the 1980s forward the government and medical associations have been periodically making official recommendations regarding cardiac risk factors. While some of these recommendations—such as getting more exercise, quitting smoking, and drinking less alcohol—have helped, others have not. Lowering cholesterol by eating less cholesterol and saturated fat and consuming more vegetable oils has had no measurable effect on improving health and preventing a future heart attack. It simply has not worked. So let's explore what does help.

> I am frustrated with the slowness of our health care system to incorporate advances in medical science into improved healthcare.

CHOLESTEROL AND PREDICTING HEART ATTACKS

Cholesterol has traditionally been measured as a part of screening for heart attack risk. But what we now know about cholesterol is much more nuanced, and recent advances have led us to different conclusions about how to approach the cholesterol issue.

After the national guidelines of the early 1980s, and early in my cardiology career, I learned from Dr. Bill Castelli, the second director of the landmark Framingham Heart Study, that the cholesterol levels of the average heart attack victim were not very different from those who did *not* experience a heart attack. This was interesting and confusing and it naturally made us ask, "Why?" Why were total cholesterol and total LDL levels such poor predictors of heart attacks?

My confusion regarding the cholesterol paradox began to clear up when I heard a lecture by Dr. Robert Superko many years ago at the annual meeting of the American College of Cardiology. He, along with Dr. Ron Kraus, were pioneers in introducing the concept that just as total cholesterol has to be broken down into LDL, HDL, and triglycerides, total LDL and HDL are made up of either small or large particles that need to be measured as well. This was discovered using a series of new technologies beginning in the 1950s that ultimately improved the accuracy and decreased the cost of testing the size and number of cholesterol particles. In the last decade, its benefits have become easily accessible to physicians and their patients.

Dr. Superko taught me and many other physicians about the cluster of lipid abnormalities associated with insulin resistance called the "atherogenic lipid profile." This is comprised of high triglycerides, low HDL, and small LDL and HDL particles and it is a much better predictor of heart disease than total or LDL cholesterol. What causes the atherogenic lipid profile? It all starts with a genetic tendency for insulin resistance and then too much sugar, refined carbs, and vegetable oils in our diet. This leads to too much fat being produced in our livers. While the triglycerides and HDL components of the atherogenic lipid profile are part of the routinely measured complete lipid profile, measuring small LDL is still not standard. It should be, and now it can be.

WHEN IT COMES TO CHOLESTEROL, SIZE MATTERS

Size here really does matter. We have learned that it is predominantly the small LDL particles that burrow into our coronary artery walls and build up the arteriosclerotic plaque that eventually causes heart attacks and strokes. Studies now confirm that, except in rare cases, large LDL particles do not get into vessel walls to deposit cholesterol and build up plaque. The measurement of large LDL particles alone does not predict heart attacks or strokes. Small LDL particles do, and the smaller they are, the more dangerous.

Once I began measuring the size of LDL particles, I found that my patients with high cholesterol but predominantly large particles were the ones with little or no arteriosclerotic plaque on coronary calcium scans. Those with predominantly small particles were the ones who had developed arteriosclerosis, even though their total cholesterol and LDL cholesterols were relatively low. Total cholesterol, it turns out, was just an indirect indicator of total LDL, which in turn was just an indirect indicator of the number of small LDL particles. Now that we can measure small LDL particles directly, this should be our main focus. And remember, it is insulin resistance associated liver fat that produces high triglycerides and small LDL particles. Cholesterol confusion is clearing up.

THE ROLE OF STATINS

An important part of our approach to treating high cholesterol is through the use of a class of drugs called statins. In the mid- to late 1980s, along came the miracle statin drugs: Zocor (simvastatin) and Pravachol (pravastatin) were the first out of the box. While they didn't affect weight, they gave us, for the first time, a tool to significantly lower cholesterol and prevent heart attacks.

You might be wondering, "If cholesterol is not a good predictor of heart attacks, why lower it?" The answer is that statins decrease the amount of small *and* large LDL particles. Therefore, when we saw total LDL drop dramatically with statin therapy in the 1980s and '90s, we did not appreciate that it was the decrease in small LDL that was making the difference. Now we do.

The statins are probably the most studied drugs in history, and all the clinical trials agree: they are safe and prevent heart attacks— though not everyone tolerates them or needs them. We have learned that the highest-risk individuals, such as those who have already experienced a heart attack, have the best results with statins. This is true whether their baseline cholesterols are high, medium, or low.

THE AGATSTON CALCIUM SCORE

With the introduction of statins, we now had a tool to prevent heart attacks. But if cholesterol was not a good predictor of heart attacks, then who should have their cholesterol lowered with a statin? We were left with a quandary: If we only treated people with high cholesterol, we would be missing the majority of those des-

tined for heart attacks. But if we treated everyone with just average cholesterols, we would be unnecessarily giving drugs to large numbers of people not destined for a heart attack. This was the dilemma at the start of the statin era.

While I was wrestling with this question in the late 1980s, a new technology came to the rescue: the ultrafast CT scanner. With this tool, we could quantify the amount of arteriosclerotic plaque in an individual's coronary arteries by imaging calcified plaque. Better yet, the procedure took about five minutes and was noninvasive, safe, and inexpensive to perform. The "calcium score," derived from the scan, I am proud to say, is also known as the "Agatston Score." The scan protocol and the score were developed with my colleagues Dr. Warren Janowitz, engineer David King, and several others. The score reflects the total amount of arteriosclerosis in the coronary arteries, known as the "plaque burden." It is, by far, the best predictor we have of a future heart attack.

THE POWER OF ZERO

Now we knew which patients should be treated with statin drugs and, just as important, whom not to treat. My colleague Dr. Khurram Nasir developed the concept of the "power of zero." With a calcium score of zero, your chance of having a heart attack in the next 10 years is so low that statins would not make a difference. This is true even in individuals with very high cholesterols and other risk factors, such as high blood pressure. Many people out there taking statins because of high cholesterol don't need them. On the other hand, if your calcium score is high, you should be treated aggressively, even if you do not have high cholesterol.

Having a calcium score is like having x-ray vision to peer into the future. With this scan, we can noninvasively look into a heart's coronary arteries to see who is really at risk and who isn't. And we can do this in the "preclinical" stage of the disease process—before the disease causes the changes in our organs that produce symptoms. It is at this stage that prevention measures are most effective. A good example of the potential of the calcium score combined with the Kraft insulin secretion test is how we can identify patients in their 30s and 40s who are insulin resistant (have abnormal Kraft tests) and have been producing small LDL particles that are building up plaque in their coronary arteries. In this way we find out who is at risk for a heart attack and why. With early detection we can stabilize their arteriosclerosis and reverse their insulin resistance without drugs many years before they are destined for a heart attack or develop type 2 diabetes.

Unfortunately, too much health care time and too many resources are applied to put out fires after disease has progressed to a point that it is causing symptoms. At that point, it is much harder to treat. Our challenge should be to identify diseases in their preclinical stage, when we can prevent them from causing misery and death, and unnecessarily consuming our economic resources as well.

SATURATED FAT, RED MEAT & HEART ATTACKS

A review of the effects of saturated fat (including coconut oil, dairy fat, and red meat) on cholesterol particles provides another excellent illustration of how new technology can solve a prior

dilemma and explains how it impacts our health. Your red-meat steak, your dark-meat chicken leg, and your whole-fat plain yogurt all contain saturated fat, long thought to be the villain because it increases your total and LDL cholesterol. These foods also increase your good HDL. Nevertheless, they were demonized, even though clinical trials failed to show they caused heart disease, diabetes, cancer, or any other chronic diseases. Sometimes we forget that one-third or more of the fat in red meat is monounsaturated, just like the fat in healthy olive oil. (Interestingly, even olive oil contains saturated fat, although it is predominantly monounsaturated.)

> Having a calcium score is like having x-ray vision to peer into the future.

More advanced cholesterol testing and recent studies have provided the answer. These saturated fat–containing foods increase the large LDL particles. Your total and LDL cholesterol go up, but not your risk of a heart attack. The early investigators were like the classic group of blind men trying to describe an elephant: each only felt one element and the real answer eluded them.

HIGH BLOOD PRESSURE

One of the first medical consequences of insulin resistance and high insulin levels is high blood pressure (hypertension), because insulin promotes salt and fluid retention in your kidneys, which raises your blood pressure. It has been recognized for decades that weight loss lowers blood pressure and gets people off their medications. Now we know that it is not just the weight loss, but the lowering of insulin levels associated with the weight loss that lowers blood pressure. Excess sugar intake causing insulin resistance also raises your uric acid levels which, besides being a risk factor for gout, also raises your blood pressure. So a keto-friendly diet can reverse insulin resistance and high blood pressure.

FATTY LIVER & LIVER FAILURE

The fat that accumulates in your liver cells (due to sugar overload and insulin resistance) does not initially cause cell damage and the abnormal liver enzymes seen in routine laboratory testing. But eventually the increasing fat disrupts and damages the structure of the cells in the fatty liver, causing inflammation that can be detected by elevated liver enzymes. This inflammation ultimately causes the death of liver cells that then heal with scarring.

Before the obesity epidemic, this scarring, called cirrhosis of the liver, was most commonly seen in alcoholics. Excessive alcohol consumption causes a fatty liver in a manner similar to fructose in sugar, by overwhelming the liver's ability to burn it. And, like fructose, alcohol cannot be stored as glycogen; its only pathway for storage is by transforming the alcohol to fat. The excess fat undergoes the same changes as fructose- and glucose-produced fat, eventually causing inflammation and then cirrhosis. Currently, nonalcoholic liver disease has overtaken alcoholic liver disease as the major cause of liver failure worldwide.

KETO-FRIENDLY DIETS & YOUR BRAIN

The use of low-carb and keto diets to help with memory problems and Alzheimer's disease has been a growing area of interest, with some early studies looking very encouraging. As I have learned from my colleague Dr. Richard Isaacson, director of the Alzheimer's Prevention Clinic at Weill Cornell Medical College, "What's good for your heart is good for your brain." We are both interested in the observation that when the Western diet comes to a region, Alzheimer's prevalence goes up along with other chronic diseases. Type 2 diabetes is a well-known risk factor for Alzheimer's; the association is so strong that Alzheimer's disease is often labeled "type 3 diabetes."

Another technological advance that has taught us a lot about memory has been pioneered by Dr. Stephen Cunnane. He uses "dual tracer quantitative PET CT" to explore the sugar and ketone metabolism of the brain. Please don't worry about the long name. What is important is that he has shown, in patients with different degrees of memory problems, that their brain cells have a problem getting enough glucose from the blood for normal brain cell function.

Patients with diabetes or prediabetes do not take up normal amounts of glucose, due to brain insulin resistance. Their brain cells may take up enough glucose to stay above the level where memory problems can be detected, but it appears that worsening insulin resistance can eventually decrease glucose uptake to levels where memory problems do occur. The implication is that reversing insulin resistance can improve glucose uptake into brain cells and help memory. There are also trials underway studying the usefulness of ketones as brain fuel. This line of research looks very promising for our metabolic understanding of memory.

> ## The implication is that reversing insulin resistance can improve glucose uptake into brain cells and help memory.

Dr. Isaacson has recently published a study showing that a low-sugar, low–refined carbohydrate, high–healthy fat diet—along with a strategy of replacing missing nutrients—can slow mental decline. It is also possible that the improved mental acuity that so many of our patients report is due to improved insulin sensitivity leading to better brain glucose utilization. It certainly seems prudent with our current knowledge to minimize sugar and refined carbohydrates, especially if there is Alzheimer's disease in the family.

CANCER PREVENTION

Cancer is another area of interest in the low-carb and keto community. At this time, there is no clinical trial evidence of low-carb, keto-friendly diets in the treatment or prevention of cancer. We do know that certain cancers are associated with obesity. Recent studies show that obesity may be just a marker for the presence of insulin resistance. In one study, overweight women without insulin resistance did not have an increased risk of breast cancer, while those with insulin resistance did. We do know that insulin is a growth factor. Remember the "little women of Loja" who are missing growth hormone receptors? They are very insulin sensitive and, despite a high rate of obesity, do not get cancer and live long, healthy lives free of diabetes or other chronic disease.

Pancreatic cancer is also associated with obesity. Studies show that a fatty pancreas, seen in insulin resistance patients, is a risk factor for developing pancreatic cancer. Finally, we know that in populations where diabetes is increasing, so is the incidence of cancer. Although it's not yet proven, I think cancer prevention is another potential benefit of lowering your insulin levels.

ATHLETIC PERFORMANCE

Much of our knowledge of athletic performance and a low-carb or keto diet is from the research and experience of Dr. Tim Noakes and Dr. Jeff Volek. Dr. Noakes is a physician specializing in exercise physiology with special expertise in marathon running. He has run many marathons himself and written books and counseled endurance athletes on how to enhance performance.

For years, to prepare for a marathon run, the conventional wisdom was to load your liver and muscles with glycogen by consuming pasta and other starchy high-carbohydrate foods. During the marathon, it took a few hours to burn through your stored glycogen, and then your body had no choice but to burn fat for energy. At that point your body, not being adapted to fat burning, would become suddenly exhausted in what is termed "hitting the wall." The rationale was that the better your carb loading, the longer it took to deplete your glycogen stores and hit the wall, and the better your performance.

Dr. Noakes had written books about this strategy. But while he was quite thin and still running, he developed type 2 diabetes, seemingly out of nowhere. Being a brilliant scientist, Dr. Noakes went back to square one. He began to research the possible causes of his diabetes in the face of an apparently healthy diet and lifestyle. He concluded that he had been eating too many carbohydrates. He went on a strict low-carb/keto diet, reversed his diabetes, and wrote a book about his experience. It seemed too many of the carbs he was consuming to keep his glycogen stores full were, unbeknownst to him, turning into fat, causing insulin resistance and eventually diabetes. He appeared thin on the outside but on the inside had accumulated fat in his liver, his viscera, and his pancreas. This is a common presentation and has been termed TOFI (thin on the outside and fat on the inside). He no doubt had excess fat in his muscles as well.

Dr. Noakes and Dr. Volek, a Ph.D., have since performed and published metabolic studies and have coached elite endurance runners about training on a low-carb diet. They have found that when runners are on a ketogenic diet with minimal glycogen stores, their bodies become adapted to burning fat efficiently and they perform better than carb loaders. Their bodies learn to readily access their huge stores of fuel in the form of fat. They don't hit the wall, and several have become leaders in super-endurance competitions including triathlons as well as 50- and 100-mile runs.

Studies of athletes such as professional soccer players have also shown better endurance on a ketogenic diet. While I am not in ketosis most of the time, as I reported earlier, my athletic endurance has improved dramatically since becoming fat adapted on my keto-friendly diet.

BENEFITS, SUMMARIZED

With so much science thrown at you, it is only fair to provide a CliffsNotes-style summary to put it all together. I hope you find this helpful.

- In the 1980s, with the advent of high-fructose corn syrup and the low-fat government recommendations, Americans started consuming much higher quantities of sugar and refined carbohydrates. This caused swings in our blood sugars and less satiety because of our significant reduction of fats and meat proteins. This made us want to eat more food, and to eat more often. This led to "supersizing" our meals and to more frequent snacking to the point of continuously "grazing," a newly recognized phenomenon that has come to mean eating almost constantly throughout the day. The decrease in protein and fat intake, with the associated increase in sugar and refined carb consumption, is continuously elevating our insulin levels. This results in overstimulating insulin receptors on our livers, muscles, fat, and other organs, causing insulin resistance.

- Our genetic susceptibility to insulin resistance determines the point at which it begins. Insulin resistance prevents the efficient transport of glucose from the blood into the liver, so the liver reacts by making its own glucose, further increasing glucose levels in the blood. Meanwhile, our unprecedented consumption of sugar, especially its fructose component, overwhelms our liver's ability to burn it or safely store it. This fructose tsunami is therefore converted into fat, some of which remains in our liver resulting in a fatty liver and exacerbating insulin resistance.

- This process, repeated across the United States, has caused our epidemic of nonalcoholic fatty liver disease and liver failure. Most of the fat, moreover, spills into the bloodstream in the form of VLDL particles that deposit fat in tissues where it doesn't belong, including in our visceral fat, pancreas, and muscle. This extra fat worsens insulin resistance in all of these tissues, aggravating the whole process.

- The excess fat produced results in VLDL particles that are overstuffed. This is manifested clinically by elevated blood triglycerides, a low "good cholesterol" (HDL), and an increase in small LDL (bad cholesterol) particles. These small LDL particles are the ones that infiltrate the walls of the coronary arteries, eventually causing heart attacks. At this early stage, pancreatic beta cells produce enough extra insulin to overcome the liver's and muscles' insulin resistance and keep blood sugar and hemoglobin A1C normal. But, all is not well.

- The best way to make the diagnosis at this stage is with the Kraft oral insulin tolerance test, which measures the higher levels of insulin in the bloodstream that are necessary to keep blood sugar normal.

- This early stage, where insulin levels have increased but blood sugar has not yet elevated, is the ideal point at which to reverse the process. This can be done simply by minimizing sugar, refined carbohydrates, and omega-6 vegetable oil intake—in other words, a keto-friendly diet.

- As fat continues to accumulate in our organs, their normal functioning becomes disturbed, although not yet producing symptoms that are currently recognized as being associated with diabetes.

- Fat that accumulates under the skin (subcutaneous fat) is "safe fat" because it doesn't alter the function of these fat cells. The subcutaneous fat cells just divide, creating more fat cells to accommodate the extra fat being produced by the liver. In contrast, the fat cells in and around your organs are dangerous. These visceral fat cells are not able to divide when overloaded. They just grow in size until their structure becomes disrupted, causing local inflammation that eventually affects the entire body.

- The inflammation of and damage to the overloaded fat cells cause the release of some of their fat into the organs and into the blood stream. This worsens insulin resistance. This is when the now-fatty pancreas is affected and begins to fail. The pancreas can no longer produce enough insulin to overcome the insulin resistance of muscle (the largest reservoir for taking up blood glucose) and other tissues. It is at this point that blood glucose and hemoglobin A1C rise and the diagnosis of prediabetes and type 2 diabetes is made. But by now, there is severe insulin resistance and pancreatic beta cell dysfunction, and much of the damage to blood vessels, the liver, and other tissues have been progressing for years.

- Our challenge as a society is to identify this process at a stage when it is easiest to treat and when organ damage can be reversed. If you have a family history of diabetes and/or heart disease, if you have gained weight in your belly as an adult, if you tend to yo-yo diet or have high blood pressure associated with weight gain, if your blood tests show high triglycerides, low HDL or small LDL particles, you should also be concerned. You are likely insulin resistant, and the Keto-Friendly South Beach Diet can be a real life changer as well as a life extender.

GET READY TO CHANGE YOUR DIET & YOUR LIFE

As you've read, there is a tremendous amount of science and clinical experience that are cause for great excitement and optimism about the ability of a keto-friendly diet to not only help you lose weight, but also prevent disease and help you feel great. Now that you have the scientific principles under your belt, let's dive in and get started.

PART II
THE PLAN

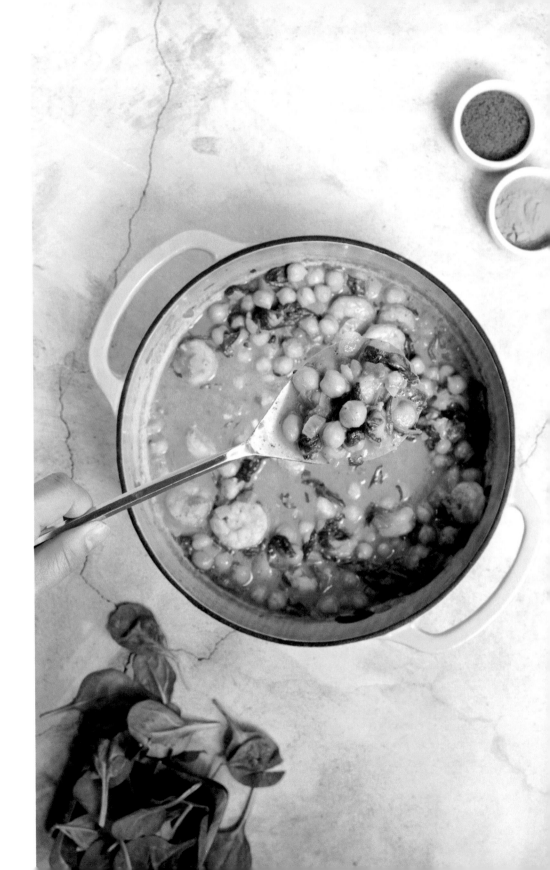

CHAPTER 6

GET READY . . .
The Plan Explained

Now that you've learned the science behind and benefits of a keto-friendly lifestyle, it's time to put that knowledge into practical use. It won't be long before you start to feel better. You will notice reduced appetite, loss of sugar cravings, more energy, improved mental clarity, and possibly the resolution of other symptoms including joint pain and acid reflux. Some of my patients report these changes within the first two weeks, and some as soon as the first three days. Of course, you'll also lose weight, especially around your belly.

In this section of the book, we outline the details of following the Keto-Friendly South Beach Diet and give you some practical tips on how to transform the diet into a lifestyle.

One of the best parts of the Keto-Friendly South Beach Diet is its flexibility. While the diet is designed around a certain macronutrient balance, these are just guidelines. The quality of your food is more important than the relative macronutrient amounts. The exception, of course, are sugars and high-glycemic carbs, which you'll want to watch very carefully. These must be minimized, particularly on Phase 1. This is the phase where you will be keeping your intake between 20 and 50 grams of net carbs per day. Otherwise, there is plenty of wiggle room.

Want all the benefits of full-fat dairy? Choose from plain yogurt, cheeses, cream, and whole milk. Prefer a more plant-based approach? Get your fats from coconut, avocado, and olive oil instead. Don't have much weight to lose? Add more higher-protein beans into Phase 1. You'll be able to decide whether you want to do a three-meals-a-day approach or see if intermittent fasting, skipping meals, or swapping out a meal for a snack or smaller meal works better for you. Healthy snacks that don't significantly raise your insulin levels are good to keep handy when you miss a meal, are stuck on a plane, or you are running late. You'll also decide on the best time to transition from Phase 1 to Phase 2, or if you want to transition at all. How you feel, as well as what your blood chemistries reveal when you review them with your doctor, will be your guide. As we've said before, one size does not fit all.

> ## The better you understand the diet principles, the better you will do; but trial and error is part of the process.

Whether your goal is weight loss, more energy, better sleep, improved mood, better athletic performance, or all the above, you can achieve it with this plan. Once you begin, you will soon notice improvement in how you look and how you feel. You'll turn your body into a fat-burning machine and burn more calories per day, depending on your baseline level of insulin resistance and your size, weight, and individual metabolism. The better you understand the diet principles, the better you will do; but trial and error is part of the process. This is an opportunity to take control of your health and your well-being.

Of course, you should consult with your physician before starting any new diet plan, especially if you have any medical issues such as high blood pressure or blood sugar

problems. I would recommend this book to your doctor, as well.

THE NEW KETO-FRIENDLY SOUTH BEACH DIET BREAKDOWN

Just like the original South Beach Diet, the Keto-Friendly South Beach Diet involves phases that you'll transition through (and can even go back and forth between) as you reach your goals and determine what works best for you. But unlike the original plan, this plan has just two phases and there are no set timelines for when to transition from Phase 1 to Phase 2.

Your insulin levels and sugar cravings will resolve quickly, but it may take one month, two months, or longer for your belly fat to disappear, depending on your starting point. You will also notice other benefits under the category of "fat adaptation," such as improved endurance. These benefits will continue to progress over many months.

As I learned from my personal experience after more than a year on this plan, I can add some fruit and whole grains to my diet without starting on a downward spiral. Importantly, I feel so good, and I am now so aware of my patterns of sugar addiction, that it is as if I'm immunized against regressing. I have almost imperceptibly transitioned to Phase 2 and a more flexible diet—especially when I travel. But when I am back at home and in my usual routine, I tend to follow Phase 1 (including with intermittent fasting) to best control my insulin level. You will find your own best balance.

THE DETAILS OF PHASE 1

Phase 1 is the more stringent "low-carb" phase. You'll stay on this phase for as long as you wish to continue more rapid weight loss and until your cravings are truly under control. There's no time restriction. You can stay on Phase 1 as long as you'd like, or you can come back to it if you feel that you've gotten carried away with additional starches. Often after a vacation with some expected refined carb indulgences, you will want to return to Phase 1.

> ## You can stay on Phase 1 as long as you'd like.

On Phase 1, your goal is to keep your net carbohydrate intake at 50 grams per day or less. Carbohydrates are not just found in sugars, starches, and grains, but are also found in healthy foods such as vegetables, nuts, and dairy products. That's where you'll be getting most of your carbohydrates in this phase, but they will make up a small percentage of your daily intake, with satiating protein and fat providing the rest.

When you're on Phase 1, you'll eat a lot of non-starchy vegetables, including broccoli, asparagus, cauliflower, and zucchini, as well as healthy fats such as full-fat dairy and olive oil. You'll also be consuming fat contained in high-quality proteins such as fish, meat, poultry, eggs, and other foods. Ultimately, you will be able to incorporate a small amount of higher-carbohydrate foods, such as lentils and black beans, into your diet.

THE DETAILS OF PHASE 2

I like to classify Phase 2 as the lifestyle phase, although you may continue to lose weight, depending on your food selections. You'll transition to Phase 2 once you reach your weight-loss goals or whenever you feel you need a little more flexibility. Depending on your level of insulin resistance, your blood test results, and your preferences, you may find that slower weight loss with the additional food options on Phase 2 is most sustainable. If you have subcutaneous fat to lose beyond your belly fat, be aware that this is a slower process and can be accomplished over a longer period on Phase 1 or Phase 2.

When on Phase 2, you'll be able to slowly increase your net carbs until you find what works best for you. Most people find their sweet spot between 75 and 100 grams of net carbs per day, although if you are still insulin resistant after Phase 1, or a postmenopausal woman, you may benefit from keeping your net carbohydrates at 50 grams or less on most days, indefinitely.

Phase 2 allows for slightly more carbohydrates than Phase 1, but it should still remain high in protein; so don't let carbohydrates push other food sources off your plate. The basics will be the same, but you will add lower glycemic whole fruits, high-protein and high-fiber grains, and a wider variety of beans, along with higher-starch veggies such as sweet potatoes. In many ways, Phase 2 is very similar to Phase 1, just more relaxed and friendly for life.

WHEN TO TRANSITION FROM PHASE 1 TO PHASE 2

How can you tell when it's time to move on from Phase 1 to Phase 2? If most of the following statements are true for you, you are likely ready to transition. This guidance is not set in stone. Like so much of the diet, the transition must be personalized for each of you. This includes those of you who have been doing blood testing with your physician. But remember, you can always return to Phase 1 if and when you feel the need or the desire.

- You have been on Phase 1 for at least one month.

- You are fat adapted: no "keto flu," increased energy and endurance.

- Cravings, frequent hunger throughout the day, and sugar addiction have all resolved.

- Weight loss has slowed because your belly fat and waist circumference have substantially decreased.

- You have evidence of metabolic improvement on blood testing: Your blood triglycerides are below 75, your Kraft test pattern has improved, your liver enzymes are normal, and your hemoglobin A1C has decreased to a reading below 5.7.

- You have reached your weight-loss goal.

TOTAL CARBS VERSUS NET CARBS

I do not count anything in my diet. If I have gained a couple of pounds, I simply become stricter about eating any starchy carbs. In other words, I keep to Phase 1 choices for a while. But many of our patients like to keep track of what they are eating every day and when it comes to starting a new eating plan, this can mean the difference between success and failure. Keeping a diary of your daily food intake has been shown to be a great help for many people revamping their eating habits. This has proven especially helpful when it comes to carbohydrates and there are some very good apps that can help you count carbs.

There are carbs in many of the foods you will be eating and these can add up quickly if you're not paying attention. Remember that "total carbohydrates" describes the entire amount of carbohydrates in a food, no matter what type of carbohydrate. "Net carbohydrates" refers only to the carbohydrates that are absorbed through your intestine into your bloodstream.

Certain types of carbohydrates, including fiber and sugar alcohols (the only sugar alcohol recommended here being erythritol), move through your digestive system without being absorbed into your bloodstream. So these carbohydrates have little or no effect on your blood sugar or insulin levels and need not be counted. All the rest of the carbohydrates—the sugar and starch components—do need to be counted. The goal is to limit your intake of insulin-raising carbohydrates so you can get your hormones under control, lose your cravings, and lose pounds.

> # The goal is to limit your intake of insulin-raising carbohydrates so you can get your hormones under control, lose your cravings, and lose pounds.

Once you transition to Phase 2, you can be more lenient with your carbohydrate sources. On Phase 2, you will still get a lot of your carbohydrates from non-starchy vegetables, but you'll be able to add in some starchy vegetables such as sweet potatoes and pumpkin because your net carbohydrate allowance will increase from 50 grams to 75 to 100 grams per day. The rest of your carbohydrates will come from a mix of legumes (including beans and lentils), whole grains, and low-glycemic whole fruits.

These whole-food carbohydrates have intact fiber skeletons that slow their digestion and achieve a favorable balance between the incretins GIP and GLP-1 released from the cells in the wall of your small intestine directly into your bloodstream. They'll raise your blood sugar and insulin levels slightly, but you won't have dramatic swings like you see with higher-glycemic carbohydrates such as French fries or a chocolate cupcake. The vitamins, minerals, and fiber found in whole foods are meant to be absorbed together.

White flour and sugar–laden sweets are not satiating and cause big swings in blood sugar. They have very little nutritional value and will likely increase your hunger, so they are not good choices even if you are within your net carbohydrate limit. Again, focus on the quality of your carbohydrates as well as the quantity.

WHAT ABOUT CALORIES?

In this plan, we don't ask you to count calories. I strongly believe that calorie counting is not helpful on its own, an opinion that has been borne out by clinical studies and years of clinical experience. Success will come with eating the right foods, and specifically watching net carbs. That said, as we always tell our patients, "Calories count, but counting calories doesn't help with long-term weight loss." The proteins, fats, and low-glycemic vegetables we recommend will satisfy your hunger. It is hard to overeat such foods. Many healthy foods have carbs, of course. You are unlikely to overdo it on high-fiber green vegetables, but foods such as nuts and dairy products may become diet busters, so watch your serving size. Even healthy oils such as avocado and olive oil can become problematic if used in excess. You can inadvertently pour a lot of oil in a pan, if you're not paying attention. When cooking or sautéing with these oils, measure the oil with a tablespoon or keep the oil in a spray bottle and spray to coat the pan. Be careful with these potential diet busters on Phase 1.

HOW TO CALCULATE NET CARBS

To calculate net carbohydrates, you subtract grams of fiber and grams of sugar alcohol (such as erythritol) from total carbohydrates (note: subtracting the total grams of sugar alcohol only applies to erythritol). For example, if a food item contains 14 grams of carbohydrates per serving, but 5 grams come from fiber and 3 grams come from erythritol, you would end up with 6 grams of net carbohydrates per serving.

Total Carbs	14
Fiber	-5
Sugar Alcohol	-3
Net Carbs	6

When it comes to sugar alcohols other than erythritol, such as maltitol, sorbitol, or xylitol, the formula changes. Those sugar alcohols are partially absorbed by your intestines, so you need to count the carbs that are absorbed and have an effect on your blood sugar. There is no standard set yet for how these sugar alcohols are calculated, but many cite the guidance of the Diabetes Education Center at University of California, San Francisco. This center suggests that half the carbs in these sugar alcohols can be subtracted from total carbs when calculating net carbs. So in this case, if a food has 14 total carbs, 5 grams of fiber, and 4 grams of maltitol, net carbs would be 7.

Total Carbs	14
Fiber	-5
Sugar Alcohol	-2
Net Carbs	7

Sugar alcohols in general have not been studied extensively, and as of the writing of this book, nutrition labels are not yet required to list sugar alcohols (though some do). It's important to note that some sugar alcohols do have an impact on blood sugar, including maltitol, the most commonly used sugar alcohol. They also are known to cause digestive upset in many people. Erythritol is the only sugar alcohol that seems to have minimal to no impact on blood sugar and does not cause digestive issues for most people. For that reason, it is the sugar alcohol we prefer. Again, if using other sugar alcohols, remember that you cannot subtract their total.

WHAT ABOUT GLUTEN?

Gluten is a protein found in wheat, barley, and rye. I became quite well versed in gluten when I wrote the *South Beach Diet Gluten Solution* a few years ago, and the science in that book has stood the test of time. My interest in gluten arose from an observation I had about South Beach Dieters: namely, that they felt great on Phase 1, seemingly independent of their weight loss. We also saw some surprising results, such as the complete resolution of a severe case of psoriasis and an unanticipated, but very welcome, pregnancy (after seven years of trying before starting the diet) and birth of a baby boy. The latter, we later learned, was because Phase 1 of the South Beach Diet had reversed the insulin resistance that was associated with polycystic ovary syndrome (PCOS), which had caused the infertility.

> You are unlikely to overdo it on high-fiber green vegetables, but foods such as nuts and dairy products may become diet busters, so watch your serving size.

And what about the relief from psoriasis? With this particular patient, when she travels and indulges in breads or pastas, her psoriasis promptly re-emerges. When she eliminates wheat, her skin completely clears. Her response was not associated with her weight—she was very thin—and she was not insulin resistant. She was just sensitive to gluten.

I started reading in depth about gluten, particularly the research and clinical experiences of Dr. Alessio Fasano and Dr. Peter Green. I soon realized that the first phase of the South Beach Diet, while intentionally grain free to prevent swings in blood sugar, was unintentionally gluten free because all grains were excluded. I started to take gluten seriously and learned that while celiac disease, an extreme form of gluten toxicity, is only found in 1 to 2 percent of Americans, gluten sensitivity is quite common. The exact prevalence of gluten sensitivity is not known because there is no reliable test for it, as there is for celiac disease.

I also learned that the adverse effects of gluten arise because, unlike the proteins in rice or corn, the gluten protein is difficult for our small intestinal enzymes to digest, especially for those who have gluten sensitivity. This difficulty with digestion ends up leaving incompletely digested fragments of gluten protein behind in the small intestine. These fragments are toxic to the small intestine and can lead directly to what is termed "leaky gut." Gluten sensitivity symptoms stem from its direct toxicity to the wall of the small intestine and from immune reactions triggered by the gluten protein fragments. This autoimmune reaction explained why my patient's psoriasis cleared up with the elimination of gluten. She was suffering from gluten-induced psoriasis, which is an autoimmune disease.

SIGNS AND SYMPTOMS OF GLUTEN SENSITIVITY

- Brain fog

- Reflux esophagitis (heartburn)

- Bloating and lower abdominal pain

- Anxiety, irritability, and mood swings

- Neuropathy

- Asthma

- Fatigue

- Joint pain

- Skin rashes

- Migraine headaches

- And other symptoms triggered by an autoimmune reaction

I developed clinical experience with patients suffering with these gluten-related symptoms and signs and improved or cured them with the removal of gluten from their diet. I was so impressed with the results that I wrote the book about it. The keto and low-carb communities have had similar experiences.

So the question is, "It is the removal of gluten that relieves these symptoms or the reversal of insulin resistance, or both?" The two cases I reported at the outset are clear, because the psoriasis patient was not overweight and not insulin resistant, so gluten was the key to her relief. The patient with PCOS was clearly cured by reversing her insulin resistance with our low-carb diet. She was including some gluten containing foods on Phase 2 and was not sensitive to small quantities of gluten.

But what about everybody else who might be insulin resistant or gluten sensitive—or both? The answer is, I don't know, unless and until I "challenge" such patients with gluten, which means they eliminate gluten for a period of time and then add gluten back into their diet and see how they feel. Another one of my patients, who I was convinced was gluten sensitive only because she was thin and not insulin resistant, challenged herself with a loaf of bakery-fresh bread when she was visiting a friend. Her symptoms, mainly stomach problems and joint pain, came roaring back in a matter of hours.

Keep in mind that gluten sensitivity varies and can depend on the quantity of gluten you are consuming. It is important to understand that the small number of those with the severe gluten problem, celiac disease, can only eat foods that are certified gluten free. For the much more common problem of gluten sensitivity, the great majority of people will not react to very small amounts of gluten. Each will find their own threshold.

Keep in mind that gluten sensitivity varies and can depend on the quantity of gluten you are consuming.

Phase I of the Keto-Friendly South Beach Diet has minimal to no gluten. So this is a good time to observe how you feel without it, or when consuming gluten in very small amounts. If you want to find out if you are gluten sensitive, monitor your reaction when gluten is reintroduced in a substantial amount. If symptoms such as a skin rash or headache improve on Phase 1, along with the reversal of insulin resistance, you can try a wheat challenge like my patient to make a diagnosis. This gluten challenge test works almost immediately, so you can observe the results and promptly return to low carb and, if sensitive, to gluten free.

WHAT ARE HEALTHY FATS?

What's considered good or bad fats has also changed with the forward progress of research and technology and our understanding of their direct effects on cholesterol particles. In the original South Beach Diet, we labeled olive oil (also known as monounsaturated fat) and omega-3 fish oils as good fats, and the subsequent medical literature continues to confirm their benefits. As you've learned, dairy fat—which is saturated but with a slightly different structure from other saturated fats—has earned its place on the list of good fats.

Dairy products are also very nutrient dense. They're high in vitamins A, B_6, B_{12}, and K as well as the minerals calcium, iodine, magnesium, potassium, phosphorus, and zinc. Of course, one of the biggest benefits of including full-fat dairy in your diet is its calcium content. Dairy is one of the richest sources of dietary calcium, with a couple of ounces of hard cheese providing around half of your daily requirement.

Many of these vitamins and minerals are found in the dairy's fat. When you remove the fat, as with low-fat and non-fat dairy products, you also remove nutrients. Additionally, full-fat dairy products are high in good-quality protein.

If you are lactose intolerant, it's helpful to focus on removing the dairy sources that contain the most lactose, such as milk, and replacing those with dairy options that are lower in lactose, including plain, whole-milk Greek yogurt; cream; and hard, fermented cheeses; as well as lactose-free whole milk. In many cases, people who don't tolerate milk well do okay with yogurt or other lower-lactose options.

Other healthy saturated fats include coconut oil and saturated fat in the form of medium-chain triglycerides, or MCTs. MCTs are found in the highest concentrations in coconut products, including full-fat coconut milk, coconut oil, and shredded coconut (unsweetened, of course). In fact, more than 50 percent of the fat in coconut products is in the form of MCTs.

MCTs have taken some flak because they're saturated fats, but they're a unique type of fat that can be used as a good source of energy because they are quickly metabolized. We are still learning about other healthy effects of MCTs.

OMEGA-3 AND OMEGA-6

You should have your omega-3 and omega-6 blood levels measured by your physician and adjust your fish intake and/or fish oil supplements accordingly. There are no formal guidelines, but we like to see an omega-3 index of greater than 6 and an omega-6 to omega-3 ratio of less than 4 to 1. This is the only way you can know for sure that the omega-3 from the fish you consume or the fish oil/omega-3 supplement you take is actually getting into your tissues.

While we prefer you get your nutrients from whole foods rather than supplements, if you do not like seafood, fish oil supplements are an exception. You should choose the fish oil supplement with the highest levels of EPA and DHA on the label. The quality of most well-known brands is good. The fish containing the highest amounts of omega-3 fatty acids are salmon, mackerel, tuna, sardines, and herring.

Walnuts contain a lot of omega-3, while most other nuts do not. Flaxseeds are another source of omega-3, but neither walnuts nor flaxseeds have the omega-3 quality and quantity of fish or fish oil supplements. Remember, too, that omega-6 in the quantities found in vegetable oils will depress your omega-3 levels and adversely impact the ratio of omega-6 to omega-3 in your blood. Your doctor can now easily test your blood levels so you will know if you are getting adequate omega-3. If your omega-3 blood level is not rising with your supplement, you are taking the wrong supplement. If your omega-3 level is low with an elevated omega-6 to omega-3 level, then omega-6 vegetable oils are sneaking into your diet.

When it comes to fat optimization, make sure you're getting plenty of omega-3 and monounsaturated fats. You also want healthy saturated fats from dairy. Other sources of saturated fat are also fine, including eggs, coconut oil, beef, pork, and poultry.

One issue often raised is the difference in the fat content of beef that is grain fed versus grass fed, or in the case of salmon, wild versus farmed. The total fat content in grain-fed beef is higher because the excess grain is readily turned into fat, and the cattle are penned and sedentary compared to range-fed cattle. But the percentage of saturated to monounsaturated fat (good fat like that found in olive oil) in grain-fed meat does not differ significantly from grass fed. True, the ratio of omega-6 to omega-3 is increased in the grain fed, but the total amounts are so small that it is unlikely to impact your omega-6 to omega-3 ratio. Grass-fed cattle are always leaner than grain fed because of the calories they burn in the fields. Grain feeding puts the animal in a fat-storage mode, just like in humans. This is why their meat is marbled in prime cuts. Similarly, farmed salmon has more fat than wild salmon, which is leaner from a lifetime of swimming upstream. The increased fat content in farmed salmon is almost all healthy omega-3, and extra omega-6 is negligible.

Therefore, as far as its effect on your omega-6 to omega-3 blood levels goes, there is not a significant difference owing to how fish or beef is fed. Ultimately, it is the total omega-3 in your cell membranes and the ratio of omega-6 to omega-3 that is important, and now this can be easily checked with a simple blood test. Then your diet or fish oil supplement can be adjusted accordingly.

There are other more complicated concerns about what might be added to grain-fed beef and farmed fish; we don't always know what and how they are fed. We also warn about certain fish that are high in mercury. If grass-fed beef and wild salmon are available, we would favor it, but the nutrient content and protein content of beef and salmon are excellent in either case.

MEETING YOUR PROTEIN NEEDS

We know that in the United States protein intake tends to decrease with age. We also know that the incidence and degree of insulin resistance increase with age as well and is known to exacerbate osteoporosis and muscle atrophy. The total percentage of fat in our bodies also increases with age, while our percentage of "lean body mass" (our muscle and bone) decreases. All of these detrimental changes worsen progressively as we age, sometimes dramatically in women after menopause, and more gradually in men as their testosterone levels decrease—a period sometimes called "andropause."

Many factors can accelerate these changes. Lack of exercise is one important factor that occurs dramatically during illness, injury, or even elective surgery such as a knee or hip replacement. In these situations, the loss of muscle and bone and its substitution with fat can occur rapidly, especially when days of bed rest are required. With more fat and less muscle

and bone, metabolism slows, and insulin resistance is increased. Insulin levels will rise while pancreatic beta cell dysfunction gets worse. These episodes of inactivity can become a downward spiral toward progressive disability and diabetes. Because they are quite common, they are often thought to be a customary part of aging—but they are not, and should not be considered normal.

This deterioration can be prevented with the right diet and exercise program. Preventing or reversing insulin resistance with the Keto-Friendly South Beach Diet, along with proper exercise, is the key. The increased protein we recommend helps prevent the loss of muscle and bone mass as we age. Dieting by just restricting calories slows your metabolism and activates your set point hormones, which increases your hunger. In contrast, when you lose weight by lowering your insulin levels with our diet, other hormones are activated that do not increase your hunger or slow your metabolism. Quite the opposite, your hunger is suppressed and your metabolism is increased.

Exercise, especially resistance training using light weights, bands, or your own body weight, as well as functional exercise like Pilates or yoga, works with the diet to maintain your muscle and bone mass. Balance practice is also critical for healthy aging.

PROTEIN QUALITY

The quality of the protein you eat and the timing of when you eat it are also important. This has been demonstrated in excellent studies performed at McMaster University by protein and exercise guru Professor Stuart M. Phillips.

His research has shown that we are constantly either building up protein or breaking it down. Some types of protein are better than others for manufacturing muscle protein. The best one appears to be the whey protein found in milk and other dairy products (another plus for dairy).

The quality of the protein you eat and the timing of when you eat it are also important.

Dr. Phillips has demonstrated that you build muscle faster with whey protein than with protein from soy or other sources, and much faster than if you are not consuming protein at all. If you exercise and consume good-quality protein, their effects are synergistic—better together than either alone. Dr. Phillips also taught us that your ingested protein decreases its muscle-building effect if you wait too long after exercise to consume it. On the Keto-Friendly South Beach Diet, you don't have to have a full meal after exercise. You can drink a whey protein shake or have a high-protein snack that gives you the protein you need to build new muscle without significant increases in blood sugar or insulin levels.

You may ask, "If I am consuming more protein than on the conventional keto diet, does that mean I won't take in enough fat to go into fat-burning mode?" The answer is no. In your weight-loss mode, you have plenty of fat to burn from your own fat stores whether or not you are in ketosis. The point to remember is that as long as you are avoiding sugar and high-glycemic carbs, your insulin levels will remain low enough to keep you in a fat-burning mode. Sometimes dieters believe they have to consume a lot of fat and be in ketosis to burn fat, but our keto-friendly diet will put you in fat-burning mode without having to be in ketosis.

Another advantage of protein is that it is the most satiating of the macronutrients, and many studies confirm that high-protein diets are effective for weight loss. The extra muscle and bone you build will also increase your resting metabolism, another benefit. So the combination of staying low in refined carbs along with eating adequate protein will help you lose weight while maintaining your muscle and bone mass—and therefore your strength. This is what we call *quality* weight loss, which leads to healthy aging.

As you have learned, you can live a long life without chronic disease while enjoying a relatively high whole-food carbohydrate and low-meat and -dairy diet, as is found in many traditional Asian societies. But remember that the high meat and high dairy–consuming Mongols conquered all the "grain eaters" of Asia. The famous Maasai warriors of Africa, who also lived on meat and dairy, were bigger, stronger, and had better teeth and jaws than their lower-protein neighbors. Interesting.

FRUITS AND VEGETABLES

The nutrition establishment and the government always seem to lump fruits and vegetables together, as in their mantras, "You should have five servings of fruits and vegetables a day" and "Fruits and vegetables prevent heart attacks." Surprisingly, few of these claims are actually evidence based. And even more importantly, fruits and vegetables should not be lumped together.

Non-starchy vegetables are whole foods containing good levels of vitamins, minerals, and fiber, and while they contain some starch, they are very low in sugar. They are good for you. Fruit, on the other hand, often has less fiber and more fructose which is why we like sweet fruits and can be tempted to overeat them.

Many people assume that all fruits and even fruit juices are healthy. Big mistake. All fruit has fructose, and many tropical fruits, such as pineapple, have enough fructose and little enough fiber that we commonly see patients' blood sugars shoot out of control if too much is eaten. When one patient's hemoglobin A1C jumped up, it was a mystery until he realized that his backyard mangos had ripened, and he had overindulged.

> # Many people assume that all fruits and even fruit juices are healthy. Big mistake.

As for fruit juices, you might as well be drinking sugary sodas. In most fruit juices, much of the fiber has been removed and all that remains is the high-fructose juice. And, even if fiber remains, the juicing process has disrupted the fibrous skeleton of the whole fruit. Therefore, you should be careful with quantities of all fruits, but especially those that are high in sugar and low in fiber. Let's stop lumping fruits and vegetables together as if they were nutritionally equivalent; they most certainly are not.

That's why non-starchy vegetables are a staple of our diet, and fruits are allowed but in more limited amounts.

SODIUM AND THE "KETO FLU"

We are always amazed by how well our patients feel as they start the diet and begin to lose their bellies—with the exception of one common side effect, the "keto flu" or the low-carb flu. This term was coined by people beginning a strict keto diet who felt fatigue and other symptoms such as weakness, decreased workout performance, headaches, dizziness, muscle cramps, and various other related symptoms. It is also common in low-carb, keto-friendly diets, and people who are not in ketosis may feel these same symptoms from a significant reduction in carbohydrates. This may happen even after listening to our advice on how to prevent it. In fact, two of my colleagues and I have experienced it along with many of our patients.

Before I relate my own experience, let me reassure you that the keto flu is not a disease and is easily relieved. It is actually a sign that your body is working the way nature intended, and that you will do well on the diet.

The reason for the keto flu comes back to our nemesis, insulin. As we related earlier, high insulin levels cause your kidneys to absorb extra salt (sodium) from your blood as it circulates through them. This salt retention increases your blood pressure by increasing your fluid volume. When you minimize sugar and high-glycemic carbs and lower your insulin level, your kidneys begin to excrete salt very efficiently through the urine, causing your fluid levels to decrease. When your fluid level drops, your blood pressure decreases as a result. The higher your insulin levels were before beginning the diet, the greater the increase in salt excretion, and the faster your blood pressure may drop when you start the diet.

HYDRATION AND THE KETO FLU

Your hydration level (the amount of fluid in your body and your bloodstream) is dependent on the amount of salt you retain or excrete. When you reabsorb salt from your kidneys so that it is not lost in your urine, or you consume more salt in your diet, your total body fluid volume goes up. The concentration of salt in your blood, which we routinely measure as sodium, does not change and is not a measure of your body's fluid level.

After vigorous exercise (as has been studied in professional athletes), even with attention to salt and water replacement, your body's salt and fluid levels fall and you become dehydrated to a degree that it usually takes several days to replenish. Your sodium concentration will remain normal the whole time because you lose fluid in proportion to your loss of salt.

The keto flu and its varied symptoms are due to your welcome drop in insulin levels causing dehydration from the loss of salt and fluid in your urine. The simple cure is the replacement of the lost salt and water.

The reason the keto flu is a good sign is that it means your previously high insulin levels have fallen enough to initiate this response, and it also means your fat stores have been unlocked. So, congratulations! The higher your insulin levels when you began and the more dramatic the fall, the more the Keto-Friendly South Beach Diet is needed for your long-term

health—and the better it is working. Your keto flu will disappear with the stabilization of your insulin levels and with adequate salt intake.

MY BOUT OF KETO FLU

Even though I was well aware of this issue, when I returned from my summer vacation to my vigorous morning boxing workouts in the south Florida heat, I misjudged how much salt I required. On several occasions, after twelve rounds with my trainer, Juan, and a quick hot shower, I came to the office to start my workday and felt the beginning of a migraine headache, as well as mild dizziness. I took one of the hard-boiled eggs I had brought for lunch, poured salt all over it and ate it, along with drinking a bottle of water. My headache and dizziness quickly resolved.

I have always drunk water in between boxing rounds, but with lower insulin levels and more efficient salt excretion, I found I needed to have salt and water before and after I trained. This solved the problem, with one more caveat: I also experienced some muscle cramping. For the cramping, salt replacement helped, but with my lower insulin levels, I had to replace magnesium as well. Magnesium is found in leafy green vegetables, nuts, sunflower seeds, fatty fish, and yogurt. But for me and several patients, taking a slow-release magnesium supplement twice a day is necessary to prevent the cramps. A warm Epsom salt bath also helps.

One common misconception is that the weakness and other symptoms associated with the keto flu are due to low blood glucose and will be cured with sugar. This is wrong and counterproductive. Attention to salt and water intake, even with a zero-calorie electrolyte drink, will solve the problem. The keto flu is most common during the first few days of a low-carb diet because that is when you experience the biggest drop in your insulin levels and the biggest increase in salt excretion. After that, it is not common and very easily recognized and treated if it does occur.

SALT INTAKE

Another myth encouraged by national guidelines is that the lower your salt intake, the healthier you will be. We all believed this until a landmark paper was published in *The New England Journal of Medicine* in 2014. It concluded that optimal sodium intake is between 4 and 6 grams per day—well above the national recommendations of 2.3 grams per day. Below 4 grams, death rates rose quickly. Above 6 grams, death rates increased gradually. For those who exercise vigorously, especially in a hot environment, sodium intake needs to be on the high side. However, for people with salt-sensitive high blood pressure or other medical issues, lower levels are needed, so talk to your doctor.

For the many Americans consuming fast food and packaged and processed foods, the associated salt intake is often too high. But for those cooking at home, total salt intake is naturally lower.

We find that patients, especially those who exercise frequently, often think they are being healthy by avoiding salt. In fact, they need more. The experience of a fitness trainer we work with illustrates this not uncommon issue. He is in outstanding shape, exercises regularly and

vigorously, with blood pressure on the normal to low side. But he was complaining of chronic fatigue. It turned out he was limiting his salt because the national guidelines recommended low salt intake for good health. By increasing the salt in his diet, his fatigue promptly resolved and his energy greatly increased.

FASTING, FOOD TIMING, SNACKING & MIXED MEALS

As we discussed in Chapter 4, fasting can be an excellent strategy for keeping your insulin levels low. We often suggest it to our patients who have trouble initiating the diet or if their weight loss has slowed at a point when they clearly have more belly fat to lose. Many patients just feel better and more alert when they are intermittently fasting. They often continue with varying degrees of fasting even when they have achieved their weight-loss goals. They report that they feel fine, are less hungry during the day, and find it easier to stay at their ideal weight. This can simply mean not eating until lunchtime, if you are not hungry.

HOW TO GET STARTED WITH FASTING

While there have always been recommendations to not skip breakfast, or to skip meals in general, there was never any solid evidence behind such advice. We do know that there is an important hunger hormone named ghrelin, which travels from your intestine to your brain to stimulate your appetite. It is often associated with a "growling" abdomen. When you first start intermittent fasting and skipping a meal, ghrelin will be secreted at your regular meal time and induce hunger. But, if you do not eat, that feeling of hunger will not persist.

I became aware of this phenomenon on busy days in the office when I was concentrating on a patient visit or a project and working right through lunch. After a hunger pang, I would forget about lunch and by the time I was no longer distracted and realized I hadn't eaten, I wasn't hungry. I am sure many of you have had similar experiences. This pattern occurs because your ghrelin blood levels go back to normal in one hour, if not sooner. You don't get hungry because you are lacking in energy stores; you have plenty of fat stores to tap into. Fortunately, the regular ghrelin secretion at your usual mealtime subsides in a few days, and so does your hunger. When this happens, it means you are using your stored fat for energy.

We find it best to begin intermittent fasting by skipping just one meal, usually breakfast (although it doesn't have to be). Once this is comfortable, you can begin delaying lunch and extending your fast into the afternoon. You will see what works for you.

It is important to keep up your fluid and mineral intake. Stay hydrated with plenty of water, salt, and magnesium supplementation. We find bone broth or bouillon cubes are helpful. Using a "light" salt that contains extra potassium is also helpful to maintain your potassium levels.

You can exercise while fasting, but pay special attention to fluids, salt, and potassium and magnesium levels, which are important. To see what your ideal supplementation is, you might have to experiment and discuss this with your doctor. While I advise finding what works best for you, if you plan to fast more than 24 hours, you should definitely discuss this with your doctor first.

SNACKING & INTERMITTENT FASTING

You can still get the benefits of intermittent fasting while enjoying a snack or two if the snack does not significantly raise your insulin levels. These snacks are sometimes referred to as "fasting equivalents." An example is "bulletproof coffee," which is black coffee with approximately a tablespoon of butter and a tablespoon of coconut oil added and blended.

Intermittent fasting is certainly the quickest strategy for lowering your insulin levels promptly and tends to work very well for many of our patients. In some, it has been a true diet saver. So feel free to experiment and determine what works best for you. Again, we do suggest that, as with any major change in your diet, you consult with your doctor. It is prudent to check your electrolyte levels including magnesium periodically.

CHAPTER 7

GET SET . . .
Plan, Prep & Shop

So you've learned all about the science behind the Keto-Friendly South Beach Diet. You've read about the basics of which foods to eat more of and which to minimize. Now the fun begins. It's time to dive in! This chapter will give you important information about how we set up the Phase 1, 28-day meal plan, along with tips and advice to help you shop for food and prepare some delicious recipes. Most importantly, though, this is when you start to put this diet into action—and in a short time, you will be feeling the positive effects.

BOOSTING YOUR SUCCESS WITH MEAL PREP

Reviewing your menu for the approaching week and making some meals ahead of time will really help increase your likelihood of success. You may be familiar with the saying, "If you fail to plan, you are planning to fail." This is especially true when it comes to your nutrition, even more so when you're starting something new. One of the biggest favors you can do for yourself is to plan your meals and prep what you can ahead of time. This takes away the uncertainty about what or when you're going to be eating, especially when you're out of the house or just short on time. We've provided some meal plans you can use as a starting point, until you're comfortable enough to design your own menus. As you're adjusting to the Keto-Friendly South Beach Diet and its two phases, use these meal plans along with the food lists at the end of this chapter for inspiration and to keep you on track.

First, we advise that you read the meal plans in advance and look over the recipes included for the week ahead. See whether any of them require special preparation, such as marinating meat, thawing frozen ingredients, or freezing a make-ahead dessert. Take special note of the tips on each day of the plan. You'll see three different types:

Plan ahead: A tip labeled "Plan ahead," gives you a heads-up that you might need to make and store an extra serving of a recipe for later in the week, for lunch the next day, or to freeze for another time. Life can be hectic and it will help save time if some meals can stretch over more than one day. Leftovers can be your friend.

Prep: In these menu plans, we have two types of meal suggestions. First are meals that come from the recipe section in this book, for which we provide a corresponding page number. Second are suggestions for simple make-it-yourself meals to help you get the hang of keto-friendly cooking without a cookbook. For these, we set out basic instructions within the meal plan. You can, and should, experiment with spices, cooking methods, and Phase 1 condiments to make these meals your own.

Variation: This tip offers some substitutions or twists on recipes or meal suggestions to give you more options.

Looking ahead at your upcoming week can help put you on the fast track to success. Of course, the timing of your meal planning and prepping will depend on your schedule, but here are a few strategies to help.

WEEKEND PREP

Over the weekend, take a look at the plan for the week ahead. Read through the ingredient lists and create a list for everything you will need for the week. Be sure to include items from the Foods to Enjoy List (see page 84) that you may want to have on hand. You can also use this time to customize or tweak the meal plan to suit your tastes. If you don't care for one of the recipes on that week's plan, you can replace it with another recipe in the same phase. Most of the recipes in the lunch and dinner categories contain similar amounts of net carbohydrates to make swapping things out easier for you. Just remember to stick to Phase 1 recipes as you get started.

> Most of the recipes in the lunch and dinner categories contain similar amounts of net carbohydrates to make swapping easier.

It's helpful to divide your shopping list into different sections, such as "produce," "canned goods," "dairy," and "meat," so you can save time when you actually do your shopping. Once you've written down all of the ingredients, check to see what you already have on hand; no need to purchase duplicates. Once your list is organized, read through the directions for each recipe and see which of them require a bit more time to prepare, as well as those best prepared in advance. Review your calendar for the week ahead and pencil in a cooking schedule. If things change, as they often do, switch one recipe for another depending on the time you have to cook or prep.

A little time spent organizing for the week ahead will make sticking to the plan much easier. You don't want to arrive home after a long day at work, probably hungry, only to have to start a recipe requiring more prep and cooking time than you're up for.

PERSONALIZING YOUR MEAL PLAN

The Phase 1 meal plan should serve as your guide to eating keto friendly for the next 28 days. However, you can still be "on plan" without including every recipe we have suggested. Remember, if you find that you want to swap out one of the recipes and make your own keto-friendly meal instead, fine! Just aim to create meals that include a combination of healthy fats, lean proteins, and non-starchy vegetables. Look at the Foods to Enjoy, Phase 1 list beginning on page 84 to see the types of foods that can be included. Ideally, you should also aim to include no more than 12 grams of net carbs at most meals, and to limit your net carbs in snacks to 5 grams or fewer. In fact, we encourage you to make your own meals several times each week, so you can really learn how to customize recipes or food choices to suit your tastes and keep them as complicated or simple as you like. You can also swap or repeat recipes from one day to the next.

For ideas on great keto-friendly ways to flavor or season your meat, fish, poultry, and vegetables, see page 82.

STAYING FLEXIBLE

The Phase 1 meal plan was designed to be flexible. It is meant as a guide to help you learn the keto-friendly way of eating. If you're creating your own meals, you may want to keep things

simple, especially in the beginning. But, if you are someone who enjoys cooking, or loves lots of intricate flavors and textures in their foods, just be sure you keep to the Foods to Enjoy list for Phase 1 and be cognizant of those ingredients that may be "diet busters." Stick to a template of protein, healthy fat, and non-starchy vegetables for Phase 1, with the occasional addition of beans or legumes, preferably after your cravings are controlled. Proteins, healthy fats, non-starchy vegetables, and an additional complex carbohydrate or occasional fruit are included later on Phase 2.

These relaxed parameters will allow you even more flexibility as you adjust and learn. A meal may consist of grilled salmon with a side of roasted, seasoned broccoli tossed in a tablespoon of olive oil, or eggs scrambled with spinach and goat cheese, topped with a slice of avocado. On Phase 2, those same meals could transition to grilled salmon and roasted broccoli with a side of quinoa, or eggs scrambled with spinach and goat cheese topped with a slice of avocado, along with a side of a few baked sweet potato fries. The additional food choices provide a lot of variety to keep you satisfied long term.

NAVIGATING THE GROCERY STORE

The next step is shopping. As you make up your shopping list, remember that you can also substitute suggested items based on your own personal preferences, as long as you follow the Foods to Enjoy lists. For example, if a recipe calls for ground beef but you'd rather use ground turkey, or if ground chicken happens to be on sale, simply swap out the beef for the turkey or chicken. You can also substitute non-starchy veggie choices based on what looks good, what's in season, or what you prefer. While recipes are designed around net grams of carbohydrates as well as fats and protein, substitutions are encouraged, particularly if they will help you stay on course and enjoy your meals. As long as you use the Foods to Enjoy lists and keep the meal nutritionally balanced with proteins, healthy fats, and non-starchy vegetables, you will be okay. Just replace protein with protein, fat with fat, and non-starchy vegetables with another non-starchy vegetable. The recipes are not written in stone.

You should be sure to allow sufficient time when shopping to carefully read food labels. As we've already discussed, while we typically recommend choosing whole foods as much as possible, sometimes convenience foods are necessary. If you're opting for packaged foods, do check the net carbohydrates and make sure they fall into the desired macronutrient balance for a meal, snack, or side. Be on the lookout for added sugars or artificial sweeteners. Remember that sugars must be kept to a minimum. The good news is that, as the keto-friendly lifestyle becomes more widespread, more low-carb, nutrient-dense options are becoming available in your grocery store. You should already be able to find cauliflower rice (fresh or frozen) and premade cauliflower crust, as well as stevia- or erythritol-sweetened chocolate at many supermarkets, and they are easy to find if you shop online.

While your shopping list will be pretty straightforward, there may be some items in the meal plan that are new to you. Here is a quick rundown of some of the most popular keto-friendly items:

Cauliflower rice: This "rice" is made from cauliflower and can be found in either the produce or frozen section of your local market and makes a great side dish. You can also make your own by grating a head of fresh cauliflower, which gives it more or less the consistency of rice.

Keto-friendly shakes: You'll see keto-friendly shakes suggested in your meal plans. This means any shake that is very low in net carbs (<5g) and higher in healthy fats. The protein in the shake doesn't necessarily have to be very high. These shakes can be a good option when you're on the run.

Whey protein shakes: Whey protein shakes should also be low in net carbs (<5g) but should also be high in protein (at least 10 grams protein, or 20 percent of the Daily Value on the nutrition label). While these shakes can be consumed as a convenient snack option, they are particularly good for recovery after a workout for helping to maintain your lean body mass.

Keto-friendly flours: The flours we recommend using in place of traditional flour for baking include almond flour and coconut flour. They are used in different ways to substitute for refined carbohydrate flours, so learn from the suggested recipes about relative amounts. You can also experiment yourself.

Keto-friendly mayonnaise: Good options on the market now include mayo made with avocado oil but be sure the mayonnaise does not include added starches or sugars.

Keto-friendly sweeteners: We recommend only three: erythritol-based sweeteners, which come in granulated, powdered, and even brown sugar form; stevia-based sweeteners; and monk fruit.

Zoodles: A low-carb staple, "zoodles" refer to the spiralized zucchini noodles that are often used in keto-friendly recipes to replace flour pasta noodles. You can find these in the produce section of the grocery store or make them at home using a spiralizer or a food processor with a spiralizer attachment.

FREQUENTLY ASKED QUESTIONS

We get lots of questions about certain types of foods to eat. Here are the answers to some common FAQs:

What can I put in my coffee or tea?
Look for higher-fat, lower-carb options to add flavor and indulgence to your morning coffee and tea. Try using one tablespoon of full-fat cream or half-and-half or butter. If you're looking for a dairy-free alternative, try one teaspoon of coconut oil. For a touch of sweetness, you can add keto-friendly sweeteners erythritol, monk fruit, or stevia.

How do I jazz up plain yogurt?
If you like a bit of sweetness in your plain whole-milk Greek yogurt, try mixing in a small amount of our suggested keto-friendly sweeteners (erythritol, monk fruit, or stevia), and perhaps a bit of vanilla extract. You might also try some walnuts and cinnamon, or some sugar-free stevia-sweetened chocolate chips.

What about snacks?
We have built these meal plans to include three main meals and two snacks each day; however, keep in mind that the fewer eating occasions you have throughout the day, the greater the opportunity to reduce the amount of insulin your body secretes. If you prefer to eat three meals a day and generally eliminate snacks, you can move the contents of the suggested snacks into one of your other meal occasions to create a larger meal. However, keep in mind that you never want to leave yourself feeling so hungry that you are likely to grab the wrong thing. In that case, have a keto-friendly snack. You may find your need to snack lessening as your insulin level drops on the plan.

Ultimately, the goal is to find what works best for you to make keto friendly a lifestyle you can maintain long term. What suits you best may on some days mean including smaller meals and a few high-fat or high-protein snacks, while on other days you will have three larger meals incorporating your snacks, or simply not snack at all. Your preference may change as you lose visceral fat and your insulin resistance resolves.

What about sodium?
Sodium is not off-limits on a keto-friendly plan. You should aim for 4,000 to 6,000 mg of sodium each day to avoid dehydration due to the lower-carb nature of the program. Be liberal with the use of salt when adding it to flavor meals and snacks, and pay particular attention if you exercise rigorously. Remember to consult with your physician if you have high blood pressure, are salt sensitive, or have other medical conditions.

GET COOKING

It's time to cook some meals in advance. A good place to start is with egg cups, soups, and other items that are easy for grab-and-go during the week. You can divide the completed recipe into individual portion sizes and store them in airtight containers in the refrigerator for a few days or freeze them as directed. This ensures that you'll have an easy, healthy option when you don't have time to cook. You can also double the quantity of certain recipes or freeze several portions of a larger recipe, which will significantly cut down on cooking time in the future. Look for notes indicating which recipes are to make in advance or freeze.

KETO-FRIENDLY COOKING TIPS

Cooking Methods

Most cooking methods are fine—you can bake, roast, grill, sauté, slow cook, and more. Just follow our advice on how to grease your pans and keep heated oils below their smoke point.

How to Grease or Spray the Pan

Olive oil is a staple, with avocado oil right behind. Coconut oil is another delicious choice. You can fill a pump or spray bottle with oil and spray your pan to grease before cooking. Alternatively, measure out one or two tablespoons of oil to grease the pan. The amount will depend on pan size, of course, which should correlate to the quantity of food (and servings) you are preparing. It's always a good idea to measure the oil, so you don't inadvertently over pour. Butter is also a great option when greasing a pan, especially for certain foods such as scrambled eggs or an omelet.

Seasoning & Spices

Spices and seasonings can help make a plain roasted meat or vegetable quite delicious. Be sure to keep your pantry stocked with your favorites and try some options that are new to you. If you like, create some combinations or rubs that you enjoy and keep them handy in an airtight bag or container. Incorporating a wide variety of herbs and spices can make all the difference in keeping your meals varied and delicious.

Dips, Dressings & Sauces

We have included several recipes that can be used as dips, as well as sauces and dressings. Tzatziki (see page 225) is a wonderful dip for meats, poultry, fish, or veggies, and guacamole (see page 253) is always a favorite and a great topping containing healthy fats. Horseradish mixed with a little mayo and yogurt makes a nice dipping sauce with a bit of heat. Add a splash of Tabasco, sriracha, or other hot sauce (with no added sugar) to spice up any low-carb combination. Chimichurri (made with lemon juice, bell pepper, chili pepper, garlic, parsley, salt, and pepper) is another wonderful low-carb topping for meats.

Once you've learned which ingredients can be incorporated in your Keto-Friendly South Beach Diet, you can experiment and develop your personal favorites. Vinaigrettes can also be made with red or white wine vinegar or apple cider vinegar and olive oil along with herbs, Dijon mustard, and a bit of pressed garlic. One particularly delicious trick is to boil a couple of peeled garlic cloves for 10 minutes and mash the softened garlic into your dressing. See the condiments in the Foods to Enjoy list for more ideas.

TIPS FOR EATING OUT

Lots of people think that following a low-carb, keto-friendly diet makes it difficult to eat outside the home, but it's easy to eat out once you understand the plan. Most restaurants offer the basics, so you can make good choices and enjoy a delicious meal when you're out with friends or family.

To start, ask your waiter which meats, poultry, or fish their chef can grill, roast, or lightly sauté with olive oil or butter. You may want to ask about the catch of the day or a recommended steak. Pesto on grilled proteins is usually a good option and many keto-friendly dips or dressings, including tzatziki in a Greek restaurant, are likely available. You should have plenty of choices. Accompany your entrée with a non-starchy vegetable such as broccoli, grilled asparagus, or sautéed spinach as a side dish.

If everyone is ordering appetizers, start your meal with a shrimp cocktail (but watch out for sugar in the cocktail sauce) or a house salad (without croutons) and ask for a side of olive oil and vinegar to create your own no-sugar-added dressing. Don't be afraid to ask several questions about the food preparation, or ingredients that might be added (like sugar). Most chefs are happy to help if your waiter doesn't know the answer.

The bottom line is that as long as you're staying within the carbohydrate recommendation of 50 grams or below on Phase 1, and somewhere between 75 and 100 grams on Phase 2, you have a lot of options to make this plan your own. What's most important is that you're able to learn and enjoy an eating plan that works for you over the long term, because the most effective diet is one that you can stick to.

EATING ON THE GO

What about when you are on the run—in the car or at an airport? The headline here is: be prepared. Be sure to take snacks and portable foods with you in case you get hungry or are traveling at mealtime. This can be as simple as throwing some whole-milk cheese sticks and some nuts (apportioned in a sealed container) in your bag. Sitting on a tarmac in a delayed airplane is a recipe for finishing off an entire jar or a 16-ounce bag of nuts, so prepacking is key. A hard-boiled egg or two in a sealed bag is also always a good choice. It's very filling and should keep you satisfied for quite a while. Another make-ahead option is a turkey and cheese roll-up with a couple of slices of meat and cheese; wrap it in plastic wrap or a sealed plastic bag and go. A small container of whole-milk Greek yogurt is a nice treat, but if you're traveling by air, you will need to buy it once you've passed the TSA checkpoint. And, you will need to watch the time it's outside the fridge, unless it is packed in a cold, insulated bag (and don't forget a spoon!).

If you're unprepared and the only options available are wrapped sandwiches and fast food, you know how to improvise . . . buy the turkey and cheese hoagie and eat the middle without the bread. Pick up a plastic knife and fork at checkout and scrape off any excess sauce that may contain added sugar. You can use the utensils to eat your snack or use your (washed) fingers to make a roll-up.

Becoming familiar with the Foods to Enjoy lists and understanding the Keto-Friendly South Beach Diet program and the science behind it will enable you to make good choices and be flexible, no matter what the circumstances. And, of course, a small indiscretion will not be a disaster. Just start fresh with your next meal!

KETO-FRIENDLY FOODS TO ENJOY

We've given you a lot of background, advice, and tips for cooking, grocery shopping, and eating out. What follows is an outline of what foods to eat on this plan, meant to give you a helpful and fairly thorough list to get you started. Take a picture with your phone or make a paper copy to bring along when you shop. The list does not include every possible allowable food and there are, no doubt, foods that could be added. But this is a strong base to work from and your new understanding, along with the lists, will guide you to make the right selections.

PHASE 1

This is a recommended list of keto-friendly foods that are ideal for Phase 1. But remember: this is recommended guidance only. You may find that you can incorporate low-sugar fruits in limited quantities beginning in week three or four, though we have placed them on the Phase 2 list. That said, if any other foods "sneak into" your diet, don't panic; just keep those to a minimum, especially in the first two weeks, and aim to keep your daily carb allowance under 50 grams. If you find your cravings returning or your appetite increasing between meals, be sure to keep a stricter watch on your Phase 1 choices.

PROTEINS

We suggest consuming a variety of meats and seafood, or if you are vegetarian or vegan, a variety of plant-based proteins.

Meat & Poultry: All types

- Bacon & sausage, all types (bacon, chorizo, turkey, etc. Note: Read the label to watch for added sugars and starches)

- Beef, all cuts and types (steak, ground beef, liver, etc.)

- Deli meats (beef, chicken, turkey, ham, etc. Note: Read the label to watch for added sugars and starches)

- Game meats, all types (venison, bison, etc.)

- Lamb, all cuts and types (chops, ground, loin, etc.)

- Pork, all cuts and types (ham, pancetta, pork tenderloin, etc.)

- Poultry, all cuts and types (chicken, Cornish hen, duck, turkey, etc.)

Seafood: All types

Limit your intake of fish high in mercury and other contaminants; these include marlin, swordfish, shark, tilefish, orange roughy, king mackerel, bigeye and ahi tuna, and canned albacore tuna—use light canned tuna instead.

- Fish: all types, especially fish high in omega-3 (mackerel, salmon, anchovies, herring)

- Shellfish, all types

Plant-Based (look for low-carb options)

- Full-fat tofu

- Pea protein

- Soy milk, unsweetened

- Soy protein crumbles

- Tempeh

- Vegan protein powder, unsweetened

Other Protein Sources

- Eggs

- Whey protein powder (5g net carbs or less, 10g protein or more)

NUTS, NUT BUTTERS & SEEDS

All nuts and nut butters are allowable but we recommend that you watch your serving size and daily intake as nuts and seeds are common diet busters.

Nuts

- Almonds (23 or about ¼ cup)

- Almond butter (all natural, no added sugar, 2 tablespoons)

- Brazil nuts (6 or about ¼ cup)

- Hazelnuts (20 or about ¼ cup)

- Macadamia nuts (10 to 12 or about ¼ cup)

- Peanuts (28 or about ¼ cup)

- Peanut butter (all natural, no added sugar, 2 tablespoons)

- Pecans (19 halves or about ¼ cup)

- Pine nuts (¼ cup)

- Walnuts (14 halves or about ¼ cup)

Seeds

- Chia seeds (¼ cup)

- Flaxseeds (¼ cup)

- Hemp seeds (¼ cup)

- Poppy seeds (¼ cup)

- Psyllium husk (¼ cup)

- Pumpkin seeds (¼ cup)

- Sesame seeds (¼ cup)

- Sunflower seeds (¼ cup)

- Tahini (2 tablespoons)

DAIRY

We recommend full-fat/whole-milk dairy. But dairy can be high in net carbs, so you will need to watch your daily intake, particularly with milk, yogurt, cottage cheese, and ricotta cheese.

- Brie
- Butter
- Cheese (with 1g net carbs or less per serving)
- Cheddar cheese
- Colby or Monterey Jack cheese
- Cottage cheese (4% milk fat)
- Cream cheese (full fat)
- Feta cheese
- Ghee
- Goat cheese or chèvre (firm or soft)
- Gorgonzola or blue cheese

- Gouda
- Greek yogurt, whole milk, plain
- Heavy cream
- Kefir (3% milk fat, plain)
- Milk (whole; limit intake)
- Mozzarella cheese (whole milk)
- Muenster cheese
- Parmesan cheese
- Provolone
- Ricotta cheese (whole milk)
- Sour cream (full fat)
- Swiss cheese

OILS

- Almond oil
- Avocado oil
- Coconut oil
- Hazelnut oil
- MCT oil

- Olive oil
- Sesame oil

VEGETABLES

- Artichoke
- Arugula
- Asparagus
- Bell peppers, all varieties
- Bok choy
- Broccoli
- Broccoli rabe
- Broccolini
- Brussels sprouts
- Cabbage (red or green)
- Cauliflower
- Carrots (limited)
- Celery
- Collard greens
- Cucumber
- Eggplant
- Fennel
- Green beans
- Hearts of palm
- Jicama
- Kale
- Leeks
- Lettuce (all varieties)
- Mushrooms (all varieties, including cremini, white, portobello)
- Okra
- Onions (all varieties)
- Peppers (all varieties)
- Pickles (dill, no added sugar)
- Pimientos
- Radicchio
- Radish
- Rhubarb
- Scallions
- Seaweed
- Shallots
- Sugar snap peas (edible pea pods)
- Snow peas (edible pea pods)
- Spinach
- Sprouts
- Squash (yellow, spaghetti, summer, zucchini)
- Swiss chard
- Tomatillos
- Tomato (fresh or canned, no added sugar)
- Turnips (and turnip greens)
- Wax beans
- Zucchini

FRUITS

- Avocado
- Coconut (shredded, with no added sugar)
- Lemon & lime (when used in limited amounts for dressing or cooking)
- Olives (black or green)

SPICES, SEASONINGS & CONDIMENTS

- Cacao nibs
- Capers
- Celery seed
- Cocoa powder
- Coconut aminos
- Crushed red pepper
- Garlic
- Ginger
- Herbs, all varieties dried (no added sugar), or fresh (chives, cilantro, dill, oregano, parsley, rosemary, thyme)
- Horseradish and horseradish sauce (no added sugar)
- Hot sauce
- Ketchup (no added sugar)
- Lemon juice
- Lime juice
- Mayonnaise (no added sugar; olive or avocado oil–based varieties)
- Mustard (Dijon or yellow)
- Peppers, hot (serrano, jalapeño)
- Pesto
- Salsa (no added sugar)
- Salt (sea salt or Himalayan pink)
- Soy sauce
- Spices, all varieties (cayenne, chili powder, cinnamon, cumin, curry powder, garlic powder, nutmeg, onion powder, pepper, turmeric, etc.)
- Tamari gluten-free soy sauce
- Tomato paste
- Vanilla extract, pure
- Vinegar (rice vinegar, red wine vinegar, white wine vinegar, apple cider vinegar)
- Wasabi

SWEETENERS

- Erythritol
- Monk fruit
- Stevia

PANTRY ESSENTIALS

- Almond flour
- Baking powder
- Baking soda
- Bone broth
- Broth or stock (beef, chicken, seafood, vegetable)
- Chili paste
- Chipotles in adobo

- Coconut flour
- Coconut milk, canned, full fat, unsweetened
- Extracts (such as pure almond, pure vanilla)
- Keto-friendly chocolate chips (no added sugar, ideally sweetened with erythritol or stevia)

BEVERAGES

- Almond milk (unsweetened)
- Club soda
- Coconut milk (full-fat rich coconut milk; from the beverage or dairy aisle in a carton or box; unsweetened)

- Coffee
- Sparkling waters (plain, or flavored without sugar)
- Tea (all varieties: herbal, green, white, black)

LEGUMES

Allowable, but in limited quantities:

- Beans, all varieties (black, garbanzo, pinto, white)
- Edamame

- Hummus
- Lentils
- Split peas

PHASE 2

On Phase 2, the idea is to open up your diet to additional food options—like high-protein grains and low-glycemic fruits—while still keeping your carbs under 100 grams per day. You may want to go lower, and this number can vary from day to day. You'll figure out what works best for you.

Phase 2 is flexible—it is meant to be a lifestyle. This means there will be occasions when you eat foods that are not on this list. It's okay. You know which foods are more or less likely to cause you to backslide. Just try to consume high-sugar and -starch foods minimally and infrequently, such as a piece of cake at a birthday party or a slice of pizza with your kids. Remember also: if you are prone to sugar addiction, be very watchful of your fruit intake and limit that to one serving daily, particularly if you are still in a weight-loss phase.

GRAINS

One serving equals ½ cup cooked. If you find you cannot limit yourself, or fear you are backsliding, minimize grains.

- Amaranth
- Buckwheat
- Oats
- Quinoa
- Wild or brown rice

VEGETABLES

Since Phase 2 is meant to be a lifestyle, feel free to add some higher-starch vegetables back into your diet. Try one serving per day and monitor any increase in hunger or return of cravings.

- Calabaza (½ cup)
- Pumpkin (¼ cup)
- Sweet potato (½ medium)
- Taro (⅓ cup)
- Winter squash (½ cup)
- Yam (½ medium)

FRUITS

We believe you can add a variety of lower-sugar fruits to Phase 2. However, we recommend limiting your daily intake. These fruits have less than 10 grams of net carbs per ½ cup serving. We have noted the lowest net-carb fruits here with an asterisk*. Be mindful to limit dried fruits as they have more concentrated sugars.

- Apples
- Apricots
- Blackberries *
- Blueberries
- Boysenberries
- Cantaloupe *
- Casaba melon
- Gooseberries *

- Grapefruit
- Honeydew melon
- Kiwi
- Peaches
- Raspberries *
- Starfruit *
- Strawberries *

ALCOHOL

Even though some spirits may have zero carbs, they are primarily metabolized in the liver and, like fructose, if not burned will be stored as fat. They may slow weight loss and contribute to fatty liver. Preferably, limit to a 1½-ounce serving of spirits, or one 4-ounce glass of wine, no more than twice a week.

- Beer (light/low carb)
- Champagne (extra-brut)
- Distilled spirits (such as bourbon, whiskey, scotch, gin, and vodka; watch for ingredients in added flavorings)

- Wine (red or white, dry wines preferable; avoid sweet dessert wines)

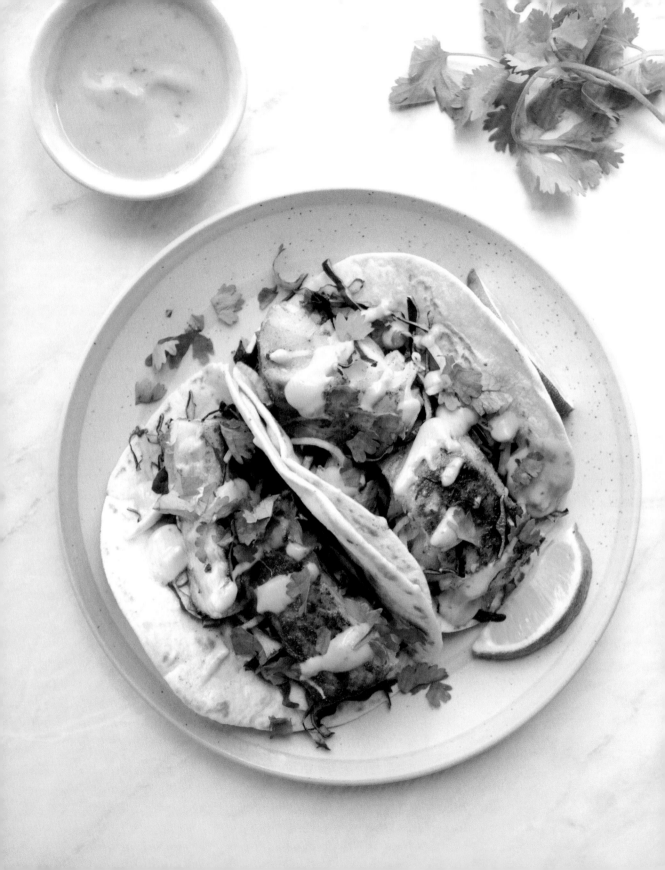

CHAPTER 8

GO! PHASE 1

A 28-DAY MEAL PLAN

DAY 1

BREAKFAST

Plain whole-milk Greek yogurt with walnuts and cinnamon (1 cup yogurt, 1 tablespoon chopped walnuts, and a dash of cinnamon)

Coffee or tea

SNACK

Chai Tea Latte (page 164)

LUNCH

Deviled Egg Salad (page 170) with cucumber slices (½ medium cucumber, sliced)

DINNER

Pan-seared salmon fillet (3 ounces) with cauliflower rice (½ cup), and Parmesan Roasted Brussels Sprouts (page 248)

Prep: Sear the salmon in a frying pan with a little bit of olive oil. For an additional boost of flavor, top with 1 to 2 tablespoons of tzatziki sauce (page 225).

Plan ahead: Prepare or save an extra serving of fish for a quick lunch on Day 3!

Prep (cauliflower): For quick and easy prep, look for a prepared version of cauliflower rice in your supermarket freezer section. Otherwise, grate cauliflower with a cheese grater. Give it a flavor boost by adding herbs, spices, or garlic.

SNACK

1 Chocolate Chip Cookie (page 283) with a glass of whole milk (8 ounces)

TOTAL DAILY NUTRITION

1,353 calories ▪ 63% fat ▪ 25% saturated fat ▪ 16% carbs ▪ 29g net carbs ▪ 25% protein

DAY 2

BREAKFAST

2 Egg Cups 3 Ways, Chive & Prosciutto version (page 138)

Plan ahead: Make the whole Egg Cups 3 Ways recipe, and keep a serving of the Bacon & Cheddar version in an airtight container in the refrigerator for a quick breakfast option tomorrow, along with a serving of the Spinach & Feta version for Day 5. You can freeze the rest on a baking sheet lined with parchment paper. Once it is frozen, transfer to a freezer-safe bag for long-term storage and future use.

Coffee or tea

SNACK

Almonds and red bell pepper slices (23 almonds, half a large bell pepper)

LUNCH

Shredded chicken breast on a green salad dressed with extra virgin olive oil and red wine vinegar

Prep: Toss in a large salad bowl 2 cups mixed salad greens, 1 cup chopped red cabbage, ½ cup cooked and chopped asparagus, and ½ cup fresh broccoli florets. Top with 3 ounces cooked and shredded chicken breast. Dress with 1 tablespoon oil and 1 tablespoon red wine vinegar.

DINNER

Keto Spaghetti & Meatballs (page 197), with 2 pieces of Keto Cloud Bread, Garlic Parmesan version (page 258)

Plan ahead: Make half of the Keto Cloud Bread using the Garlic Parmesan topping for tonight's dinner, and put the Everything Bagel topping on the other half as a make-ahead for breakfast on Day 7.

SNACK

1 Salted Tahini Dark Chocolate Fudge Cup (page 272)

Plan ahead: Make these at the start of the week and stash them in the freezer for a quick, indulgent snack that is still on plan! They keep, frozen, for up to 2 weeks.

TOTAL DAILY NUTRITION

1,427 calories ▪ 60% fat ▪ 18% saturated fat ▪ 13% carbs ▪ 33g net carbs ▪ 27% protein

DAY 3

BREAKFAST

2 Egg Cups 3 Ways, Bacon & Cheddar version (page 138)

Coffee or tea

SNACK

Sweet & Salty Trail Mix (page 267)

LUNCH

Salmon salad over mixed greens, tomatoes, and cucumbers

Prep: Make a quick and easy salmon salad by mixing 3 ounces of chopped leftover salmon fillet with 1 tablespoon keto-friendly mayonnaise and 1 tablespoon chopped scallions. Serve over mixed greens with 1 cup cherry tomatoes and 1 cup sliced cucumbers. Season with salt and pepper.

SNACK

Plain whole-milk Greek yogurt (1 cup)

DINNER

Buffalo Chicken Zucchini Boats, version without beans (page 198), steamed broccoli, and sugar snap peas in the pod

Prep: To prepare the side dish, steam 1 cup broccoli and 1 cup sugar snap peas.

TOTAL DAILY NUTRITION

1,250 calories ▪ 55% fat ▪ 21% saturated fat ▪ 13% carbs ▪ 29g net carbs ▪ 31% protein

DAY 4

BREAKFAST

Tomato and spinach omelet served with avocado and a glass of whole milk (8 ounces)

Prep (omelet): Very lightly coat a small pan with olive oil or butter and place it over medium heat. Add ¼ cup chopped spinach. Sauté until the spinach is wilted, about 2 to 3 minutes. Remove the spinach from the pan. Beat 2 large eggs and cook them in the pan. Add the cooked spinach and ¼ cup chopped tomatoes. Garnish with ½ avocado.

Variation: Short on time? Grab previously prepared hard-boiled eggs and a handful of almonds instead of the omelet and avocado as you head out the door.

Coffee or tea

SNACK

8 Herbed Seed Crackers (page 256) with hummus and goat cheese

Prep: Mix together 2 tablespoons hummus and 2 tablespoons goat cheese as a spread or dip with crackers.

Variation: If you're looking to reduce net carbs even further during your first week, try substituting hummus for a lower-carb option, such as tzatziki sauce (page 225).

Plan ahead: Be sure to save another serving of crackers for lunch on Day 7!

LUNCH

Grilled Buffalo Chicken Salad (page 184)

SNACK

1 Salted Tahini Dark Chocolate Fudge Cup (page 272)

DINNER

Pan-seared chicken breast (3 ounces) with Garlic & Parmesan Mashed Cauliflower (page 254)

Prep: To cook the chicken, lightly grease a skillet with olive oil over medium-high heat, place the chicken breast in the pan, and cook for about 5 minutes or until golden brown on that side. Then flip and cook on the other side until cooked through, about another 4 to 5 minutes.

Plan ahead: When preparing the chicken breast for tonight's dinner, make the breaded chicken cutlets for Day 5's Almond Flour Chicken Piccata (page 201). Tomorrow night's dinner is now halfway complete!

TOTAL DAILY NUTRITION

1,474 calories ▪ 54% fat ▪ 21% saturated fat ▪ 15% carbs ▪ 36g net carbs ▪ 28% protein

DAY 5

BREAKFAST

2 Egg Cups 3 Ways, Spinach & Feta version (page 138)

Coffee or tea

SNACK

Gouda cheese with cucumber slices (1 ounce full-fat cheese, ½ medium cucumber, sliced)

LUNCH

Shrimp & Avocado Salad with Cilantro Vinaigrette (page 180)

Prep: Buy fresh, precooked shrimp from a seafood shop or the seafood section at your grocery store. If you like, buy precooked frozen shrimp to save on some of the prep time. Store shrimp and salad greens separately in airtight containers in the refrigerator, combining with cut avocado immediately before serving.

DINNER

Almond Flour Chicken Piccata (page 201) with zucchini sautéed with white beans and garlic

Prep: Lightly coat a small sauté pan with olive oil and sauté 1 cup chopped zucchini, 1 clove minced garlic, and ¼ cup canned white beans, rinsed and drained.

SNACK

Plain whole-milk Greek yogurt with cashews (½ cup yogurt, 2 tablespoons chopped cashews)

TOTAL DAILY NUTRITION

1,374 calories ▪ 54% fat ▪ 17% saturated fat ▪ 12% carbs ▪ 36g net carbs ▪ 33% protein

DAY 6

BREAKFAST

Goat cheese and tomato omelet with a keto-friendly shake

Prep: Beat 2 large eggs and cook in a small sauté pan lightly coated with olive oil. Add 2 tablespoons goat cheese and ¼ cup chopped tomato.

Variation: In a morning rush? Skip the omelet and head out the door with 2 hard-boiled eggs, cherry tomatoes, and a whole-milk mozzarella cheese stick.

Coffee or tea

SNACK

Sweet & Salty Trail Mix (page 267)

LUNCH

Almond Flour Chicken Piccata (page 201) with baby spinach

Prep: Place leftovers from last night's dinner on top of 2 cups of baby spinach. Dress with 1 tablespoon extra virgin olive oil and a dash of apple cider vinegar.

SNACK

1 Salted Tahini Dark Chocolate Fudge Cup (page 272)

DINNER

Roast pork tenderloin with steamed asparagus (3 ounces pork, 1 cup asparagus)

Prep: Season the pork tenderloin with salt and pepper (and any other spices or herbs you desire) and roast in the oven at 400°F until golden brown and an instant-read thermometer inserted into the center reaches 145°F (approximately 20 to 30 minutes), flipping halfway through.

TOTAL DAILY NUTRITION

1,408 calories ▪ 63% fat ▪ 21% saturated fat ▪ 9% carbs ▪ 17g net carbs ▪ 28% protein

DAY 7

BREAKFAST

Broccoli, Swiss cheese, and Canadian bacon omelet with 2 pieces of Keto Cloud Bread with Everything Bagel topping (page 258)

Prep: Beat 2 large eggs and cook in a small sauté pan lightly coated with olive oil. Add ¼ cup chopped broccoli, 2 tablespoons full-fat cheese, and 1 slice Canadian bacon.

Coffee or tea

LUNCH

8 Herbed Seed Crackers (page 256) with turkey deli meat, fresh mozzarella, red bell pepper slices, and hummus

Prep: Lunch includes 2 ounces deli meat; 1 ounce fresh, whole-milk mozzarella cheese; half a large bell pepper, sliced; and 2 tablespoons hummus.

SNACK

Whey protein shake

DINNER

Seared Steak with Gorgonzola Cream Sauce (page 202) served with roasted cherry tomatoes (½ cup tomatoes)

Prep: Toss ½ cup cherry tomatoes lightly with olive oil, salt, pepper, and thyme. Spread on a baking sheet or in a baking dish and roast in the oven at 425°F for 20 minutes.

Plan ahead: Set aside a serving of steak for tomorrow's lunch. Store the steak and cream sauce separately in the refrigerator and combine right before eating.

SNACK

1 Chocolate Chip Cookie (page 281)

TOTAL DAILY NUTRITION

1,340 calories ▪ 62% fat ▪ 26% saturated fat ▪ 12% carbs ▪ 24g net carbs ▪ 32% protein

DAY 8

BREAKFAST

2 Egg Cups 3 Ways, Spinach & Feta version (page 138)

Coffee or tea

SNACK

Tuna salad and cucumber slices

Prep: Combine ½ cup canned tuna (packed in oil, drained) with 1 teaspoon keto-friendly mayonnaise. You can also add chopped celery and scallions if desired. Add ½ medium cucumber, sliced, on the side.

LUNCH

Seared Steak with Gorgonzola Cream Sauce (page 202) left over from last night's dinner, served over green salad

Prep: Place a serving of leftover steak (3 ounces) and cream sauce over 2 cups mixed greens, 1 cup diced tomatoes, and 1 cup sugar snap peas. If fresh sugar snap peas are not in season, use frozen ones, steaming them just a bit before adding them to your salad, or use a different green vegetable of your choice.

SNACK

8 Herbed Seed Crackers (page 256) with Camembert cheese (1 ounce full-fat cheese)

DINNER

Chicken Fajita Bowl (page 205)

TOTAL DAILY NUTRITION

1,456 calories ▪ 59% fat ▪ 22% saturated fat ▪ 10% carbs ▪ 27g net carbs ▪ 33% protein

DAY 9

Plain whole-milk Greek yogurt with almonds (½ cup yogurt, 23 almonds)

Coffee or tea

LUNCH

Chockfull of Veggie Chili (page 183) topped with half an avocado cut into cubes.

Plan ahead: You can prepare this recipe 3 to 4 days ahead of time and refrigerate it in an airtight container.

SNACK

Whey protein shake

DINNER

Broiled scallops with Parmesan Roasted Broccoli Rabe (page 261)

Prep: Turn the broiler on to high heat. Place 3 ounces scallops in an oven-safe dish lightly coated with olive oil and season with salt and pepper. Melt 1 tablespoon butter and drizzle it over the scallops. Broil the scallops until cooked through, approximately 6 to 10 minutes.

SNACK

1 square Chocolate Freezer Fudge (page 276)

Tip: Make this recipe ahead of time and store it in your freezer for up to 1 month.

TOTAL DAILY NUTRITION

1,259 calories • 59% fat • 16% saturated fat • 15% carbs • 31g net carbs • 27% protein

DAY 10

BREAKFAST

Mushroom, spinach, and feta omelet

Prep: Very lightly coat a small pan with olive oil or butter and place it over medium heat. Add ¼ cup chopped spinach and ¼ cup sliced mushrooms. Sauté until the spinach is wilted and excess liquid evaporates from the mushrooms, about 4 to 5 minutes. Remove the spinach and mushrooms from the pan. Beat 2 large eggs and cook them in the pan. Add the cooked spinach and mushrooms and ¼ cup feta cheese. Season with salt and pepper to taste.

Coffee or tea

SNACK

Savory Pesto Yogurt Bowl (page 262)

LUNCH

Tuna salad with celery sticks and a keto-friendly shake

Prep: Combine ½ cup canned tuna with 1 tablespoon keto-friendly mayonnaise and 1 tablespoon scallions. Serve with 2 medium celery sticks on the side.

DINNER

Roast chicken with brussels sprouts and Camembert cheese (3 ounces chicken, 1 cup brussels sprouts halved, 1 ounce full-fat cheese)

Prep (chicken): Preheat the oven to 350°F. Place 3 ounces chicken thighs in a baking dish and add 2 to 3 tablespoons chicken broth. Season the chicken with salt and pepper. Cover the baking dish and bake until the chicken is cooked through and no longer pink in the center, approximately 25 to 30 minutes. For extra zest, feel free to add a little parsley, sage, rosemary, or thyme.

Prep (brussels sprouts): Very lightly coat a baking sheet with olive oil. Season 1 cup brussels sprouts with salt and pepper and very lightly drizzle with more olive oil. Roast the sprouts in the preheated oven for approximately 20 to 25 minutes. Remove them from the oven and top with sliced Camembert cheese. Return them to the oven for 2 to 3 minutes longer, or until the cheese is melted.

Plan ahead: Prepare an extra serving of roast chicken for a quick lunch tomorrow. You can also use a precooked rotisserie chicken. Just remember that 3 ounces of meat is about the size of a deck of cards. And be sure to read the ingredients or ask questions at the supermarket about preparation methods to ensure the chicken was not basted with any sauces or seasonings that contain added sugars or additives.

SNACK

1 Chocolate Chip Cookie (page 283) with a glass of whole milk (8 ounces)

TOTAL DAILY NUTRITION

1,365 calories ▪ 58% fat ▪ 24% saturated fat ▪ 15% carbs ▪ 34g net carbs ▪ 29% protein

DAY 11

BREAKFAST

Hard-boiled eggs with cheddar cheese

Prep: Hard boil 2 large eggs; peel and slice in half. Top with salt and pepper if desired, or for an extra kick, add a dash of hot sauce or smoked paprika. Add a 1-ounce serving of full-fat cheddar cheese on the side.

Coffee or tea

SNACK

Chai Tea Latte (page 164)

LUNCH

Roast chicken with cooked broccoli and cauliflower

Prep: Use 3 ounces of leftover roast chicken from last night's dinner. Serve 1 cup cooked broccoli and cauliflower medley as a side dish. For a quick, convenient option, look for a microwaveable, steamable broccoli and cauliflower medley in the frozen section of the supermarket.

Plain whole-milk Greek yogurt mixed with fresh dill and lemon juice, plus cucumber and bell pepper slices for dipping

Prep: Cut ½ medium cucumber and ½ large bell pepper into slices. For the dipping sauce, combine ½ cup yogurt, 1 to 2 teaspoons finely chopped dill, and a squeeze of lemon juice or make tzaziki sauce (page 225).

Make Ahead: Make extra tzazaki sauce to use as a dip or condiment in the upcoming days.

DINNER

Beef & Vegetable Stew, version without beans (page 214), and roasted asparagus (½ cup)

Prep: Preheat the oven to 400°F. Lightly coat a baking dish with olive oil. Lay the asparagus in the dish, season with salt and pepper, and brush or very lightly drizzle with more olive oil. Bake for approximately 15 to 20 minutes.

Variation: Looking to add a flavor twist to your asparagus? After taking it out of the oven, sprinkle it with grated Parmesan cheese and a squeeze of fresh lemon juice.

Plan ahead: Save a serving of stew for tomorrow's lunch.

SNACK

1 square Chocolate Freezer Fudge (page 276)

TOTAL DAILY NUTRITION

1,276 calories ▪ 56% fat ▪ 27% saturated fat ▪ 12% carbs ▪ 29g net carbs ▪ 32% protein

DAY 12

BREAKFAST

Coconut Chia Pudding (page 141)

Plan ahead: This pudding is a great make-ahead breakfast for mornings on the run! Feel free to prepare it the night before. Double the recipe and store 1 serving in an airtight container in the refrigerator to use for breakfast on Day 14.

Coffee or tea

SNACK

Pistachios (¼ cup, approximately 50 kernels)

LUNCH

Beef & Vegetable Stew (page 214) left over from last night's dinner

SNACK

Mozzarella cheese stick and cucumber slices (1 whole-milk cheese stick, ½ medium cucumber, sliced)

DINNER

Portobello Shakshuka (page 206) with 2 Cheesy Garlic Cauliflower Breadsticks (page 268)

TOTAL DAILY NUTRITION

1,469 calories ▪ 61% fat ▪ 25% saturated fat ▪ 12% carbs ▪ 30g net carbs ▪ 26% protein

DAY 13

BREAKFAST

Smoked Salmon Bowl (page 142)

Coffee or tea

SNACK

Goat cheese with cucumber slices (1 ounce cheese, ½ medium cucumber, sliced)

LUNCH

Cauliflower Tahini Rice Bowl (page 192) plus hummus with celery sticks (2 tablespoons hummus, 2 medium celery sticks)

Plan ahead: You can prepare the Cauliflower Tahini Rice Bowl the night before and store it in an airtight container in the refrigerator. Toss in the tahini sauce right before eating.

SNACK

Whey protein shake

DINNER

Prosciutto & Gouda Pizza (page 210) served with a green side salad

Prep: To make the salad, toss 2 cups mixed greens with 1 tablespoon extra virgin olive oil and 1 tablespoon red wine vinegar.

TOTAL DAILY NUTRITION

1,420 calories ▪ 63% fat ▪ 16% saturated fat ▪ 12% carbs ▪ 29g net carbs ▪ 25% protein

DAY 14

BREAKFAST

Coconut Chia Pudding (page 141)

Coffee or tea

SNACK

Plain whole-milk Greek yogurt (1 cup)

LUNCH

Deviled Egg Salad (page 170)

Plan ahead: If you plan to make the egg salad ahead of time, wait until just before eating to add the bacon so it stays crisp. Store the egg salad and the bacon in the refrigerator separately in airtight containers.

Quick green beans (1 cup)

Prep: Blanch the green beans by adding them to salted, boiling water and letting them boil for 3 to 4 minutes. Remove pot from heat, drain, and quickly immerse beans in ice water for 5 minutes. This will result in crisp, tender beans that also hold their bright green color. For a quick, convenient option, look for microwaveable, steamable green beans in the frozen section of the supermarket.

DINNER

Sticky Sesame Chicken (page 213) with sugar snap peas, raw or steamed (1 cup peas)

SNACK

Almond Flour Tortilla Chips with Homemade Guacamole (page 253)

TOTAL DAILY NUTRITION

1,418 calories ▪ 58% fat ▪ 19% saturated fat ▪ 13% carbs ▪ 31g net carbs ▪ 27% protein

DAY 15

BREAKFAST

1 Spinach & Artichoke Quiche Cup (page 145)

Plan ahead: Freeze the extra cooled quiche cups in an airtight container. You will include these in your meal plan again for breakfast on Day 19 and a snack on Day 20.

Coffee or tea

SNACK

Mocha Frappé (page 166)

LUNCH

Bento box lunch: Ham and Swiss cheese roll-ups, cashews, bell pepper slices, and celery sticks
Prep: Assemble 1 ounce deli ham (approximately 2 slices), 1 ounce full-fat Swiss cheese (approximately 1 to 2 slices), 1 teaspoon Dijon mustard, 16 to 18 cashews, half a bell pepper cut into slices, and 2 medium celery stalks cut into sticks.

SNACK

5 Spicy Parmesan Crisps (page 266)

Plan ahead: Crisps can be stored in an airtight container for up to 2 days. You will enjoy these again as a snack tomorrow.

DINNER

Stuffed Chicken Breast with Zucchini Fettuccine (page 216)

TOTAL DAILY NUTRITION

1,249 calories ▪ 61% fat ▪ 29% saturated fat ▪ 19% carbs ▪ 41g net carbs ▪ 26% protein

DAY 16

BREAKFAST

1 Coffee & Hazelnut Muffin (page 146) with full-fat (4% milkfat) cottage cheese (½ cup)

Plan ahead: Store extra muffins in an airtight container in the refrigerator to use for a quick breakfast later this week (Day 18).

Coffee or tea

SNACK

5 Spicy Parmesan Crisps (page 266)

LUNCH

Thai Chopped Chicken Salad (page 173)

SNACK

Hummus and fresh vegetables (2 tablespoons hummus, 1 cup non-starchy veggies of choice such as celery, broccoli, cauliflower, bell pepper)

DINNER

Cod with Almond-Basil Relish (page 218) and roasted asparagus (1 cup)

Prep: Preheat the oven to 400°F. Very lightly coat a baking dish with olive oil. Lay the asparagus in the baking dish, season with salt and pepper, and drizzle very lightly with more olive oil. Bake for approximately 15 to 20 minutes.

TOTAL DAILY NUTRITION

1,265 calories ▪ 57% fat ▪ 22% saturated fat ▪ 17% carbs ▪ 34g net carbs ▪ 28% protein

DAY 17

BREAKFAST

Warm Avocado with Egg (page 150)

Coffee or tea

SNACK

Whey protein shake

LUNCH

Beef Burrito Bowl (page 174) with steamed broccoli (½ cup)
Prep: Assemble the bowls ahead of time, adding the avocado and salsa when you are ready to eat.

DINNER

Roasted turkey breast (3 ounces) served with Radicchio & Mushroom Gratin (page 257)

Prep: Preheat the oven to 350°F. Place a turkey breast tenderloin in a baking dish very lightly coated with olive oil and season with salt, pepper, and any additional desired herbs and spices. Bake for approximately 1 hour.

Variation: For a quick dinner option, rotisserie chicken can be substituted for the roasted turkey. See the note on page 103 about being careful with hidden ingredients.

SNACK

1 Chocolate Chip Cookie Dough Bite (page 286)

Plan ahead: Make a whole batch! You will enjoy this snack again on Days 19 and 21, and remaining cookie bites can be stored in the freezer for up to one month.

TOTAL DAILY NUTRITION

1,287 calories ▪ 56% fat ▪ 19% saturated fat ▪ 12% carbs ▪ 27g net carbs ▪ 29% protein

DAY 18

BREAKFAST

1 Coffee & Hazelnut Muffin (page 146) with plain whole-milk Greek yogurt (½ cup)

Coffee or tea

SNACK

Hard-boiled egg (1 large egg)

LUNCH

Curried Chicken Salad with Cucumber Dressing (page 172)

Plan ahead: You can prepare the chicken and salad the night before and dress it with salad dressing immediately prior to eating.

SNACK

Feta cheese and cherry tomatoes (¼ cup cheese, 1 cup tomatoes)

DINNER

1 Cilantro-Lime Turkey Burger (page 221) served with roasted eggplant, portobello mushrooms, and yellow summer squash

Prep: To prepare the veggies, preheat the oven to 400°F. Roast ½ cup diced eggplant, ½ cup diced mushrooms, and ½ cup diced squash on a pan or baking sheet very lightly coated with olive oil for approximately 20 minutes or until golden brown.

Plan ahead: Prepare an extra turkey burger for tomorrow's lunch.

TOTAL DAILY NUTRITION

1,308 calories ▪ 61% fat ▪ 25% saturated fat ▪ 15% carbs ▪ 33g net carbs ▪ 27% protein

DAY 19

BREAKFAST

1 Spinach & Artichoke Quiche Cup (page 145)

Plan ahead: Keep an extra quiche cup in the refrigerator for tomorrow's snack!

Creamy Protein Latte (page 167)

SNACK

Plain whole-milk Greek yogurt (1 cup)

LUNCH

1 Cilantro-Lime Turkey Burger (page 221) left over from last night's dinner served over spinach salad.

Prep: Toss 2 cups baby spinach, 1 large hard-boiled egg, chopped, and half an avocado in a salad bowl. Top the salad with the burger. Add a squeeze of fresh lime juice over the salad to taste.

DINNER

Chicken Shepherd's Pie with Cauliflower (page 222), and sautéed asparagus with cherry tomatoes and garlic

Prep: Add ½ cup chopped asparagus to boiling water and blanch for about 2 minutes. Place a sauté pan over medium heat, very lightly coat with olive oil and add the parboiled asparagus, 1 minced clove of garlic, and ½ cup halved cherry tomatoes. Sauté until warmed through, approximately 4 to 5 minutes.

SNACK

1 Chocolate Chip Cookie Dough Bite (page 286)

TOTAL DAILY NUTRITION

1,392 calories ▪ 63% fat ▪ 23% saturated fat ▪ 13% carbs ▪ 36g net carbs ▪ 26% protein

DAY 20

BREAKFAST

Keto-friendly shake with 2 hard-boiled eggs

Coffee or tea

SNACK

1 Spinach & Artichoke Quiche Cup (page 145)

LUNCH

Cream of Broccoli Soup (page 179), with 2 Cheesy Garlic Cauliflower Breadsticks (page 268) and sautéed spinach (½ cup cooked spinach)

Prep: Heat a small sauté pan on medium heat. Very lightly coat it with olive oil. Add the spinach and cook for approximately 3 to 5 minutes, or until the spinach is wilted. Season with salt and pepper to taste. Note: About 3 cups of raw fresh spinach will be needed to prepare ½ cup cooked.

SNACK

Full-fat (4% milkfat) cottage cheese with a dash of cinnamon (½ cup cottage cheese)

DINNER

Creamy Cauliflower & Chicken (page 209) served with steamed green beans (1 cup)

TOTAL DAILY NUTRITION

1,315 calories ▪ 57% fat ▪ 24% saturated fat ▪ 15% carbs ▪ 43g net carbs ▪ 30% protein

DAY 21

BREAKFAST

Full-fat (4% milkfat) cottage cheese with walnuts and cinnamon (1 cup cottage cheese, 14 walnut halves, and a dash of cinnamon)

Coffee or tea

LUNCH

Bento box lunch: Turkey breast deli meat with almonds, olives, and bell pepper slices

Prep: Assemble 2 ounces deli meat (approximately 4 thin slices), 23 almonds, ¼ cup olives, and half a bell pepper cut into slices.

SNACK

Whey protein shake

DINNER

Spiced Lamb Loaf (page 225) with roasted cauliflower

Prep: For the side dish, preheat the oven to 400°F. Very lightly coat a baking sheet with olive oil and place 1 cup cauliflower florets on the sheet. Very lightly drizzle the cauliflower with more olive oil and roast for approximately 20 to 25 minutes.

Plan ahead: Set aside a serving of this meatloaf for tomorrow's lunch.

SNACK

1 Chocolate Chip Cookie Dough Bite (page 286)

TOTAL DAILY NUTRITION

1,233 calories ▪ 58% fat ▪ 15% saturated fat ▪ 13% carbs ▪ 32g net carbs ▪ 30% protein

DAY 22

BREAKFAST

Ham, Swiss, and spinach omelet

Prep: Sauté 1 cup fresh spinach in a small sauté pan very lightly coated with olive oil. Beat 2 large eggs and add to pan. Add 1 ounce ham and ½ ounce Swiss cheese.

Coffee or tea

SNACK

Full-fat (4% milkfat) cottage cheese (½ cup), with cherry tomatoes (1 cup)

LUNCH

Spiced Lamb Loaf (page 225) left over from last night's dinner over a bed of romaine lettuce

Prep: Place 1 slice of the Spiced Lamb Loaf on 2 cups of chopped romaine lettuce and dress with 1 tablespoon olive oil and 1 tablespoon red wine vinegar.

Variation: This lamb loaf is great served with a side of tzatziki sauce.

DINNER

Kale Caesar Salad with Creamy Cashew Dressing (page 237) topped with beef tenderloin and a side of green beans

Prep: Preheat the oven to 400°F. Line a roasting pan with aluminum foil and set a rack on top. Season the beef with salt and pepper (and any other herbs or spices desired) and place it on the rack. Roast for approximately 35 minutes. Meanwhile, sauté 1 cup green beans in 1 teaspoon olive oil. Serve 3 ounces of beef with the salad and the side of green beans.

Variation: If you'd like a substitute for beef tenderloin, some alternative cuts of beef include flank steak (marinated overnight) or sirloin.

SNACK

1 Peanut Butter & Tahini Protein Bite (page 279)

TOTAL DAILY NUTRITION

1,406 calories ▪ 62% fat ▪ 18% saturated fat ▪ 13% carbs ▪ 36g net carbs ▪ 26% protein

DAY 23

BREAKFAST

Warm Avocado with Egg (page 150)

Coffee or tea

SNACK

Gouda cheese with almonds (½ ounce full-fat cheese, 12 almonds)

LUNCH

Lemon-Rosemary Braised Chicken Breasts (page 189) with Zucchini Feta Salad (page 251)

SNACK

Celery sticks with almond butter and a glass of whole milk (2 medium celery stalks cut into sticks, 1 tablespoon almond butter, 8 ounces whole milk)

DINNER

Sesame-Glazed Beef & Veggie Bowl (page 229) with edamame

Prep: Steam ½ cup edamame in the shell and serve with a side of 1 tablespoon tamari sauce for dipping.

Plan ahead: Prepare an extra serving of beef and set it aside to incorporate into tomorrow's lunch.

TOTAL DAILY NUTRITION

1,543 calories ▪ 59% fat ▪ 15% saturated fat ▪ 12% carbs ▪ 39g net carbs ▪ 28% protein

DAY 24

BREAKFAST

Mexican Breakfast Bake (page 160)

Plan ahead: Make extra and store in the refrigerator for 3 to 4 days; you will enjoy this for breakfast again on Day 26.

Coffee or tea

SNACK

Greek yogurt dip with veggies

Prep: Prepare 1 cup fresh non-starchy vegetables of your choice (celery, bell pepper, broccoli, cauliflower) and dip in a yogurt dip made from ½ cup plain whole-milk Greek yogurt, 1 teaspoon fresh finely chopped dill, and lemon juice to taste.

LUNCH

Greek-inspired bento box lunch: Beef, olives, feta, almonds, and tzatziki sauce

Prep: Assemble 3 ounces of leftover beef from last night's dinner, cut into small bite-sized pieces. Add ¼ cup pitted Kalamata olives, ¼ cup feta cheese cubes, 23 almonds, and ¼ cup tzatziki sauce (page 225) for dipping.

DINNER

Home-Style Chicken & "Rice" (page 233) with green beans and almonds

Prep: Blanch 1 cup green beans and set them aside. Very lightly coat a small sauté pan with olive oil and heat over medium-high heat. Add 1 tablespoon sliced almonds to the pan and toast for 1 minute. Add the blanched green beans to the toasted almonds in the sauté pan and cook for another 30 seconds to 1 minute, until heated through.

Plan ahead: Prepare an extra chicken breast for tomorrow's lunch.

SNACK

1 Peanut Butter & Tahini Protein Bite (page 279)

TOTAL DAILY NUTRITION

1,428 calories ▪ 57% fat ▪ 22% saturated fat ▪ 11% carbs ▪ 31g net carbs ▪ 32% protein

DAY 25

BREAKFAST

Keto-friendly shake, scrambled egg with cheddar cheese and broccoli

Prep: Beat 1 large egg and pour into a small sauté pan lightly coated with olive oil. Scramble. Add ½ ounce full-fat cheese and ¼ cup broccoli.

Coffee or tea

LUNCH

Chicken breast over a bed of sautéed spinach, garlic, and mushrooms

Prep (chicken): Sauté or roast 3 ounces chicken breast.

Prep (vegetables): Heat 1 tablespoon olive oil in a medium sauté pan over medium heat. Add 1 clove chopped garlic to the pan and sauté for 30 seconds. Add ½ cup sliced mushrooms and cook for 2 to 3 minutes. Add 3 cups fresh baby spinach to the mushroom and garlic mixture and cook until the spinach is wilted, about 3 to 5 minutes.

Variation: Look for precooked grilled or roasted chicken breast in the prepared food section of your supermarket.

SNACK

Gouda cheese with bell pepper slices and hummus (1 ounce full-fat cheese, ½ bell pepper cut into slices, ¼ cup hummus)

DINNER

2 Mini Taco Salads with Cilantro-Lime Yogurt Dip (page 234)

Plan ahead: Make enough to have leftovers for tomorrow's lunch!

SNACK

1 Keto Brownie (page 280)

TOTAL DAILY NUTRITION

1,372 calories ▪ 61% fat ▪ 27% saturated fat ▪ 20% carbs ▪ 29g net carbs ▪ 27% protein

DAY 26

BREAKFAST

Mexican Breakfast Bake (page 160)

Coffee or tea

SNACK

Plain whole-milk Greek yogurt (½ cup yogurt)

LUNCH

2 Mini Taco Salads with Cilantro-Lime Yogurt Dip (page 234) left over from last night's dinner (version in a jar)

SNACK

1 Smoky Goat Cheese & Almond Ball (page 265) with cucumber slices (1 medium cucumber, sliced)

DINNER

Heirloom Tomato Lasagna (page 238) with a side salad

Prep: To make the salad, combine 2 cups mixed greens with ¼ cup cherry tomatoes and ¼ medium cucumber, sliced. Dress with 1 tablespoon extra virgin olive oil and 1 tablespoon red wine vinegar.

Plan ahead: Store an extra portion in the fridge overnight for an easy lunch tomorrow.

TOTAL DAILY NUTRITION

1,290 calories ▪ 64% fat ▪ 27% saturated fat ▪ 11% carbs ▪ 29g net carbs ▪ 26% protein

DAY 27

BREAKFAST

1 Chocolate Peanut Butter Mug Muffin (page 156)
Coffee or tea

SNACK

Hard-boiled eggs (2 large eggs)

LUNCH

Heirloom Tomato Lasagna (page 238) left over from last night's dinner

1 Smoky Goat Cheese & Almond Ball (page 265)

SNACK

Celery sticks with peanut butter (2 medium celery stalks cut into sticks, 2 tablespoons peanut butter)

DINNER

Spice-Rubbed Salmon with Creamy Dill Dressing (page 244) and summer squash
Prep: Sauté 1 cup yellow summer squash in a small sauté pan very lightly coated with olive oil.
Plan ahead: Save a portion of the salmon for lunch tomorrow!

TOTAL DAILY NUTRITION

1,297 calories ▪ 64% fat ▪ 22% saturated fat ▪ 17% carbs ▪ 28g net carbs ▪ 26% protein

DAY 28

BREAKFAST

2 pieces Keto Cloud Bread with Everything Bagel topping (page 258), avocado, and poached eggs

Prep: Poach 2 large eggs and add ½ avocado on the side. For an extra kick of flavor and spice, add a dash of chili flakes.

Coffee or tea

SNACK

Whey protein shake

LUNCH

Spice-Rubbed Salmon with Creamy Dill Dressing (page 244) left over from last night's dinner, over a side salad.

Prep: To make the salad, combine 2 cups mixed greens with ¼ cup cherry tomatoes and ¼ cup medium cucumber, sliced. Dress with 1 tablespoon extra virgin olive oil and 1 tablespoon red wine vinegar. Top your salad with 3 ounces leftover salmon.

DINNER

Moroccan Lentil Stew (page 242) and roasted cauliflower florets (½ cup cauliflower)

Prep: Preheat the oven to 400°F. Very lightly coat a baking dish with olive oil. Add cauliflower florets to the baking dish and season with salt and pepper. Brush the cauliflower with a little additional olive oil and roast for approximately 15 to 20 minutes.

SNACK

1 Keto Brownie (page 280)

TOTAL DAILY NUTRITION

1,494 calories ▪ 58% fat ▪ 21% saturated fat ▪ 20% carbs ▪ 36g net carbs ▪ 28% protein

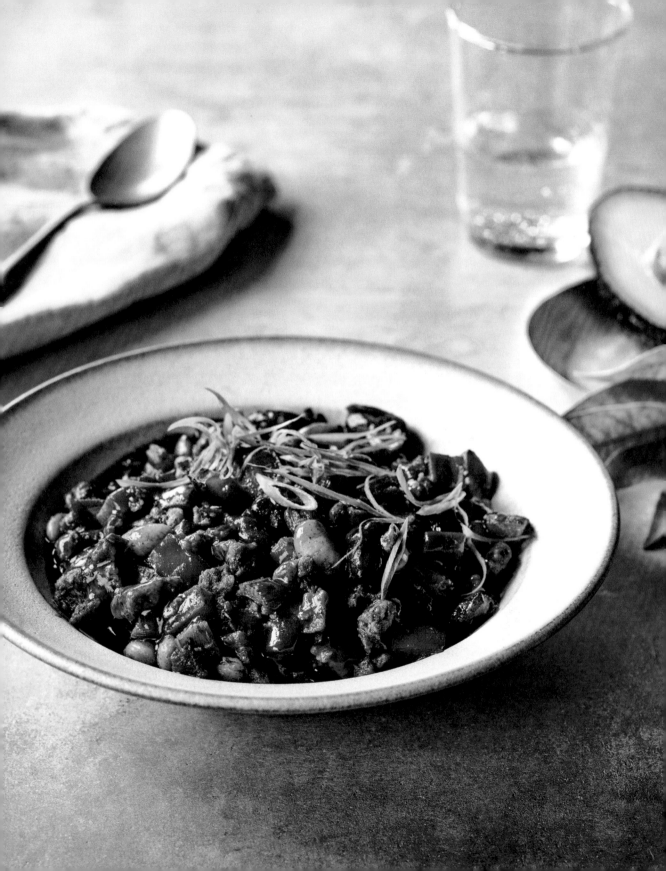

CHAPTER 9

KEEP GOING! PHASE 2

A 7-DAY MEAL PLAN

DAY 1

BREAKFAST

3 Sweet Potato Egg Cups (page 154) with a glass of whole milk (8 ounces)

Coffee or tea

Plan ahead: You can freeze the remainder of the egg cups to have on hand for breakfasts and snacks in the coming weeks. Place them in the freezer on a baking sheet lined with parchment paper. Once they are frozen, transfer them to a freezer-safe bag for long-term storage and future use.

SNACK

Plain whole-milk Greek yogurt with raspberries (½ cup yogurt, ¼ cup berries)

Variation: Frozen raspberries are a convenient option if fresh are not available; however, be sure to read the label and avoid added sugars.

LUNCH

Grilled chicken with tzatziki sauce (page 225) and roasted broccoli (6 ounces chicken breast, 2 tablespoons sauce, 1 cup broccoli)

Prep (chicken): Grill or sauté the chicken breast in a pan very lightly coated with olive oil. Cook over medium-high heat for 5 minutes. Turn the chicken over and continue cooking for another 4 to 5 minutes, or until cooked through (until internal temperature reaches 165°F).

Prep (broccoli): Preheat the oven to 400°F. Toss 1 cup broccoli florets in 2 teaspoons olive oil, add salt and pepper to taste, and spread the broccoli on a baking sheet very lightly greased with olive oil. Roast for approximately 15 minutes.

SNACK

Whey protein shake

DINNER

Blackened Salmon with Mango Quinoa (page 226) and green beans sautéed in olive oil and garlic

Prep (green beans): Sauté 1 cup green beans in a pan with 1 tablespoon olive oil at medium-high heat for 3 to 5 minutes. Season to taste with salt, pepper, and garlic powder.

TOTAL DAILY NUTRITION

1,660 calories ▪ 45% fat ▪ 19% saturated fat ▪ 17% carbs ▪ 63g net carbs ▪ 36% protein

DAY 2

BREAKFAST

Plain whole-milk Greek yogurt, fresh strawberries, kiwi, and pistachio nuts (½ cup yogurt, ¼ cup sliced berries, ¼ cup sliced kiwi, 1 ounce or about 3 to 4 tablespoons pistachios, chopped)

Coffee or tea

SNACK

Swiss cheese and cucumber slices (1 ounce cheese, 1 medium cucumber)

LUNCH

Thai Chickpea Curry (page 186) with roasted baby carrots

Prep (carrots): Preheat the oven to 400°F. Toss ½ cup baby carrots with 1 teaspoon olive oil and salt and pepper to taste. For a twist, add a little thyme or garlic powder. Spread the carrots on a baking sheet and roast for approximately 15 to 20 minutes.

SNACK

Tuna salad with celery sticks

Prep (tuna salad): Mix ½ cup canned tuna with 1 tablespoon keto-friendly mayo and 1 green onion, chopped. Serve with 2 medium celery stalks, cut into sticks.

DINNER

Sesame-Glazed Beef & Veggie Bowl (page 229) with steamed, deshelled, and salted edamame (1 cup)

TOTAL DAILY NUTRITION

1,674 calories ▪ 51% fat ▪ 18% saturated fat ▪ 18% carbs ▪ 59g net carbs ▪ 30% protein

DAY 3

BREAKFAST

2 Egg Cups 3 Ways, Bacon & Cheddar version (page 138) and plain whole-milk Greek yogurt with blueberries (½ cup yogurt, ¼ cup berries)

Coffee or tea

SNACK

Walnuts (14 halves)

LUNCH

Kale Caesar Salad with Creamy Cashew Dressing (page 237) topped with grilled chicken breast (6 ounces chicken)

Prep (chicken): Skip the prep! Buy precooked chicken breast in the supermarket for a quick, protein-packed salad topper!

DINNER

Baked firecracker salmon with asparagus and sweet potato (6 ounces salmon, 6 spears asparagus, ½ small sweet potato)

Prep (salmon): Whisk together 1 tablespoon soy sauce, 1 tablespoon olive oil, ½ tablespoon erythritol brown sugar sweetener, ¼ teaspoon red pepper flakes, 1 tablespoon chopped scallion, 1 tablespoon fresh, finely grated ginger, and salt to taste. Marinate the salmon in this mixture in a glass baking dish in the refrigerator for at least 1 hour.

Preheat the oven to 400°F and bake the salmon for 15 to 20 minutes.

Prep (asparagus): Sauté the asparagus in 1 tablespoon olive oil and garnish with fresh lemon zest.

Prep (sweet potato): Preheat the oven to 400°F. Bake the sweet potato for about 45 minutes. Serve with a dash of cinnamon. For another option, melt 1 teaspoon of butter on the potato.

Plan ahead: Store extra potatoes in the refrigerator for up to 4 days.

SNACK

1 Peanut Butter Cup (page 284)

TOTAL DAILY NUTRITION

2,020 calories ▪ 60% fat ▪ 19% saturated fat ▪ 14% carbs ▪ 51g net carbs ▪ 31% protein

DAY 4

BREAKFAST

Mushroom, spinach & feta omelet with 2 pieces Keto Cloud Bread, Everything Bagel version (page 258), and blueberries (¼ cup berries)

Prep (omelet): Very lightly coat a small pan with olive oil or butter and place it over medium heat. Add ¼ cup chopped spinach and ¼ cup sliced mushrooms. Sauté until the spinach is wilted and excess liquid evaporates from the mushrooms, about 4 to 5 minutes. Remove the spinach and mushrooms from the pan. Beat 2 large eggs and cook them in the pan. Add the cooked spinach and mushrooms and ¼ cup feta cheese. Season with salt and pepper to taste.

Coffee or tea

SNACK

Keto-friendly shake

LUNCH

Grilled Buffalo Chicken Salad (page 184)

8 Herbed Seed Crackers (page 256) with hummus (¼ cup hummus)

SNACK

Full-fat (4% milkfat) cottage cheese (1 cup)

Variation: To spice up your cottage cheese, try topping it with raspberries, blackberries, or chopped pecans mixed with cinnamon and a sprinkle of granulated erythritol.

DINNER

Pepperoni & Goat Cheese Pizza (page 241) with roasted brussels sprouts

Prep (brussels sprouts): Preheat the oven to 400°F. Toss 2 cups brussels sprouts with 2 tablespoons olive oil and salt and pepper to taste. Spread evenly on a baking sheet very lightly greased with olive oil. Roast for 25 minutes.

Plan ahead: This recipe makes 2 servings. To get a jump on tomorrow's dinner, store half the brussels sprouts in an airtight container in the refrigerator for easy reheating.

Variation (brussels sprouts): For a twist, try seasoning your brussels sprouts with lemon and garlic. Squeeze lemon juice over the brussels sprouts, and very lightly drizzle with olive oil, garlic powder, and salt and pepper to taste.

TOTAL DAILY NUTRITION

1,816 calories ▪ 54% fat ▪ 19% saturated fat ▪ 16% carbs ▪ 57g net carbs ▪ 27% protein

DAY 5

BREAKFAST

1 serving of Grab-and-Go Nut & Berry Yogurt Bark (page 153) with a keto-friendly shake

Coffee or tea

LUNCH

Pumpkin & Black Bean Chili (page 176) with a side salad

Prep (salad): Toss 2 cups mixed greens with 1 tablespoon extra virgin olive oil and 1 tablespoon apple cider vinegar.

SNACK

1 hard-boiled egg

DINNER

Rotisserie chicken (6 ounces)

Tip: Rotisserie chicken, cooked and ready to pick up at your local grocery store, makes a quick and easy dinner option. Just be mindful to look at the ingredients and check for any extra sugars or additives.

Garlic & Parmesan Mashed Cauliflower (page 254)

Roasted brussels sprouts (1 cup) from last night's leftovers, reheated

SNACK

2 Chocolate Chip Cookie Dough Bites (page 286)

TOTAL DAILY NUTRITION

1,775 calories ▪ 58% fat ▪ 21% saturated fat ▪ 14% carbs ▪ 47g net carbs ▪ 27% protein

DAY 6

BREAKFAST

Half of a Blueberry Waffle with Lemon Cream Cheese Frosting (page 159) and full-fat (4% milkfat) cottage cheese (½ cup) with dash of cinnamon

Coffee or tea

SNACK

Whey protein shake

LUNCH

Open-faced ham & cheese sandwich with slices of bell pepper (½ large bell pepper)

Prep (sandwich): Assemble 2 ounces ham deli meat, 1 ounce Swiss cheese, and 1 teaspoon Dijon mustard between 2 pieces Keto Cloud Bread, version of your choice (page 258)

SNACK

¼ cup Cinnamon Roasted Chickpeas (page 271)

DINNER

Fish Tacos with Creamy Avocado Sauce (page 230), Almond Flour Tortilla Chips with Homemade Guacamole (page 253), and Warm Raspberry Crisp (page 275)

Plan ahead: Save a serving of guacamole for tomorrow's snack. Squeeze a dash of lime juice on top of the guacamole and store it in an airtight container in the refrigerator to avoid it turning brown.

TOTAL DAILY NUTRITION

1,782 calories ▪ 69% fat ▪ 23% saturated fat ▪ 28% carbs ▪ 60g net carbs ▪ 26% protein

DAY 7

BREAKFAST

Coconut Berry Yogurt Parfait (page 149) with a Mocha Frappé (page 166)

SNACK

Greek feta salad

Prep (salad): Toss ¼ cup cherry tomatoes, halved, ¼ cup diced cucumber, and ¼ cup Kalamata olives together in a small bowl. Serve the veggie and olive mixture over 2 cups chopped romaine lettuce dressed with 1 tablespoon extra virgin olive oil and 1 tablespoon red wine vinegar.

LUNCH

Spiced Turkey & Sweet Potato Bowl (page 200) with almonds (23 nuts)

SNACK

Grilled chicken strips with Guacamole (page 253) left over from last night's dinner (3 ounces chicken, ¼ cup Guacamole)

Prep (chicken): Look for prepared chicken breast strips or grilled chicken breast in the meat or deli aisle of your supermarket or at a salad bar for a quick snack option to pair with dips or fresh vegetables.

DINNER

Roasted pork tenderloin with asparagus (6 ounces pork, 6 spears asparagus)

Prep (pork): In a small bowl, mix 2 tablespoons olive oil, 2 tablespoons freshly squeezed lemon juice, 2 garlic cloves, pressed, 1 tablespoon fresh rosemary, 1½ teaspoons Dijon mustard, and salt and pepper to taste. Brush the mixture over the tenderloin and then marinate it in the refrigerator, covered, for an hour.

Preheat the oven to 450°F. Very lightly coat a shallow baking dish with olive oil. Heat a skillet over medium-high heat and sear the tenderloin all over, for just a minute or two on each side. Place the seared tenderloin in the prepared baking dish. Add the asparagus and then season both the pork and asparagus with salt and pepper to taste. Roast for approximately 20 to 25 minutes, or until the internal temperature of the pork reaches 145°F. Rest the pork for 3 to 5 minutes before slicing.

Variation: Pork pairs well with a variety of herbs and spices, including curry powder, garlic, rosemary, dill, sage, and thyme—experiment!

TOTAL DAILY NUTRITION

1,787 calories ▪ 60% fat ▪ 23% saturated fat ▪ 13% carbs ▪ 39g net carbs ▪ 28% protein

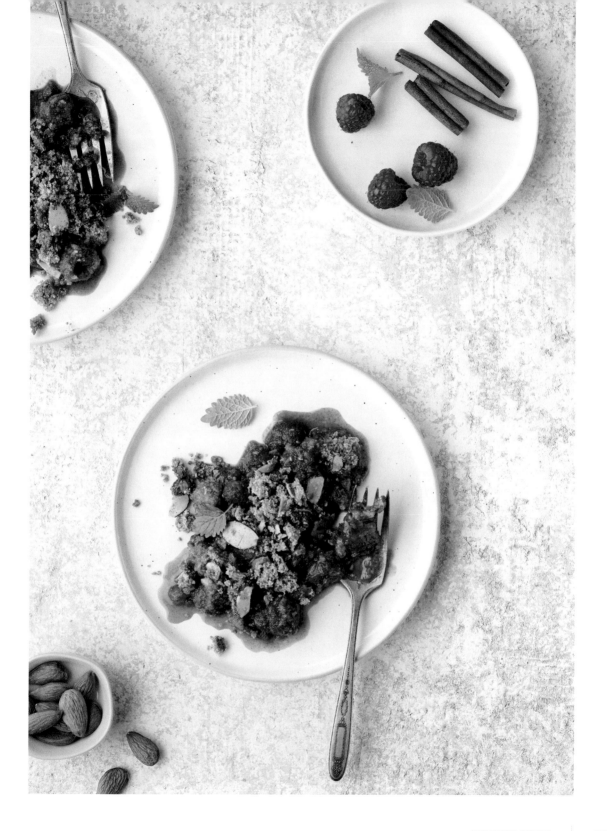

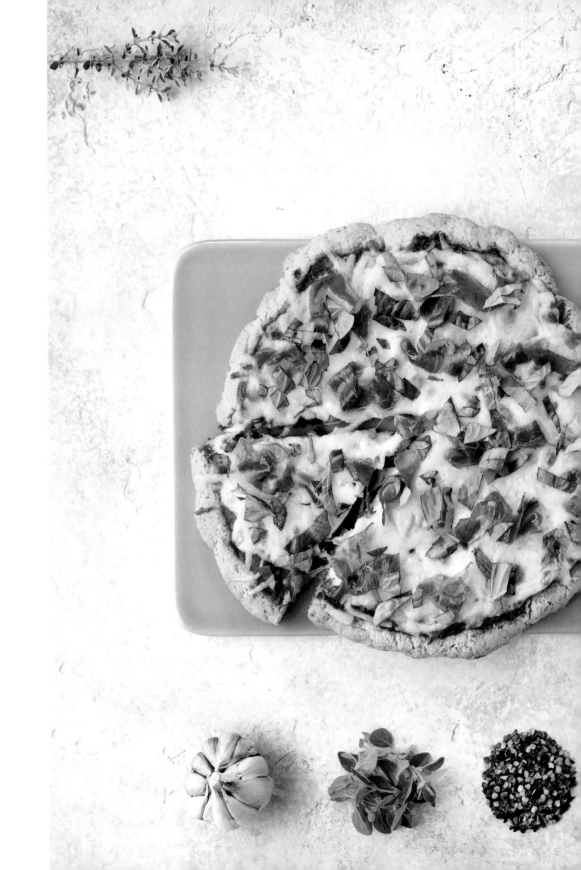

RECIPES

BREAKFAST

DRINKS

LUNCH

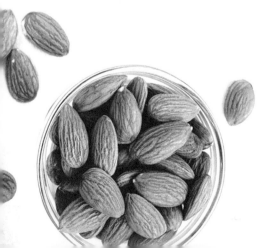

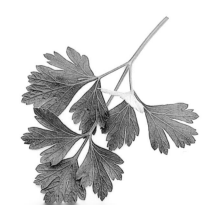

DINNER

SIDES, SNACKS & SWEETS

▪ = PHASE 1   ▪ ▪ = PHASE 2

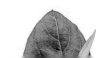

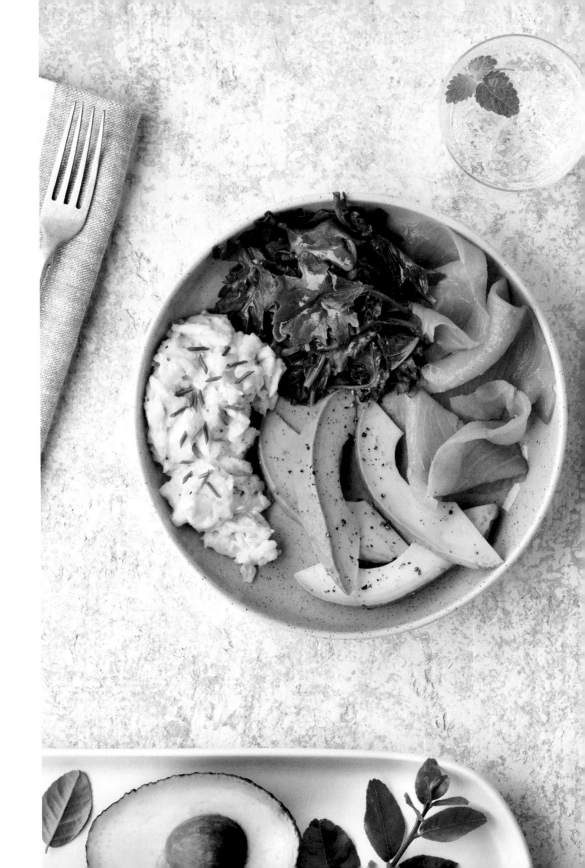

BREAKFAST

EGG CUPS 3 WAYS

YIELDS 24 EGG CUPS (2 EGG CUPS PER SERVING)

Start your morning with these easy, savory egg cups. Made with whole buttermilk and Greek yogurt, they are fluffy clouds of goodness filled with your favorite ingredients, such as prosciutto and chives, cheddar and bacon, or spinach and feta. This is a versatile recipe, so feel free to be creative and try different vegetable, meat, cheese, and seasoning combinations.

INGREDIENTS

20 eggs
1 cup whole buttermilk
1 cup plain whole-milk Greek yogurt
½ cup shredded whole-milk mozzarella cheese

For chive and prosciutto filling

¼ cup chopped chives
2 ounces chopped prosciutto

For spinach and feta filling

½ cup chopped spinach
¼ cup crumbled feta cheese

For bacon and cheddar filling

⅓ cup cooked and crumbled bacon
¼ cup shredded full-fat cheddar cheese

DIRECTIONS

Preheat the oven to 350°F.

Lightly grease with butter two 12-count muffin tins (for 24 total muffins) and set aside.

Whisk the eggs, buttermilk, yogurt, mozzarella, and salt and pepper to taste in a large mixing bowl.

Divide the mixture evenly between 24 prepared muffin cups.

Divide the chives and prosciutto among 8 egg cups.

Divide the chopped spinach and crumbled feta among 8 egg cups.

Divide the bacon and cheddar among 8 egg cups.

Transfer to the oven and bake for 20 to 25 minutes, until the eggs are set.

Cool for 5 to 10 minutes in muffin tins and then gently slide a butter knife around the edges to release the egg cups. Remove them to a wire rack.

Serve warm or store in an airtight container in the refrigerator for 3 to 4 days.

Note: You may freeze the individual cups on a baking sheet lined with parchment paper. Once they are frozen, transfer them to a freezer-safe bag. When you are ready to eat, reheat them in a 350°F oven for 8 to 10 minutes, or in the microwave for about 30 seconds.

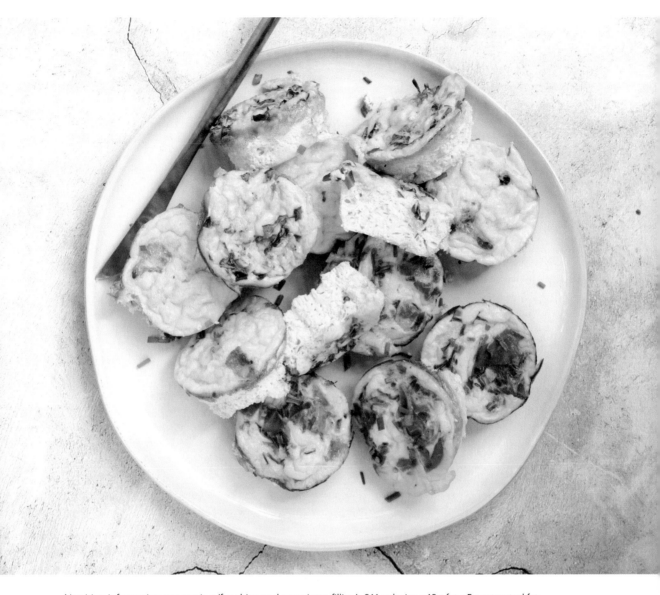

Nutrition information per serving (for chive and prosciutto filling): 211 calories ▪ 13g fat ▪ 5g saturated fat ▪ **18g protein** ▪ **4g carbs** ▪ **3g sugar** ▪ 0g sugar alcohol ▪ 0g fiber ▪ 3g net carbs ▪ 321mg cholesterol ▪ 619mg sodium

Nutrition information per serving (for spinach and feta filling): 214 calories ▪ 15g fat ▪ 7g saturated fat ▪ **16g protein** ▪ **3g carbs** ▪ **3g sugar** ▪ 0g sugar alcohol ▪ 0g fiber ▪ 3g net carbs ▪ 335mg cholesterol ▪ 309mg sodium

Nutrition information per serving (for bacon and cheddar filling): 225 calories ▪ 15g fat ▪ 7g saturated fat ▪ **17g protein** ▪ **3g carbs** ▪ **2g sugar** ▪ 0g sugar alcohol ▪ 0g fiber ▪ 3g net carbs ▪ 337mg cholesterol ▪ 434mg sodium

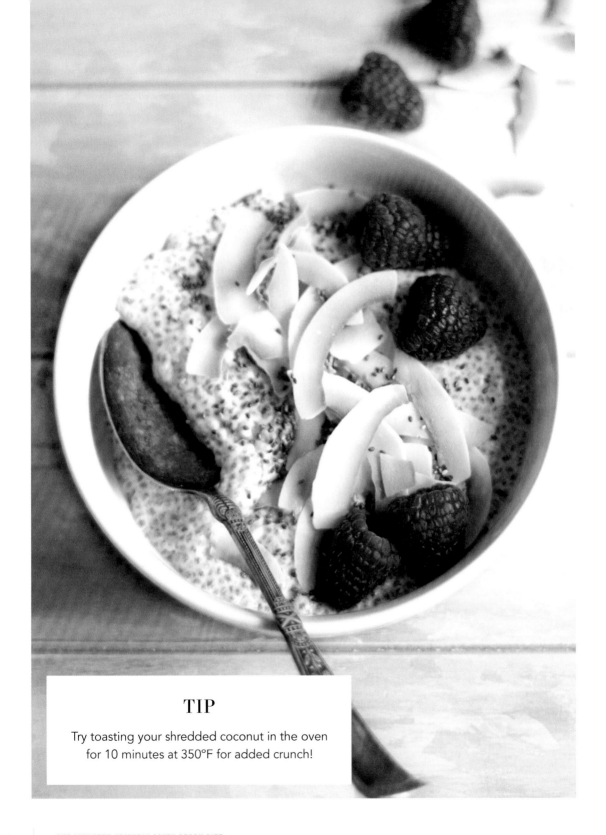

TIP

Try toasting your shredded coconut in the oven
for 10 minutes at 350°F for added crunch!

COCONUT CHIA PUDDING

YIELDS 1 SERVING

This chia pudding is a great make-ahead breakfast, and can be easily doubled or tripled to be enjoyed throughout the week. It is naturally thickened by collagen, an increasingly popular protein source that contributes to improved bone and skin health and is often added to baking mixes and smoothies.

INGREDIENTS

1 cup unsweetened coconut milk

2 tablespoons chia seeds

1 scoop (or about 2 tablespoons) collagen peptides

1 teaspoon granulated erythritol sweetener (optional)

2 tablespoons shredded unsweetened coconut

¼ cup raspberries (optional, for Phase II)

DIRECTIONS

Whisk together the coconut milk, chia seeds, collagen peptides, and erythritol sweetener (if using) in a small bowl.

Cover the bowl and place it in the refrigerator for at least 2 hours and for up to 5 days. When you are ready to serve it, top with the shredded coconut and raspberries (if using).

Nutrition information per serving: 357 calories ▪ 21g fat ▪ 13g saturated fat ▪ **25g protein** ▪ **20g carbs** ▪ **2g sugar** ▪ 2g sugar alcohol ▪ 13g fiber ▪ 4g net carbs ▪ 0mg cholesterol ▪ 221mg sodium

SMOKED SALMON BOWL

YIELDS 1 SERVING

Enjoy a hearty, protein-packed breakfast bowl full of scrambled eggs, smoked salmon, sautéed kale, and avocado. This single-serving recipe can easily be multiplied for a fun low-carb Sunday brunch spread!

INGREDIENTS

1 cup packed baby kale

¼ teaspoon olive oil

2 large eggs

⅛ teaspoon sea salt

⅛ teaspoon ground black pepper

2 ounces smoked salmon

¼ avocado, pitted and sliced

DIRECTIONS

Preheat a nonstick pan on the stove over medium heat.

Add the kale and olive oil to the pan and cook for 2 to 3 minutes, or until the kale is wilted. Season with a pinch each of salt and pepper to taste, and transfer to a serving bowl. Place the skillet back on the stove to cook the eggs.

Whisk together the eggs, salt, pepper, and 1 tablespoon of milk. Add this mixture to the pan and scramble to your desired firmness.

Place the scrambled eggs in the bowl with the kale, top with smoked salmon and sliced avocado, and serve.

Nutrition information per serving: 337 calories ▪ 21g fat ▪ 5g saturated fat ▪ **27g protein** ▪ **14g carbs** ▪ **1g sugar** ▪ 0g sugar alcohol ▪ 5g fiber ▪ 9g net carbs ▪ 385mg cholesterol ▪ 625mg sodium

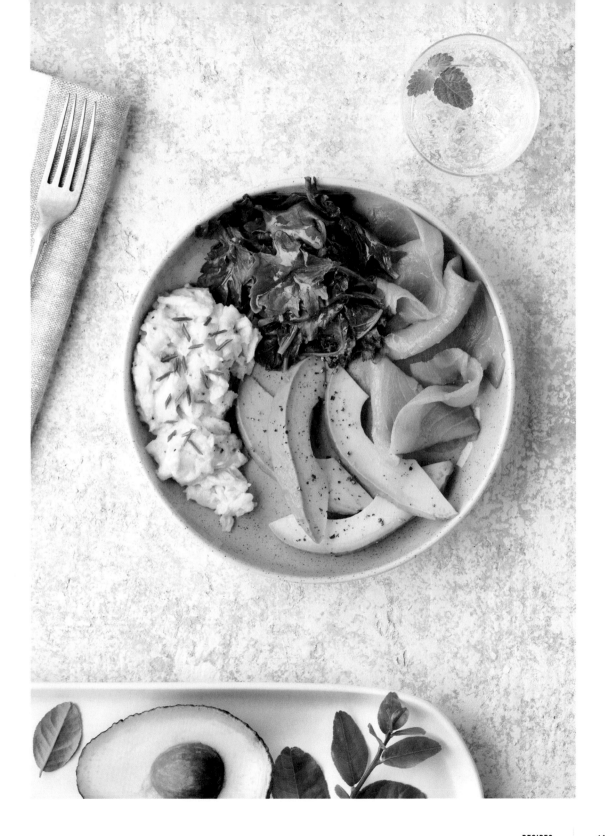

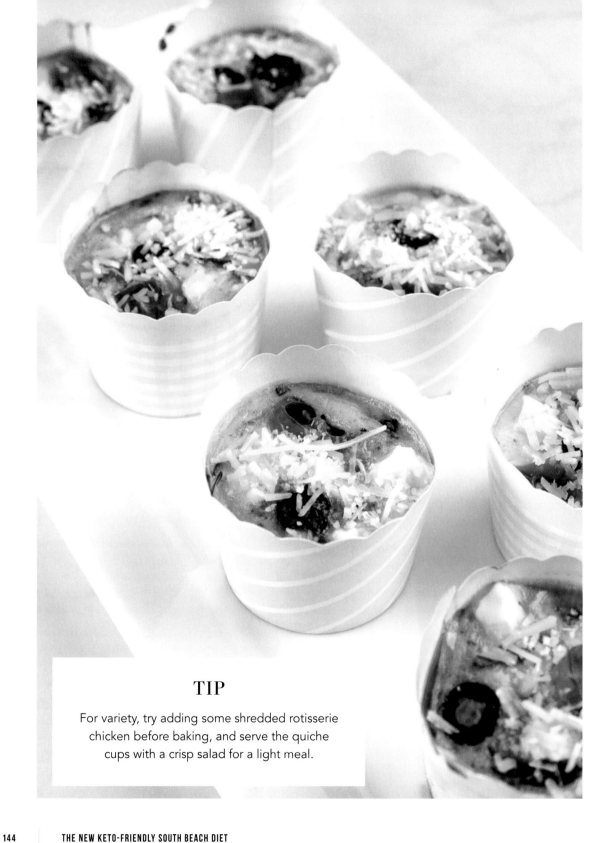

TIP

For variety, try adding some shredded rotisserie chicken before baking, and serve the quiche cups with a crisp salad for a light meal.

SPINACH & ARTICHOKE QUICHE CUPS

YIELDS 6 QUICHE CUPS (1 QUICHE CUP PER SERVING)

These colorful mini quiche cups filled with Mediterranean flavors are perfectly portable for breakfast on the run or to include in lunch boxes. Kefalotiri is a Greek hard cheese; you can substitute Parmesan.

INGREDIENTS

3 large eggs, lightly beaten

½ cup heavy cream

2 tablespoons olive oil

½ cup cherry tomatoes, halved

3 scallions, thinly sliced

⅓ cup canned chopped artichoke hearts

⅓ cup cooked chopped bacon (5 or 6 slices) or pancetta (optional)

⅓ cup roasted red peppers, chopped

2 cups baby spinach

⅓ cup pitted and sliced Kalamata olives

1 tablespoon fresh chopped oregano (can substitute 1 teaspoon dried oregano if needed)

⅓ cup crumbled feta cheese

4 tablespoons shredded kefalotiri or Parmesan cheese

DIRECTIONS

Preheat the oven to 375°F.

Line a 6-cup muffin tin with paper cupcake liners (or grease lightly with butter) and set aside.

Whisk together the eggs and heavy cream in a large bowl.

Heat the olive oil in a large skillet over medium heat. Add the cherry tomatoes and scallions and cook for 2 to 3 minutes, stirring often. Add the artichoke hearts, bacon (if using), roasted peppers, and spinach. Cook for 1 minute until the spinach has just wilted.

Add the mixture to the bowl with the eggs and cream. Stir in the olives, oregano, and feta and season with salt and pepper to taste. Using a ¼ cup measure, divide the mixture among the prepared cups, filling about ¼ inch from the top. Sprinkle the shredded kefalotiri or Parmesan on top.

Bake for 15 to 18 minutes, or until golden and the eggs are set.

Remove from the oven and let cool slightly before serving.

Note: You may store the cooled quiche cups in an airtight container in the refrigerator for up to 2 days.

Nutrition information per serving: 230 calories ▪ 21g fat ▪ 9g saturated fat ▪ **8g protein** ▪ **12g carbs** ▪ **5g sugar** ▪ 0g sugar alcohol ▪ 2g fiber ▪ 11g net carbs ▪ 129mg cholesterol ▪ 424mg sodium

COFFEE & HAZELNUT MUFFINS

YIELDS 6 LARGE MUFFINS (1 MUFFIN PER SERVING)

These gorgeous nutty muffins taste as good as they look. They will get you started in the morning and also make a great pick-me-up snack to pack in your lunch box.

INGREDIENTS

For the muffins

3 large eggs

¼ cup strong coffee

¼ cup powdered erythritol sweetener

⅓ cup unsalted butter, softened to room temperature

2 tablespoons hazelnut oil (or substitute more butter)

2 tablespoons ground flaxseeds or ground chia seeds

¼ cup coconut flour

⅓ cup plus 2 tablespoons lightly toasted hazelnuts, ground (reserve the 2 tablespoons for garnish)

½ teaspoon baking soda

½ teaspoon baking powder

¼ teaspoon Himalayan pink salt

1 teaspoon cinnamon (optional)

For the frosting

½ cup heavy cream

¼ cup powdered erythritol sweetener

½ cup full-fat cream cheese

2 tablespoons instant coffee, mixed with 2 tablespoons water

1 teaspoon vanilla extract

DIRECTIONS

Preheat the oven to 350°F.

Line a 6-cup muffin tin with silicone cups or paper cupcake liners (or grease them with butter) and set aside.

Whisk the eggs, coffee, and powdered erythritol sweetener together in a large bowl. Add all the remaining muffin ingredients to the bowl and whisk until thoroughly mixed.

Divide the batter among the prepared cups and bake for about 18 to 20 minutes, or until a toothpick inserted in the center of the cups comes out clean.

Transfer the muffins to a wire rack and let them cool to room temperature.

Whisk together all the frosting ingredients until creamy and smooth and frost the cooled muffins. Sprinkle the muffins with the remaining 2 tablespoons of ground toasted hazelnuts and serve.

Note: The muffins will keep in an airtight container in the refrigerator for up to 3 days, or you may freeze the muffins—without the frosting—for up to 2 months.

Nutrition information per serving: 371 calories ▪ 35g fat ▪ 17g saturated fat ▪ **8g protein** ▪ **19g carbs** ▪ **3g sugar** ▪ 9g sugar alcohol ▪ 5g fiber ▪ 5g net carbs ▪ 165mg cholesterol ▪ 286mg sodium

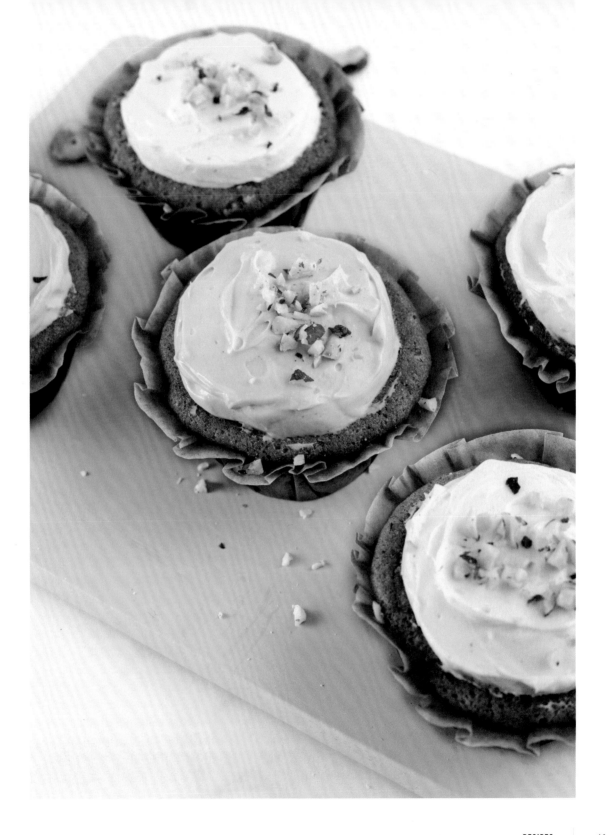

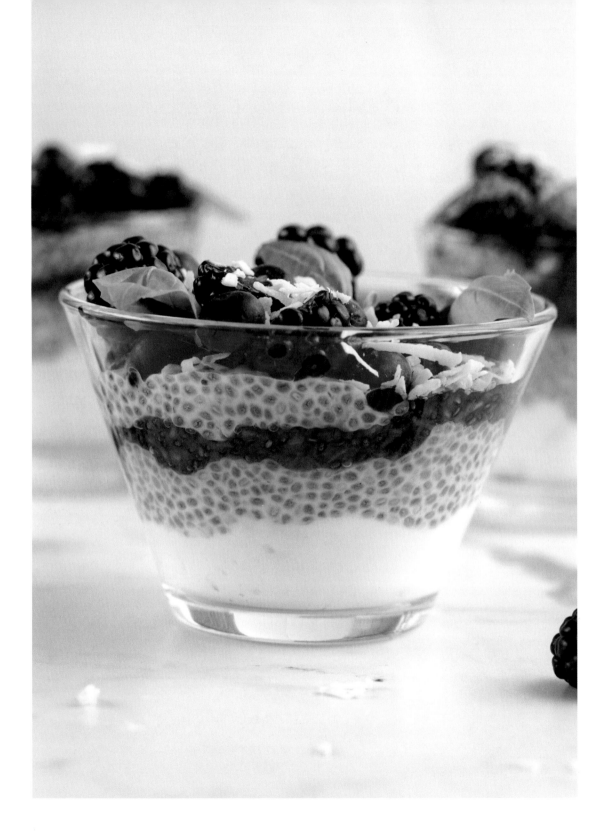

COCONUT BERRY YOGURT PARFAIT

YIELDS 4 SERVINGS (1 PARFAIT PER SERVING)

Cool and creamy, this is the ultimate guilt-free pick-me-up
for a satisfying breakfast, snack, or dessert.

INGREDIENTS

1 cup unsweetened coconut-milk yogurt

1 tablespoon powdered erythritol sweetener

For the raspberry coulis

1 cup fresh or frozen raspberries

2 tablespoons powdered erythritol sweetener

½ teaspoon arrowroot powder

For the chia coconut yogurt layer

⅓ cup chia seeds

1 cup unsweetened coconut-milk yogurt

1 teaspoon vanilla

2 tablespoons powdered erythritol sweetener

To decorate

¼ cup fresh mixed berries

2 tablespoons shredded unsweetened coconut, lightly toasted

A few fresh basil leaves (optional)

DIRECTIONS

Stir together the yogurt and powdered erythritol sweetener in a small bowl and set it aside.

Place all the raspberry coulis ingredients in a small saucepan and bring them to a boil over medium-high heat. Cook until the raspberries have softened, about 1 to 2 minutes. If desired, strain the mixture through a fine mesh sieve to remove the seeds before setting it aside to cool.

Stir together all the chia coconut layer ingredients in a bowl.

Layer the coconut yogurt, raspberry coulis, and chia yogurt into 4 small glasses or cups. Cover them with plastic food wrap and refrigerate for 4 to 6 hours, or until set (preferably overnight).

Just before serving, top each parfait with the mixed berries and sprinkle with the toasted coconut. Garnish with the basil leaves, if desired. This parfait will keep refrigerated for up to 2 days.

Nutrition information per serving: 155 calories ▪ 9g fat ▪ 5g saturated fat ▪ **3g protein** ▪ **36g carbs** ▪ **3g sugar** ▪ 19g sugar alcohol ▪ 8g fiber ▪ 9g net carbs ▪ 0mg cholesterol ▪ 26mg sodium

WARM AVOCADO WITH EGG

YIELDS 4 SERVINGS (½ STUFFED AVOCADO PER SERVING)

This speedy breakfast, made with only a handful of ingredients, will set you up for
the day and keep you satisfied until lunch, thanks to the healthy fats in the avocado.
Lime juice adds a touch of zing and prevents the avocado from browning.

INGREDIENTS

2 large avocados, halved,
pits removed

Juice of 1 lime

2 tablespoons chopped
sun-dried tomatoes

¼ cup pitted and chopped
black or green olives

2 scallions, thinly sliced

2 tablespoons chopped fresh
cilantro

2 eggs, lightly beaten

1 tablespoon olive oil

2 tablespoons shredded
whole-milk mozzarella cheese

Large handful of microgreens,
or baby arugula, to garnish

DIRECTIONS

Preheat the oven to 400°F.

Place the avocado halves on a baking sheet and drizzle with
the lime juice; set it aside.

Combine the sun-dried tomatoes, olives, scallions, and
cilantro in a bowl. Add the lightly beaten egg and olive oil
and mix well.

Fill the avocado cavities with the mixture and sprinkle with
the shredded mozzarella. Add salt and pepper to taste.

Bake for about 5 to 7 minutes, or until the eggs have set.

Serve warm, topped with microgreens or baby arugula.

Nutrition information per serving: 219 calories ▪ 18g fat ▪ 3g saturated fat ▪ **6g protein** ▪ **10g carbs** ▪ **2g sugar**
▪ 0g sugar alcohol ▪ 5g fiber ▪ 5g net carbs ▪ 95mg cholesterol ▪ 139mg sodium

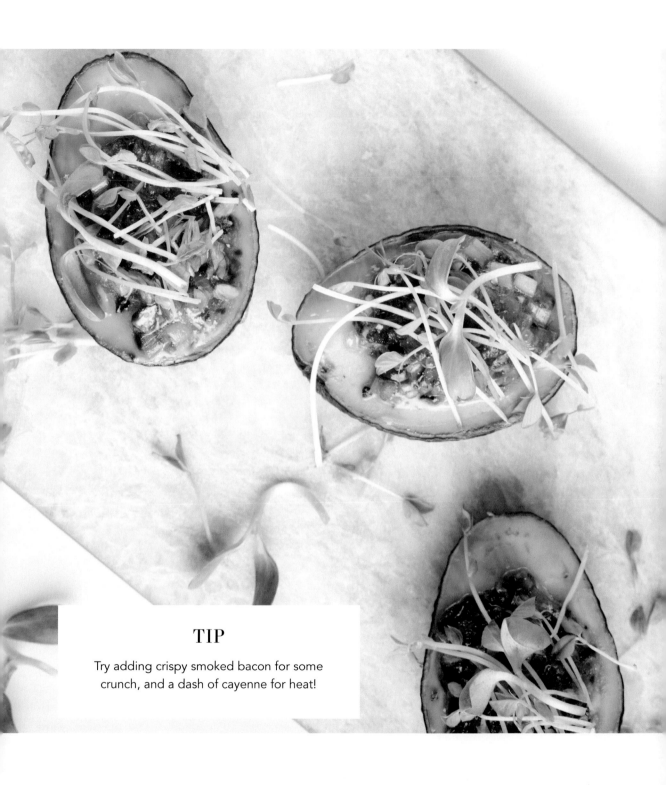

TIP

Try adding crispy smoked bacon for some crunch, and a dash of cayenne for heat!

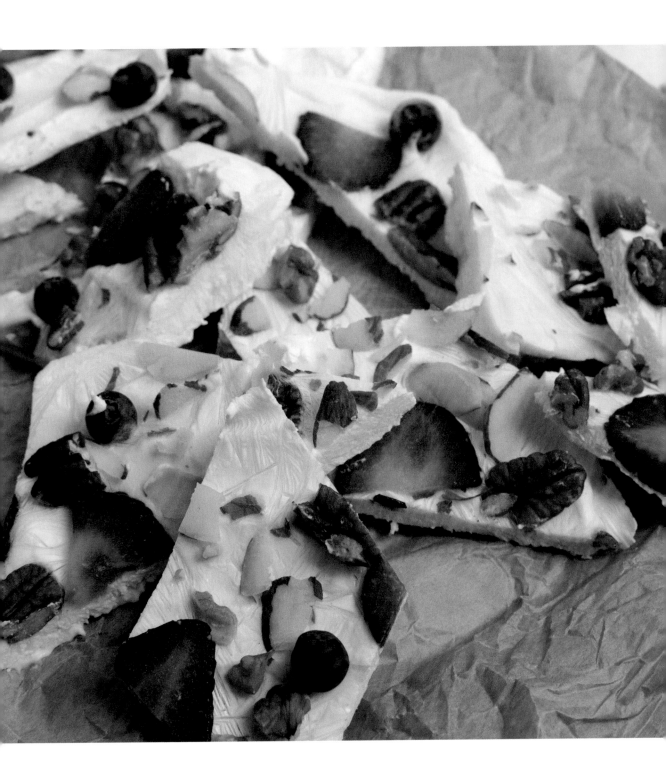

GRAB-AND-GO NUT & BERRY YOGURT BARK

YIELDS 6 PIECES OF BARK (1 PIECE PER SERVING)

Take your Greek yogurt to go with this delicious yogurt bark. It's the perfect on-the-move breakfast or snack, packed with protein and flavor.

INGREDIENTS

2 cups plain whole-milk Greek yogurt
½ teaspoon vanilla extract
2 tablespoons chopped pecans
2 tablespoons sliced almonds
2 tablespoons chopped walnuts
2 tablespoons blueberries
2 tablespoons sliced strawberries

DIRECTIONS

Line a 9 x 13-inch baking dish with parchment paper and set it aside.

In a large mixing bowl, whisk together the yogurt and vanilla extract.

Transfer the mixture to the prepared baking dish and spread it into an even layer.

Top with the pecans, almonds, and walnuts, as well as the blueberries and strawberries (if using). Gently press the toppings into the yogurt mixture.

Cover the yogurt bark and transfer it to the freezer for 3 hours, until firm.

Cut or break the bark into 6 pieces. These may be stored in the freezer for up to a month in an airtight container.

Nutrition information per serving: 113 calories ▪ 7g fat ▪ 2g saturated fat ▪ **8g protein** ▪ **4g carbs** ▪ **3g sugar** ▪ 0g sugar alcohol ▪ 1g fiber ▪ 3g net carbs ▪ 15mg cholesterol ▪ 28mg sodium

SWEET POTATO EGG CUPS

YIELDS 12 EGG CUPS (3 EGG CUPS PER SERVING)

Egg cups are an excellent addition to your menu plan for several reasons.
They're an easy, portable source of protein; you can customize them with any
combination of vegetables and cheese you like; and you can make them in advance!

INGREDIENTS

For the crust

1 medium sweet potato, peeled and shredded

¼ teaspoon sea salt

2 teaspoons coconut oil, melted

¼ teaspoon ground black pepper

¼ teaspoon garlic powder

For the egg cups

12 large eggs

½ cup heavy cream

¼ teaspoon sea salt

½ teaspoon ground black pepper

¼ cup chopped spinach

¼ cup chopped tomatoes

¼ cup crumbled full-fat feta cheese

¼ cup shredded full-fat cheddar cheese

DIRECTIONS

Preheat the oven to 400°F. Line a 12-cup muffin tin with silicone cups or paper cupcake liners and set aside.

Combine the sweet potato and sea salt in a strainer and toss to coat. Let the mixture sit for 20 minutes to release any excess water. Transfer the sweet potato to a piece of cheesecloth and squeeze out the water.

Put the sweet potatoes in a bowl and add the coconut oil, black pepper, and garlic powder. Toss to combine.

Divide the sweet potato mixture evenly between the 12 muffin cups and press the mixture down into the bottoms of the muffin cups with the tip of a spoon.

Bake for 15 minutes. Remove the muffin tin from the oven.

While the sweet potatoes are cooking, prepare the egg cups by adding the eggs, heavy cream, salt, pepper, spinach, and tomatoes to a bowl and whisk to combine.

Pour equal amounts of the egg mixture into the baked sweet potato cups. Top with the feta and cheddar.

Bake for 15 to 20 minutes, or until the eggs are set.

Remove from the oven and allow the egg cups to cool slightly before serving. They are freezer friendly and great for make-ahead meals and snacks.

Nutrition information per serving: 331 calories ▪ 21g fat ▪ 10g saturated fat ▪ **24g protein** ▪ **10g carbs** ▪ 2g sugar ▪ 0g sugar alcohol ▪ 1g fiber ▪ 9g net carbs ▪ 572mg cholesterol ▪ 740mg sodium

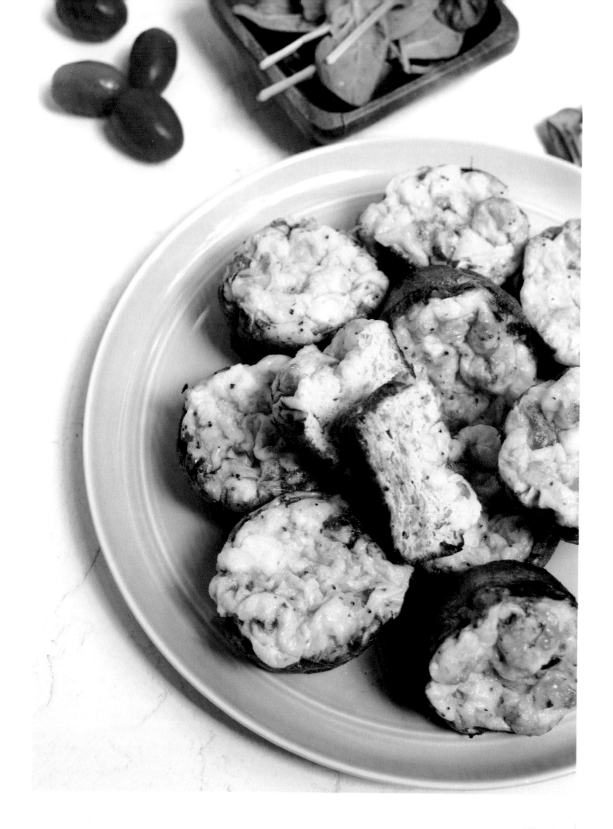

CHOCOLATE PEANUT BUTTER MUG MUFFINS

YIELDS 2 MUFFINS (1 MUFFIN PER SERVING)

Ready in just a few minutes, this mug muffin is a welcome treat before or after your morning workout and will also satisfy your sweet cravings at any time during the day.

INGREDIENTS

2 tablespoons creamy unsalted and unsweetened natural peanut butter

1½ tablespoons unsalted butter or ghee

1 tablespoon ground flaxseeds

1 scoop (about 2 tablespoons) keto-friendly vanilla protein powder

¼ teaspoon baking powder

2½ tablespoons full-fat sour cream or plain whole-milk Greek yogurt

1 large egg

2 teaspoons powdered erythritol sweetener

2 tablespoons sugar-free chocolate chips

DIRECTIONS

Split all ingredients except the chocolate chips between two large mugs and whisk with a fork until well combined. Stir in the chocolate chips.

Cook in the microwave for about 1 to 1½ minutes, until the mixture is set in the center.

TIP

For even more chocolaty muffins, add ½ tablespoon cacao or unsweetened cocoa powder, increase the sour cream to 3 tablespoons, and use keto-friendly chocolate protein powder instead of vanilla protein powder.

Nutrition information per serving: 371 calories ▪ 29g fat ▪ 12g saturated fat ▪ **21g protein** ▪ **28g carbs** ▪ **3g sugar** ▪ 20g sugar alcohol ▪ 3g fiber ▪ 4g net carbs ▪ 133mg cholesterol ▪ 163mg sodium

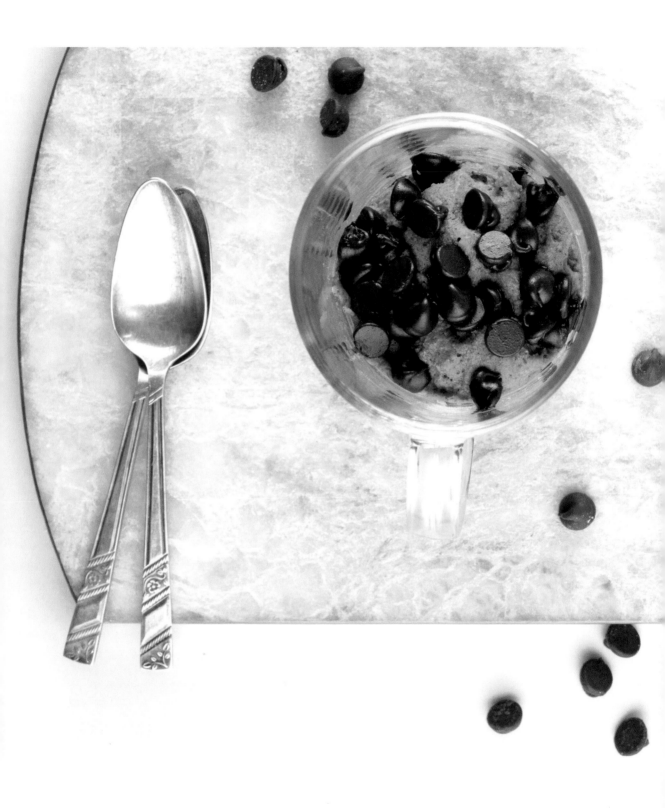

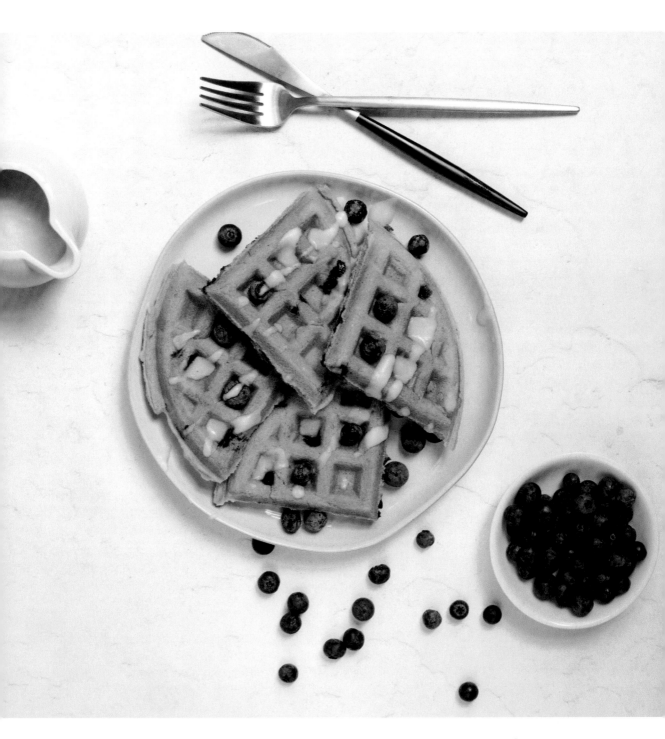

Nutrition information per serving: 517 calories ▪ 43g fat ▪ 17g saturated fat ▪ **25g protein** ▪ **50g carbs** ▪ **5g sugar** ▪ 39g sugar alcohol ▪ 3g fiber ▪ 7g net carbs ▪ 204mg cholesterol ▪ 558mg sodium

BLUEBERRY WAFFLES

WITH LEMON CREAM CHEESE FROSTING

YIELDS 2 LARGE WAFFLES (HALF A WAFFLE PER SERVING)

To make the frosting, you'll need powdered erythritol sweetener, which has a texture similar to powdered sugar. If all you have is granulated erythritol, you can turn it into powder by processing it in a blender or a food processor for about 20 to 30 seconds.

INSTRUCTIONS

3 large eggs

½ cup unsweetened vanilla almond milk

5 tablespoons unsalted butter, melted

1 teaspoon vanilla extract

¾ cup almond flour

¼ cup tapioca flour

½ cup unflavored whey protein powder

½ teaspoon baking soda

1 teaspoon baking powder

¼ teaspoon sea salt

1 tablespoon granulated erythritol sweetener

½ cup frozen wild blueberries

For the frosting

2 tablespoons unsalted butter, softened

3 tablespoons cream cheese, softened

1 teaspoon vanilla extract

2 teaspoons lemon juice

¼ teaspoon lemon zest

¾ cup powdered erythritol

1 to 2 tablespoons unsweetened vanilla almond milk

DIRECTIONS

Preheat a waffle iron to medium-high heat.

Separate the egg yolks from the whites and place in separate bowls. Add the egg yolks to one bowl with the milk, butter, and vanilla. Whisk until combined. Set the mixture aside.

In a separate bowl, combine the flour, whey protein powder, baking soda, baking powder, sea salt, and erythritol.

Fold the dry ingredients into the wet ingredients, stirring just enough to combine them.

Beat the reserved egg whites with a handheld mixer until stiff peaks form, about 3 minutes. Fold the egg whites into the batter.

Gently stir in the blueberries.

Use a ¼ cup measure to pour the batter into the center of the waffle iron. Bake according to your waffle iron's instructions.

Repeat with the remaining batter.

While the waffles are cooking, make the frosting by combining the butter and cream cheese in a bowl and beating them with a handheld mixer for 1 minute, or until smooth. Add the vanilla, lemon juice, and lemon zest and beat until combined, about 20 seconds. Beat in the powdered erythritol until incorporated.

Beat in the almond milk, 1 tablespoon at a time, until the frosting reaches the desired consistency.

Spread the frosting evenly over the waffles. Serve them immediately.

MEXICAN BREAKFAST BAKE

YIELDS 8 SERVINGS (1 PIECE PER SERVING)

Elevate your morning with this Mexican-inspired breakfast bake.
Fluffy eggs are stuffed with savory chorizo sausage, sautéed veggies,
and a duo of cheeses for a satisfying and flavorful morning.

INGREDIENTS

½ pound bulk chorizo sausage

¼ cup diced onions

1 cup diced bell peppers

½ cup sliced white mushrooms

2 tablespoons minced garlic

2 cups packed chopped baby kale

12 eggs

½ cup whole milk

1 cup shredded full-fat cheddar cheese

1 cup shredded Colby Jack cheese

¼ cup chopped fresh cilantro

DIRECTIONS

Preheat the oven to 375°F. Lightly coat with butter a 9 x 13-inch baking dish and set it aside.

Heat the sausage in a large sauté pan over medium-high heat for 6 to 8 minutes, breaking it up with a spatula as it cooks, until it is cooked through.

Remove the sausage, reserving the grease in the pan. Add the onions, bell peppers, and mushrooms to the pan and cook for 3 to 4 minutes, until the mushrooms are browned. Add the garlic and cook for 1 minute, until fragrant. Add the kale and stir until wilted. Remove the pan from the heat and set it aside for 5 minutes to cool slightly.

Whisk together the eggs, whole milk, and salt and pepper to taste in a large bowl. Add to the bowl the cooled vegetable and sausage mixture, half the cheddar, and half the Colby Jack. Stir to combine.

Transfer the mixture to the prepared baking dish. Top with the remaining cheese.

Bake for 30 to 40 minutes, until the eggs are set and the cheese is bubbling.

Cut into 8 pieces. Serve warm, garnished with cilantro.

Note: This will keep in the refrigerator 3 to 4 days. For long-term storage, freeze the entire casserole or individual portions.

Nutrition information per serving: 378 calories ▪ 28g fat ▪ 13g saturated fat ▪ **24g protein** ▪ **6g carbs** ▪ **4g sugar** ▪ 0g sugar alcohol ▪ 1g fiber ▪ 5g net carbs ▪ 335mg cholesterol ▪ 626mg sodium

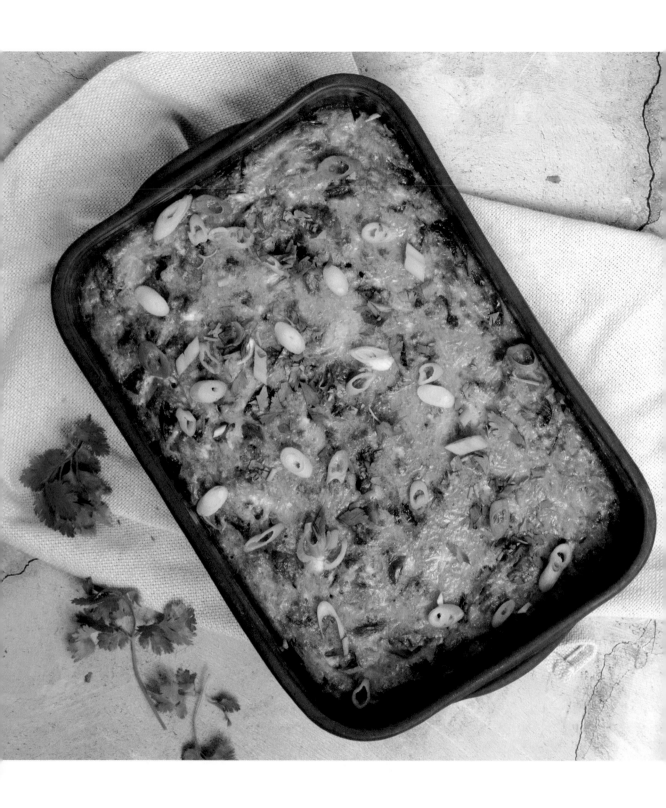

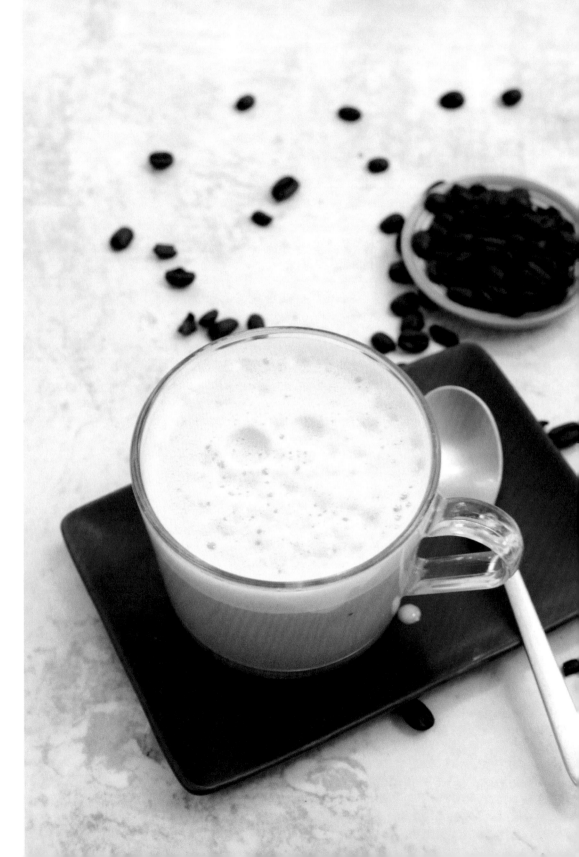

DRINKS

CHAI TEA LATTE

YIELDS 2 SERVINGS (1 MUG PER SERVING)

Transform your kitchen into your favorite coffeehouse with this easy chai tea latte. A fragrant blend of bold spices combine with creamy, frothed whole milk and a dash of coconut oil for a smooth and satisfying drink. Try it hot or cold!

INGREDIENTS

1 cup whole milk

1 tablespoon coconut oil

1 stick cinnamon

1 teaspoon minced ginger

¼ teaspoon ground allspice

½ teaspoon fennel seeds

4 cardamom pods

2 star anise pods

1 teaspoon ground black pepper

½ teaspoon vanilla extract

3 to 4 tablespoons loose black tea

½ teaspoon ground cinnamon

DIRECTIONS

Combine all the ingredients except the ground cinnamon together with ½ cup water in a small pot. Heat the mixture over medium-low heat for 5 to 7 minutes. If it begins to boil, reduce the heat to low.

Strain the mixture through a fine mesh sieve and then transfer to a blender. Blend 1 minute on medium speed, until frothy.

Divide the latte between 2 mugs. Top with the ground cinnamon.

TIP

To enjoy this latte cold, make it as directed and then transfer it to the refrigerator to cool. Although the froth will settle, the flavors will amplify with time; simply pour it over ice to serve. For a hot drink, you can also make the spice blend ahead of time, but wait until just before serving to froth the milk.

Nutrition information per serving: 137 calories ▪ 11g fat ▪ 8g saturated fat ▪ **4g protein** ▪ **6g carbs** ▪ **6g sugar** ▪ 0g sugar alcohol ▪ 0g fiber ▪ 6g net carbs ▪ 12mg cholesterol ▪ 52mg sodium

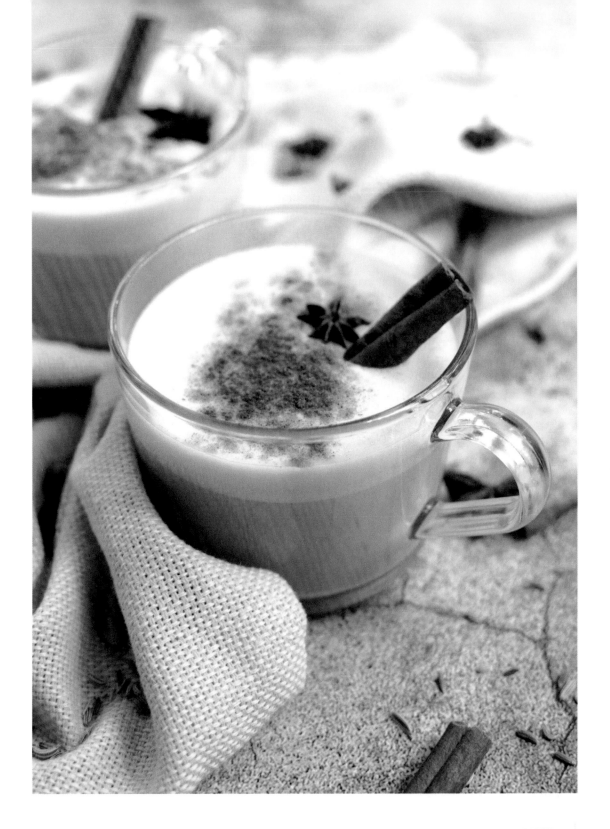

MOCHA FRAPPÉ

YIELDS 1 SERVING

This is a delicious, frothy iced coffee with a touch of chocolate,
fortified with healthy fats from MCT oil.

INGREDIENTS

1 cup cold-brewed coffee

¼ cup whole milk

1 tablespoon MCT oil

1 tablespoon cacao or unsweetened cocoa powder

2 teaspoons powdered erythritol sweetener

½ cup ice cubes

1 tablespoon cacao nibs (optional)

Dash of cinnamon

DIRECTIONS

Add all the ingredients to a blender and blend for 30 seconds to 1 minute.

TIP

You can make your own cold-brewed coffee at home! Add ⅓ cup ground coffee to a jar with 1½ cups cold water. Cover and leave on the counter overnight; then pour through a sieve lined with a coffee filter. Or you can buy bottled cold-brewed coffee at the grocery store.

Nutrition information per serving: 216 calories ▪ 17g fat ▪ 15g saturated fat ▪ **6g protein** ▪ **23g carbs** ▪ **3g sugar** ▪ 10g sugar alcohol ▪ 6g fiber ▪ 7g net carbs ▪ 6mg cholesterol ▪ 33mg sodium

CREAMY PROTEIN LATTE

YIELDS 2 SERVINGS

Add a dose of healthy protein to your morning coffee routine with this creamy protein latte. You don't need a fancy milk frother to get the perfect foam. Skip the coffeehouse and whip this one up in your blender in just a few minutes.

INGREDIENTS

4 ounces whole milk

1 scoop (about 2 tablespoons) collagen peptides

4 ounces brewed espresso

DIRECTIONS

Heat the milk over medium heat in a small pot until warm but not boiling.

Transfer the warm milk to a blender, add the collagen, and blend on medium speed for 1 minute, until frothy.

Pour the espresso into 2 cups. Top with the frothed milk. Enjoy warm.

Nutrition information per serving: 61 calories ▪ 2g fat ▪ 1g saturated fat ▪ **7g protein** ▪ **4g carbs** ▪ **3g sugar** ▪ 0g sugar alcohol ▪ 0g fiber ▪ 4g net carbs ▪ 6mg cholesterol ▪ 51mg sodium

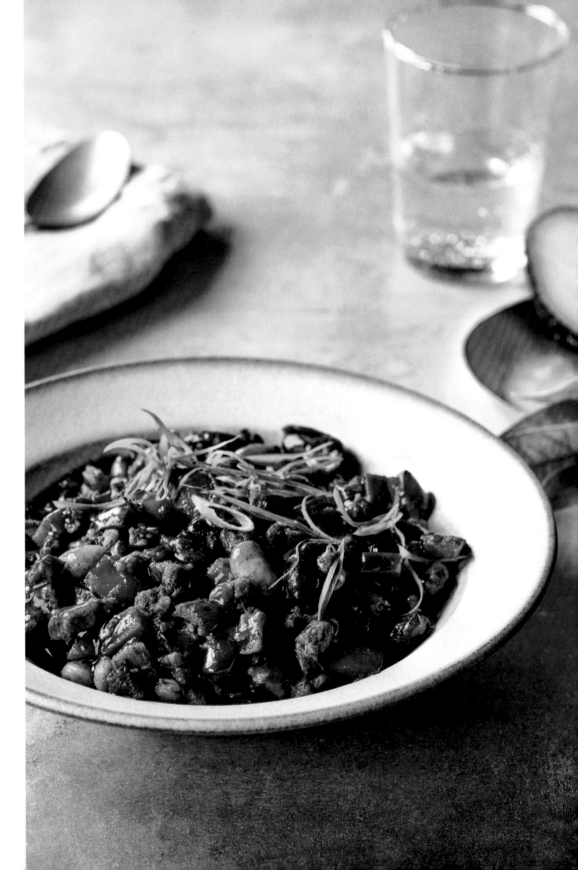

LUNCH

DEVILED EGG SALAD

YIELDS 4 SERVINGS

This salad has the classic flavors of deviled eggs with added protein from the addition of creamy raw almond butter. A dash of hot sauce lends to the sweet and spicy flavor. Top this salad with savory crumbled bacon and you've got a medley of flavors that can't be beat.

INGREDIENTS

8 hard-boiled eggs, peeled

1 teaspoon Dijon mustard

3 tablespoons mayonnaise

2 tablespoons unsweetened raw almond butter

1 tablespoon lemon juice

½ teaspoon hot sauce

¼ cup chopped scallions

¼ cup chopped celery

2 tablespoons minced shallots

½ teaspoon paprika

1 tablespoon chopped parsley

4 slices cooked and crumbled bacon

DIRECTIONS

Slice the eggs in half lengthwise. Carefully remove the yolks, place them in a medium mixing bowl, and mash them.

Roughly chop the egg whites and set aside.

To the hard boiled egg yolks, add the Dijon, mayonnaise, almond butter, lemon juice, and hot sauce. Mix until completely combined.

Fold in the cooked egg whites, scallions, celery, shallots, half the paprika, and half the parsley.

Divide into 4 portions, topping each with the crumbled bacon and remaining paprika and parsley. If you are preparing this dish in advance, store the dressing (the mustard, mayonnaise, almond butter, lemon juice, and hot sauce) and salad separately in airtight containers and toss together when you are ready to serve.

Nutrition information per serving: 343 calories ▪ 27g fat ▪ 6g saturated fat ▪ 18g protein ▪ 6g carbs ▪ 2g sugar ▪ 0g sugar alcohol ▪ 2g fiber ▪ 4g net carbs ▪ 385mg cholesterol ▪ 377mg sodium

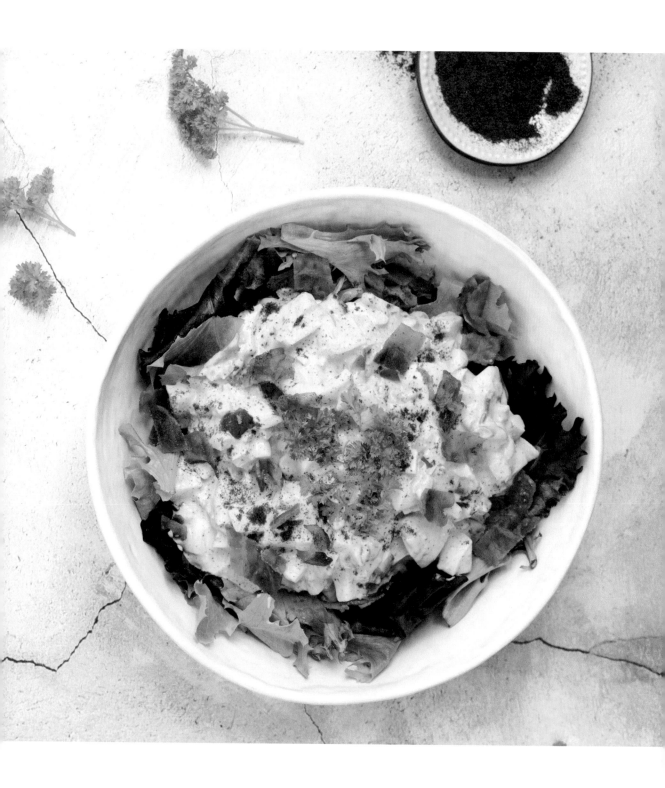

CURRIED CHICKEN SALAD
WITH CUCUMBER DRESSING

YIELDS 4 SERVINGS

This mildly spiced, flavorful salad is easily packed for a filling lunch on the go. The oven-baked strips of chicken tenderloins tossed with creamy Greek yogurt dressing burst with flavor. This recipe also makes a satisfying high-protein after-work meal or can be doubled to serve at a buffet for a crowd.

INGREDIENTS

1 pound chicken tenderloins

2 teaspoons curry powder

2 teaspoons paprika

2 tablespoons olive oil

¼ teaspoon cayenne pepper or chili powder (optional)

For the dressing

½ cup plain whole-milk Greek yogurt

1 shallot, finely chopped

¼ cup chopped cilantro

½ teaspoon curry powder

2 garlic cloves, minced

Zest and juice of 1 lemon

A pinch garam masala

For the salad

3 cups shredded lettuce of your choice

3 mini sweet peppers, cut into thin strips

1 celery heart (1 of the inner stalks), chopped

1 jalapeño, deseeded and cut into thin strips

4 radishes, thinly sliced

½ medium red onion, thinly sliced

3 tablespoons chopped toasted cashews or hazelnuts

DIRECTIONS

Preheat the oven to 400°F. Line a rimmed baking sheet with aluminum foil lightly brushed with olive oil.

Combine the chicken tenderloins with the curry powder, paprika, olive oil, and cayenne (if using) in a large bowl and mix well to coat. Season with salt and pepper to taste and transfer to the prepared baking sheet.

Bake for 18 to 20 minutes, or until the chicken is cooked through. Let the chicken cool slightly before cutting it into bite-size pieces.

Meanwhile, blend together all the dressing ingredients and season to taste. Cover the dressing and place it in the refrigerator while you prepare the salad. *Note:* The dressing can be made ahead and will keep refrigerated for up to 2 days.

Combine all the salad ingredients except the toasted cashews in a large bowl before dividing among 4 salad bowls. Top with the cooked chicken and drizzle with the dressing. Sprinkle with the toasted cashews and serve.

Nutrition information per serving: 420 calories ▪ 26g fat ▪ 7g saturated fat ▪ **33g protein** ▪ **14g carbs** ▪ **5g sugar** ▪ 0g sugar alcohol ▪ 3g fiber ▪ 11g net carbs ▪ 9mg cholesterol ▪ 46mg sodium

THAI CHOPPED CHICKEN SALAD

YIELDS 4 SERVINGS

A creamy peanut dressing adds loads of flavor to this fresh, crisp salad. If you'd like an alternative to peanuts, feel free to substitute cashews and cashew butter.

INGREDIENTS

2 heads romaine lettuce, chopped

2 cups shredded red cabbage

1 cup shredded carrots

2 cups shredded cooked chicken breast

¼ cup crushed peanuts

¼ cup scallions, sliced

For the dressing

¼ cup unsweetened natural peanut butter

¼ cup full-fat coconut milk

2 tablespoons gluten-free tamari

2 tablespoons rice vinegar

2 tablespoons lime juice

1 teaspoon sesame oil

DIRECTIONS

Place the romaine lettuce, red cabbage, carrots, chicken, peanuts, and scallions in a large bowl.

Whisk together the peanut butter, coconut milk, tamari, rice vinegar, lime juice, and sesame oil in a small bowl.

Pour the dressing over the salad, toss, and divide equally into 4 smaller bowls. If you are preparing this dish in advance, store the dressing and salad separately in air-tight containers and toss them together when you are ready to serve.

Nutrition information per serving: 359 calories ▪ 20g fat ▪ 6g saturated fat ▪ **27g protein** ▪ **20g carbs** ▪ **7g sugar** ▪ 0g sugar alcohol ▪ 9g fiber ▪ 11g net carbs ▪ 50mg cholesterol ▪ 110mg sodium

BEEF BURRITO BOWLS

YIELDS 4 SERVINGS

These burrito bowls are a great make-ahead recipe for a quick and easy lunch or dinner. Assemble the bowls ahead of time and add the avocado and salsa when you are ready to eat.

INGREDIENTS

For the beef

1 pound ground beef
2½ tablespoons chili powder
1 teaspoon ground cumin
½ teaspoon smoked paprika
1 teaspoon onion powder
1 teaspoon garlic powder
¼ teaspoon sea salt
¼ teaspoon ground black pepper

For the bowls

2 teaspoons avocado oil
4 cups cauliflower rice (1 medium head, grated or finely chopped)
1 red onion, diced
1 head romaine lettuce, chopped
½ cup cherry tomatoes, halved
1 cup salsa
1 avocado, sliced
¼ cup fresh cilantro, chopped
1 lime, sliced

DIRECTIONS

Heat a large skillet over medium-high heat and add the beef. Cook for 2 to 3 minutes, until no longer pink.

Add the chili powder, cumin, smoked paprika, onion powder, garlic powder, salt, and pepper. Continue to cook, stirring frequently, until the beef is fully browned, about 5 minutes.

In a separate skillet, heat the avocado oil over medium heat and add the cauliflower rice. Cook until tender, about 5 minutes.

Assemble 4 bowls with equally distributed cauliflower rice and beef, adding the red onion, lettuce, cherry tomatoes, salsa, avocado, and cilantro. Serve with the lime slices. If you are making this dish ahead of time, leave off the salsa, avocado, cilantro, lettuce, and lime slices until you are ready to eat.

Nutrition information per serving: 438 calories ▪ 31g fat ▪ 9g saturated fat ▪ **22g protein** ▪ **12g carbs** ▪ **3g sugar** ▪ 0g sugar alcohol ▪ 6g fiber ▪ 6g net carbs ▪ 80mg cholesterol ▪ 362mg sodium

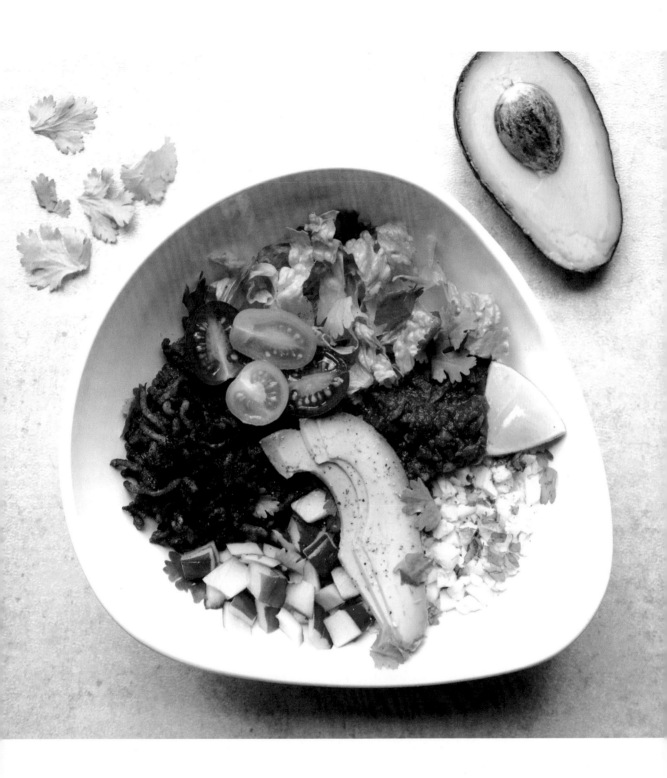

PUMPKIN & BLACK BEAN CHILI

YIELDS 6 SERVINGS

The pumpkin purée in this chili adds a subtle sweetness that nicely offsets the traditional chili spiciness. Make sure you're choosing pumpkin purée and not pumpkin pie filling, which contains loads of added sugar.

INGREDIENTS

½ teaspoon sea salt

2 tablespoons chili powder

2 teaspoons ground cumin

1 teaspoon dried oregano

½ teaspoon ground cinnamon

1 teaspoon unsweetened cocoa powder

¼ teaspoon ground allspice

2 tablespoons unsalted butter

1 small yellow onion, diced

3 cloves garlic, minced

1 pound ground beef

One 15-ounce can pumpkin purée

One 15-ounce can black beans, rinsed and drained

1 cup diced tomatoes

2 cups beef broth

6 tablespoons full-fat sour cream

1 medium avocado, peeled and sliced

Cilantro (optional)

Black olives (optional)

DIRECTIONS

Combine the salt, chili powder, cumin, oregano, cinnamon, cocoa powder, and allspice in a small bowl and set it aside.

Heat the butter in a large stockpot over medium heat. When the butter is melted, add the onion and cook for 4 minutes, or until softened. Stir in the garlic and cook for another minute.

Add the beef and cook, stirring occasionally to break up the meat, for about 4 to 5 minutes.

Stir in the prepared spice mixture, pumpkin purée, beans, and tomatoes and mix until incorporated. Pour in the beef broth and stir to combine.

Bring the mixture to a boil and then reduce the heat to low. Simmer uncovered for about 40 minutes, until thickened.

Remove the chili from the heat and divide among 6 bowls, topping each serving with 1 tablespoon of the sour cream and equal parts of the avocado. Add the cilantro and black olives, if desired, and serve.

Nutrition information per serving: 450 calories ▪ 26g fat ▪ 9g saturated fat ▪ **28g protein** ▪ **29g carbs** ▪ **5g sugar** ▪ 0g sugar alcohol ▪ 9g fiber ▪ 20g net carbs ▪ 76mg cholesterol ▪ 795mg sodium

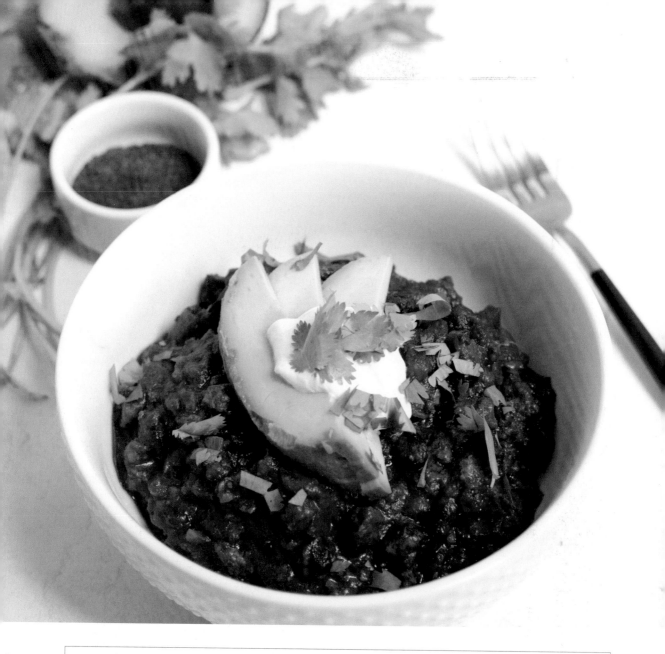

TIP

This recipe is great to make ahead; sitting in the refrigerator gives its flavors time to build. It is also easy to portion individually into resealable bags and freeze for a fast and easy lunch or dinner. You can even turn this chili into a dip for South Beach Diet keto-friendly nachos paired with the Almond Flour Tortilla recipe (page 253) for the chips!

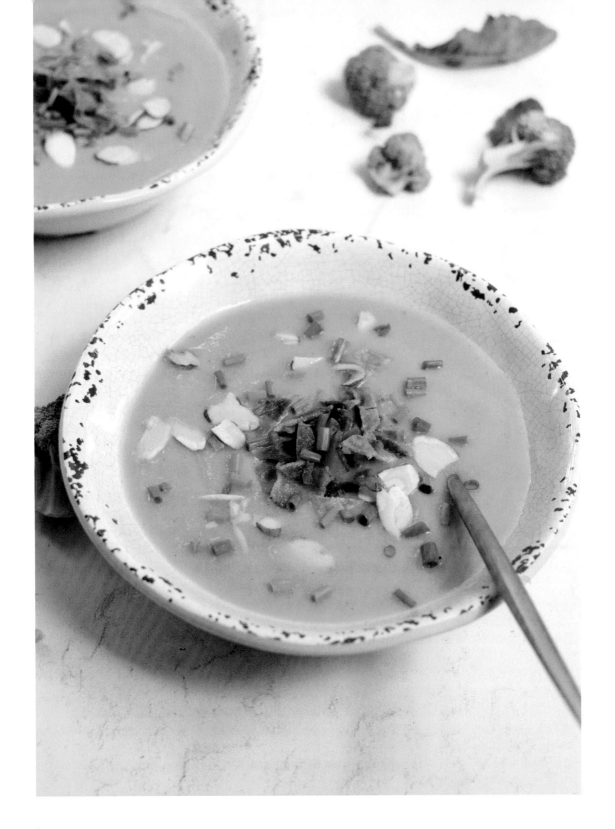

THE NEW KETO-FRIENDLY SOUTH BEACH DIET

CREAM OF BROCCOLI SOUP

YIELDS 4 SERVINGS

A warm bowl of creamy broccoli soup, topped with chives, sliced almonds, and crispy bacon, brings a smile to any day.

INGREDIENTS

6 slices raw bacon, chopped

2 tablespoons butter

2 cups broccoli florets

¼ cup chopped shallots

1 tablespoon minced garlic

½ cup plain whole-milk Greek yogurt

1 cup whole milk

2 cups chicken broth

2 tablespoons lemon juice

2 tablespoons chopped chives

¼ cup sliced almonds

DIRECTIONS

In a large stockpot, heat the chopped bacon over medium heat for 5 to 7 minutes, cooking until crisp. Remove the bacon and set aside, reserving the grease in the pan.

Add the butter to the bacon grease and melt.

Add the broccoli florets and cook for 4 to 5 minutes, until browned. Add the shallots and garlic and cook for 1 minute, until fragrant.

Add the yogurt, whole milk, chicken broth, and lemon juice. Stir to combine. Bring to a boil, then reduce the heat to medium-low. Simmer for 5 to 6 minutes, until the broccoli is tender.

Transfer the soup to a food processor and purée until smooth, or use an immersion blender.

Divide the soup evenly among 4 bowls. Garnish with the bacon, chives, and sliced almonds.

If you are preparing this dish in advance, once cool, store the soup and bacon separately in airtight containers in the refrigerator; they will keep for 4 to 5 days. Or freeze the soup in a resealable bag and defrost it in the refrigerator overnight before reheating.

Nutrition information per serving: 280 calories ▪ 19g fat ▪ 8g saturated fat ▪ **17g protein** ▪ **13g carbs** ▪ **7g sugar** ▪ 0g sugar alcohol ▪ 2g fiber ▪ 11g net carbs ▪ 44mg cholesterol ▪ 300mg sodium

SHRIMP & AVOCADO SALAD
WITH CILANTRO VINAIGRETTE

YIELDS 4 SERVINGS

This refreshing salad features fresh shrimp, tomatoes, and avocado in a lime and savory cilantro sauce.

INGREDIENTS

1 pound peeled and deveined shrimp
¼ cup extra virgin olive oil
¼ cup lime juice
¼ cup fresh cilantro, chopped
2 tablespoons chopped chives
1 avocado, pitted and diced
½ cup diced tomatoes
¼ cup thinly sliced red onion
2 tablespoons chopped jalapeño
2 cups salad greens

DIRECTIONS

Bring a large pot of water to a boil.

Add the shrimp to the boiling water and cook for 2 to 3 minutes, until pink. Drain, and run the shrimp under cold water until cool. Remove the tails (if any), roughly chop, and set aside.

Vigorously whisk together the olive oil and lime juice in a large bowl until the mixture is slightly thickened. Add the cilantro and chives and stir to combine.

Combine the shrimp, avocado, tomatoes, red onion, jalapeño, and salt and pepper to taste. Toss to coat.

Serve the shrimp mixture over the salad greens divided into 4 equal portions. The shrimp mixture may be made in advance and stored for 3 to 4 days in the refrigerator in an airtight container, separate from the salad greens.

Nutrition information per serving: 308 calories ▪ 19g fat ▪ 3g saturated fat ▪ **29g protein** ▪ **8g carbs** ▪ **2g sugar** ▪ 0g sugar alcohol ▪ 4g fiber ▪ 4g net carbs ▪ 214mg cholesterol ▪ 139mg sodium

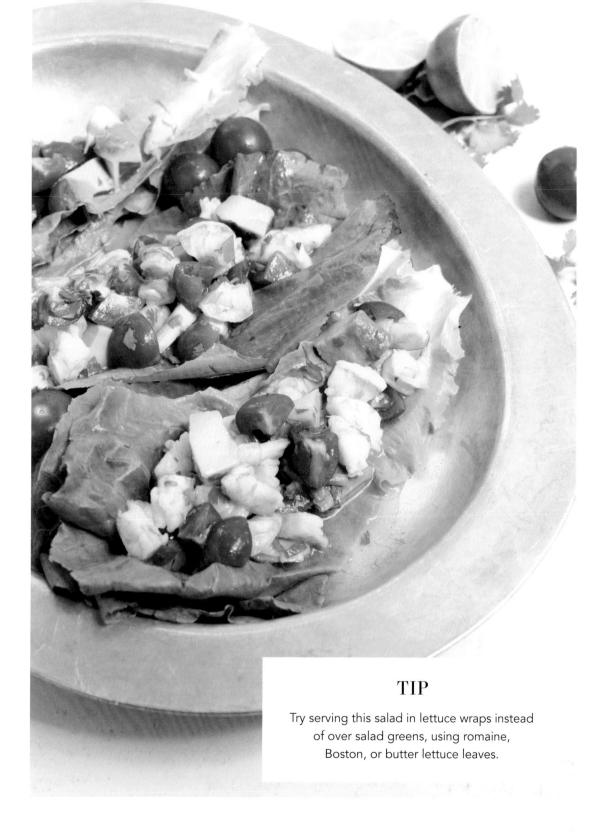

TIP

Try serving this salad in lettuce wraps instead
of over salad greens, using romaine,
Boston, or butter lettuce leaves.

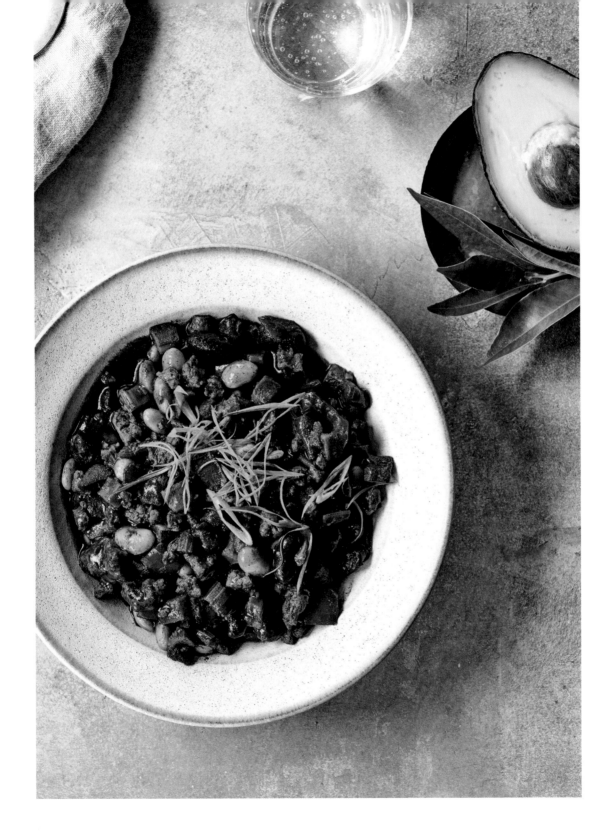

CHOCKFULL OF VEGGIE CHILI

YIELDS 2 SERVINGS

Enjoy all the meatiness of chili without the meat! Veggie crumbles add texture to this recipe, one bursting with fresh vegetables, kidney beans, and edamame.

INGREDIENTS

2 tablespoons olive oil

¼ cup diced onion

¼ cup diced carrots

¼ cup diced celery

½ cup diced zucchini

½ cup diced bell peppers

1 tablespoon minced garlic

1 teaspoon paprika

½ teaspoon chili powder

½ cup diced tomatoes

½ cup chicken broth

¼ cup canned kidney beans, rinsed and drained

¼ cup shelled edamame

¾ cup veggie crumbles (textured soy protein)

2 tablespoons chopped scallions

DIRECTIONS

Heat the olive oil over medium heat in a large saucepan.

Add the onion, carrots, celery, and salt and pepper to taste. Cook for 3 to 4 minutes, until the onions are translucent. Add the zucchini and bell peppers and cook for 2 to 3 minutes. Add the garlic, paprika, and chili powder and cook for 1 minute, until fragrant.

Add the diced tomatoes and chicken broth to the pot and stir to combine.

Add the kidney beans, edamame, and veggie crumbles. Bring the mixture to a boil and then reduce the heat to low; simmer for 8 to 10 minutes, until slightly thickened.

Divide chili evenly between 2 bowls and serve garnished with the chopped scallions.

Note: If you are preparing this dish in advance, it may be stored in an airtight container in the refrigerator for 3 to 4 days. For long-term storage, freeze individual portions and defrost them overnight in the refrigerator before reheating.

Nutrition information per serving: 308 calories ▪ 17g fat ▪ 2g saturated fat ▪ **17g protein** ▪ **25g carbs** ▪ **10g sugar** ▪ 0g sugar alcohol ▪ 9g fiber ▪ 16g net carbs ▪ 1mg cholesterol ▪ 499mg sodium

GRILLED BUFFALO CHICKEN SALAD

YIELDS 4 SERVINGS

Greek yogurt ranch dressing balances out the spice in this buffalo chicken salad. The chicken and dressing can be prepared ahead of time, making this recipe easy to put together for a quick lunch.

INGREDIENTS

2 large boneless skinless chicken breasts

¼ cup hot sauce

3 heads romaine lettuce, chopped

4 stalks celery, chopped

1 cup cherry tomatoes, halved

½ medium red onion, sliced

For the dressing

1 cup plain whole-milk Greek yogurt

1 teaspoon garlic powder

1 teaspoon onion powder

½ tablespoon chopped fresh chives

½ teaspoon dried dill

1 teaspoon lemon juice

¼ teaspoon sea salt

¼ teaspoon plus a dash of ground black pepper

DIRECTIONS

Place the chicken breasts and hot sauce in a large zip-top bag and toss until the chicken is well coated. Marinate them in the refrigerator for at least 30 minutes.

Whisk together the dressing ingredients in a small bowl and store the mixture in the refrigerator while you prepare the rest of the salad.

Lightly grease with olive oil and preheat a grill or grill pan. Add the chicken, pouring any remaining hot sauce over the top. Cook for 4 to 5 minutes per side or until the chicken is cooked through.

Transfer the chicken to a plate and let it rest before slicing.

Combine the romaine lettuce, celery, cherry tomatoes, and red onion and divide into 4 bowls. Place the sliced chicken on top of each portion and drizzle with the ranch dressing.

Nutrition information per serving: 294 calories ▪ 7g fat ▪ 2g saturated fat ▪ **31g protein** ▪ **15g carbs** ▪ **6g sugar** ▪ 0g sugar alcohol ▪ 10g fiber ▪ 5g net carbs ▪ 83mg cholesterol ▪ 633mg sodium

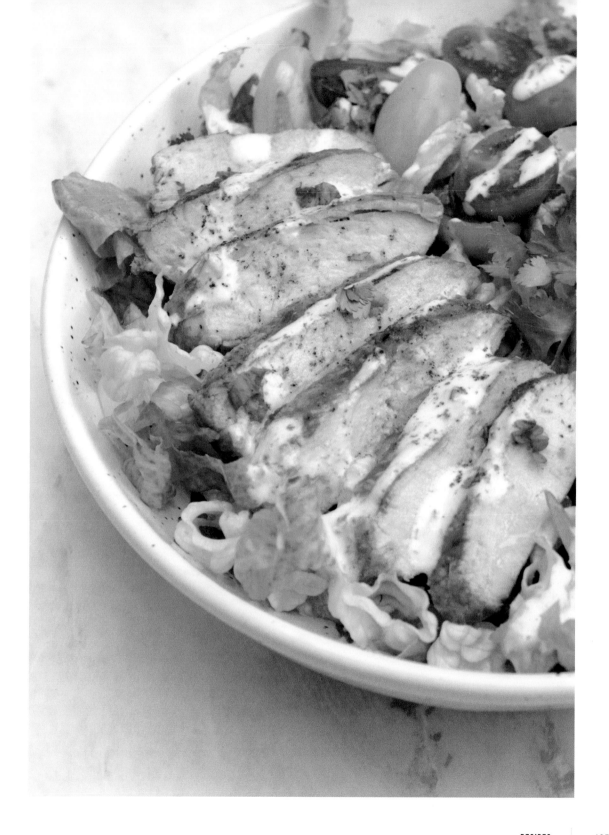

THAI CHICKPEA CURRY

YIELDS 6 SERVINGS

You can dial the spice of this curry up or down, depending on your preference, by adding a little more or a little less cayenne pepper. If you want to really let the spices meld, make this recipe the day before you want to eat it. The flavors develop as it sits in the refrigerator.

INGREDIENTS

2 tablespoons coconut oil

1 small yellow onion, finely chopped

2 cloves garlic, minced

1 teaspoon minced fresh gingerroot

1 tablespoon garam masala

½ teaspoon ground turmeric

½ teaspoon sea salt

½ teaspoon ground black pepper

¼ teaspoon cayenne pepper

¾ cup diced tomatoes

1½ cups full-fat coconut milk

Two 16-ounce cans chickpeas, rinsed and drained

24 large shrimp, deveined

2 cups chopped spinach

DIRECTIONS

Heat the coconut oil in a Dutch oven or large stockpot over medium heat. Add the onion and cook until translucent, about 4 minutes. Add the garlic and ginger root and cook for another minute.

Add the garam masala, turmeric, salt, pepper, and cayenne to the pot and stir until combined and fragrant, about 1 minute. Stir in the tomatoes, coconut milk, and chickpeas. Bring the mixture to a boil and then reduce the heat to low.

Simmer for 30 minutes, then add the shrimp. Cook for an additional 7 minutes, or until the shrimp turn opaque.

Add the spinach and cook until wilted, about 2 minutes. Remove the curry from the heat, divide into 6 portions, and serve.

Note: To prep in advance, you can cook the chickpeas in the curry broth and refrigerate. Before serving, reheat the curry over medium heat for 8 to 10 minutes and then add the shrimp and spinach as directed above.

Nutrition information per serving: 360 calories ▪ 14g fat ▪ 11g saturated fat ▪ **23g protein** ▪ **34g carbs** ▪ **3g sugar** ▪ 0g sugar alcohol ▪ 9g fiber ▪ 25g net carbs ▪ 85mg cholesterol ▪ 455mg sodium

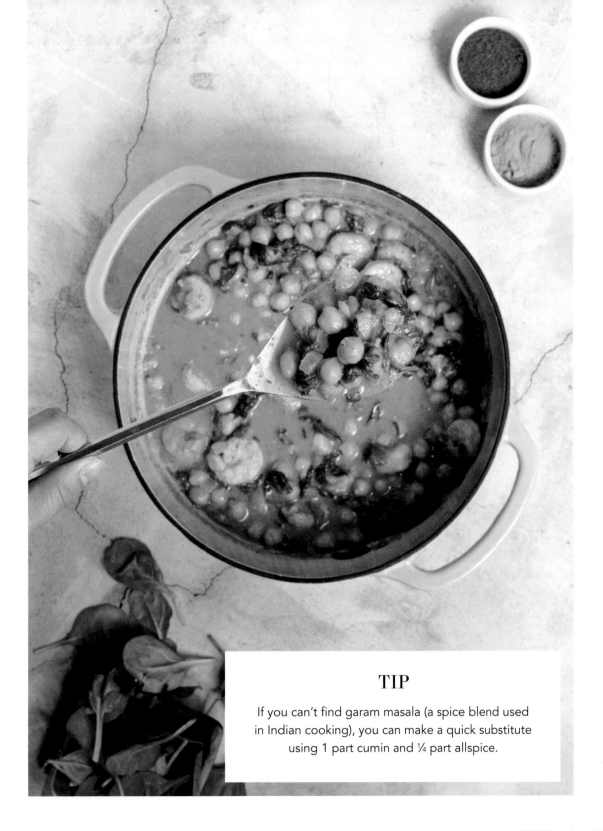

TIP

If you can't find garam masala (a spice blend used in Indian cooking), you can make a quick substitute using 1 part cumin and ¼ part allspice.

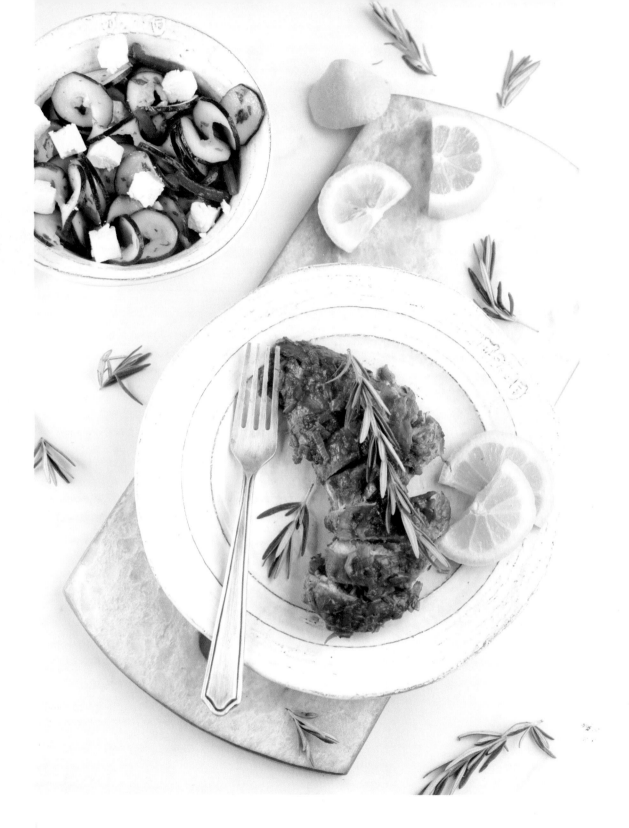

LEMON-ROSEMARY BRAISED CHICKEN BREASTS

YIELDS 4 SERVINGS

This easy-to-prepare, succulent chicken dish is full of aromatic flavors. Pair this with a simple Zucchini Feta Salad (page 251) as the perfect accompaniment to the chicken.

INGREDIENTS

3 tablespoons olive oil, divided

4 medium (about 4 ounces each) boneless skinless chicken breasts (you can also use thighs)

2 leeks, white parts only, chopped

3 to 4 cloves garlic, smashed

2 slices pancetta or bacon, diced (optional)

2 tablespoons white balsamic vinegar

2 cups (10 ounces) cherry tomatoes, cut in half (or one 14.5-ounce can diced tomatoes, drained)

2 lemons, 1 zested and juiced, the other cut into wedges

2 to 3 sprigs fresh rosemary

2 sprigs fresh sage (optional)

1 cup chicken broth (more as needed)

DIRECTIONS

Heat 2 tablespoons of the olive oil in a large, heavy-bottomed skillet over medium-high heat. Add the chicken breasts and cook, turning, until golden brown all over, about 7 to 10 minutes. Transfer them to a plate and set it aside.

Add the remaining tablespoon of olive oil and the leeks to the skillet and sauté for 3 to 4 minutes, until softened. Stir in the garlic and pancetta (if using) and cook for 2 to 3 minutes.

Deglaze the pan with the white balsamic vinegar. Add the tomatoes, lemon zest, lemon juice, rosemary, and sage (if using), and return the chicken breasts to the skillet. Season with salt and pepper to taste and then pour in the chicken broth.

Reduce the heat to medium-low and cook, covered, for about 20 minutes or until the sauce is reduced by half and the chicken is fully cooked (an instant-read thermometer placed in the center of the breast should read 165°F). If the pan gets dry during cooking, add a splash of broth or water as needed.

Slice the chicken breasts and spoon the sauce on top; serve with lemon wedges along with the zucchini salad.

Note: These chicken breasts are a great make-ahead meal and will keep in an airtight container in the refrigerator for up to 3 days. They are also freezer friendly.

Nutrition information per serving: 363 calories ▪ 17g fat ▪ 5g saturated fat ▪ **40g protein** ▪ **12g carbs** ▪ **5g sugar** ▪ 0g sugar alcohol ▪ 2g fiber ▪ 11g net carbs ▪ 103mg cholesterol ▪ 191mg sodium

SPICED TURKEY & SWEET POTATO BOWL

YIELDS 4 SERVINGS

Bowls are a great one-dish lunch option at the end of the week when you're looking for a way to use up extra veggies before your next shopping trip. You can add any non-starchy vegetables you have on hand, swap out the sweet potatoes for roasted butternut squash or pumpkin, or make it vegetarian by using chickpeas or quinoa in place of the turkey.

INGREDIENTS

1 large sweet potato, peeled and cubed

1 small yellow onion, sliced

2 small radishes, sliced

2 tablespoons coconut oil, divided

½ teaspoon sea salt, divided

½ teaspoon ground black pepper, divided

¼ teaspoon paprika

1 pound ground turkey, at least 93 percent lean

1 teaspoon garlic powder

½ teaspoon onion powder

1 cup packed chopped kale

1 small zucchini, diced

For the dressing

1 medium avocado, pitted and peeled

¼ cup plain whole-milk Greek yogurt

2 tablespoons olive oil

1½ tablespoons lemon juice

1 clove garlic

¼ teaspoon sea salt

⅛ teaspoon ground black pepper

⅛ teaspoon cayenne pepper

2 tablespoons chopped fresh cilantro

DIRECTIONS

Preheat the oven to 400°F. Line a baking sheet with parchment paper.

Spread out the sweet potato, onion, and radishes in a single layer on the prepared baking sheet. Melt 1 tablespoon of the coconut oil and drizzle it over the vegetables. Sprinkle with ¼ teaspoon salt, ⅛ teaspoon pepper, and the paprika.

Roast for 25 minutes, turning the potatoes over once halfway through the roasting.

While the potatoes are cooking, heat the remaining coconut oil in a large skillet over medium heat. Add the ground turkey, remaining salt and pepper, garlic powder, and onion powder. Cook, stirring occasionally, until the turkey is no longer pink, about 7 minutes. Stir in the kale and cook until wilted, about 2 minutes.

Divide up the turkey evenly among 4 bowls. Top with equal amounts of roasted sweet potatoes and onions, zucchini, and kale.

To make the dressing, combine all the dressing ingredients in a food processor and process until smooth, about 1 minute. If you want to make the dressing thinner, add a little water or a touch more olive oil.

Drizzle the dressing over the bowl ingredients and serve.

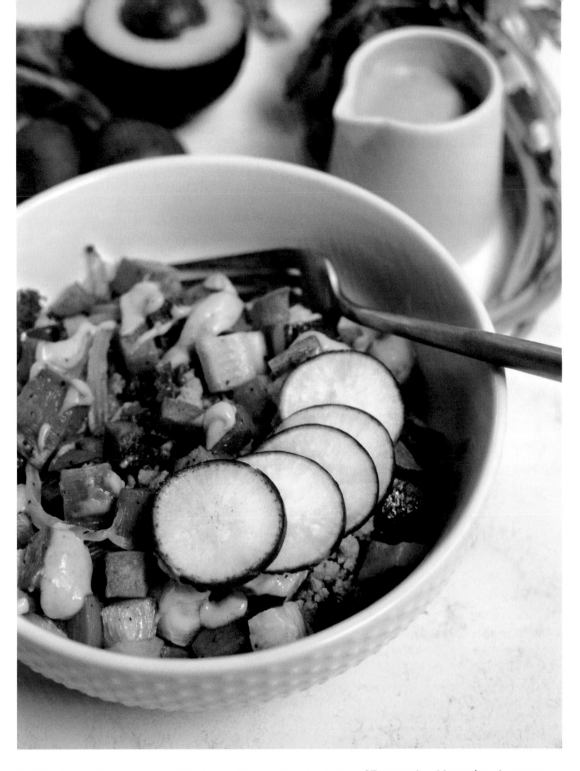

Nutrition information per serving: 437 calories ▪ 31g fat ▪ 11g saturated fat ▪ **27g protein** ▪ **16g carbs** ▪ **4g sugar** ▪ 0g sugar alcohol ▪ 5g fiber ▪ 11g net carbs ▪ 80mg cholesterol ▪ 250mg sodium

CAULIFLOWER TAHINI RICE BOWL

YIELDS 1 SERVING

This veggie-loaded lunch bowl is filled with cauliflower rice, baby spinach, avocado, and a soft-boiled egg, all topped with a homemade turmeric tahini sauce.

INGREDIENTS

½ cup cauliflower rice

⅛ teaspoon sea salt

1 cup baby spinach

½ avocado, sliced

1 soft-boiled egg, peeled

For the sauce

1 tablespoon tahini

¼ teaspoon ground turmeric

⅛ teaspoon sea salt

⅛ teaspoon ground black pepper

⅛ teaspoon garlic powder

DIRECTIONS

Preheat a nonstick pan on the stove over medium heat and lightly grease with olive oil.

Add the cauliflower and sea salt to the pan and sauté for 2 to 3 minutes, until the cauliflower is heated through.

Transfer the cauliflower to a serving bowl and top with spinach, sliced avocado, and soft-boiled egg, cut in half.

Stir together the tahini, turmeric, salt, pepper, and garlic powder in a small bowl. Add 1 tablespoon of water and stir again until completely smooth. Drizzle the sauce over the cauliflower mixture and serve immediately.

TIP

For an added boost of protein, swap out the egg with grilled chicken breast or salmon!

Nutrition information per serving: 324 calories ▪ 26g fat ▪ 5g saturated fat ▪ **12g protein** ▪ **14g carbs** ▪ **2g sugar** ▪ 0g sugar alcohol ▪ 9g fiber ▪ 5g net carbs ▪ 186mg cholesterol ▪ 550mg sodium

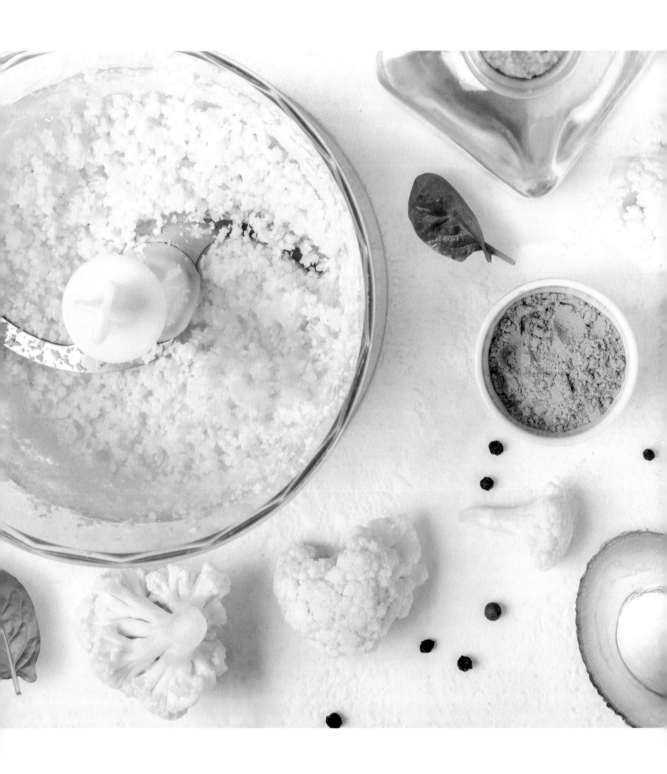

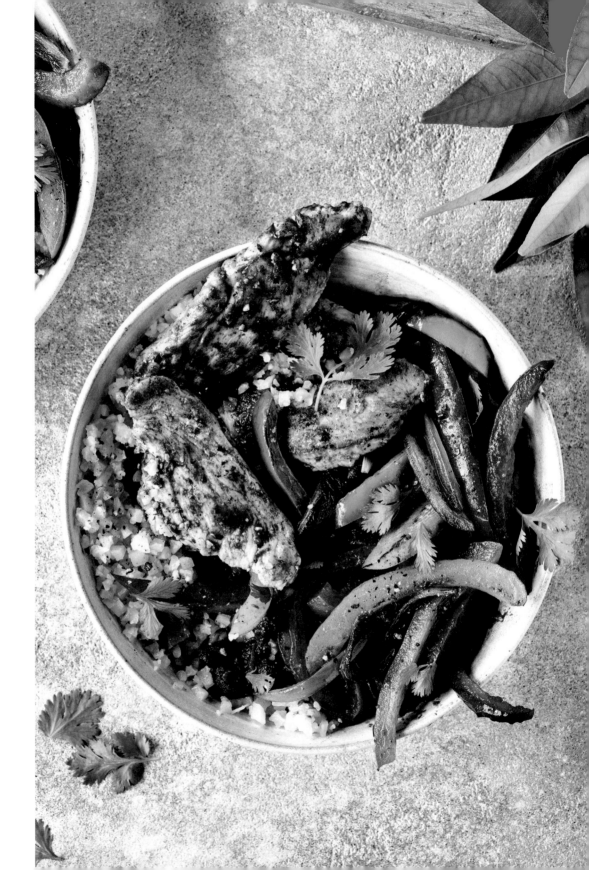

DINNER

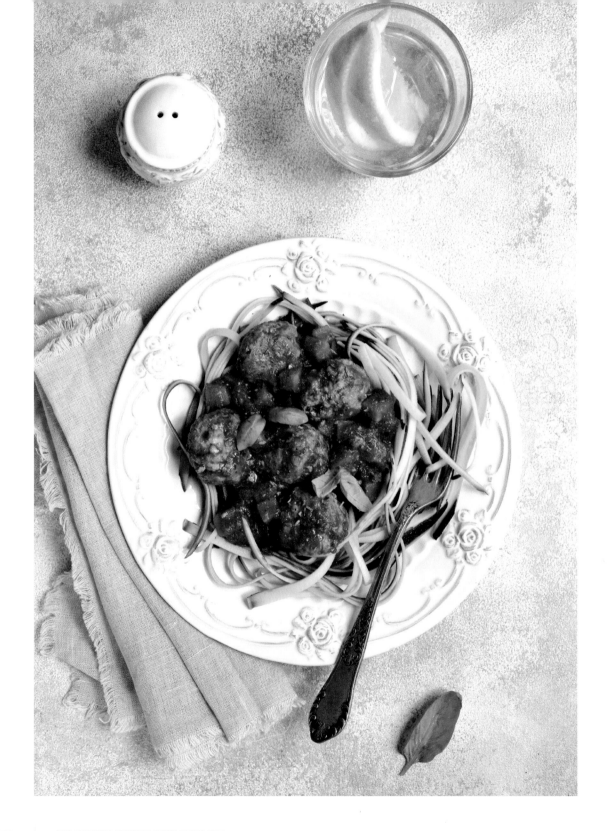

KETO SPAGHETTI & MEATBALLS

YIELDS 4 SERVINGS (3 MEATBALLS PER SERVING)

Enjoy the classic flavors of spaghetti and meatballs. These al dente zucchini noodles are topped with moist and savory meatballs and an herbed tomato sauce.

INGREDIENTS

For the meatballs

½ pound ground beef

¼ pound ground pork

2 tablespoons fresh minced garlic, divided

½ cup almond flour

2 tablespoons shredded Parmesan cheese

1 egg

For the sauce

1 tablespoon olive oil

1¼ cup crushed tomatoes

1 teaspoon dried basil

1 teaspoon dried thyme

½ teaspoon dried oregano

For the noodles

5 cups zucchini noodles

¼ cup chopped parsley

DIRECTIONS

In a large mixing bowl, combine the beef, pork, 1 table-spoon of the garlic, almond flour, Parmesan cheese, egg, and salt and pepper to taste.

Form the mixture into 12 meatballs.

Heat the olive oil in a large saucepan or Dutch oven over medium-high heat. Add the meatballs and cook for 2 to 3 minutes on all sides, until browned. Work in batches to avoid overcrowding, if needed.

Remove the meatballs and set aside.

Reduce the heat to medium. Add the remaining 1 table-spoon of garlic to the pan and sauté for 1 minute.

Add the crushed tomatoes, ½ cup water, basil, thyme, oregano, and salt and pepper to taste. Bring to a boil and then reduce heat to medium-low. Add meatballs back to the sauce and simmer covered for 10 to 12 minutes, until the meatballs are cooked through.

Turn off the heat. Add the zucchini noodles to the pot and toss to warm. If you are planning ahead, the meatballs and sauce will keep in an airtight container in the refrigerator for 3 to 4 days (longer if frozen). Reheat and toss with fresh zuc-chini noodles. Top with fresh chopped parsley and serve.

Scoop the noodles, meatballs, and sauce onto 4 plates and garnish with chopped parsley.

Nutrition information per serving: 424 calories ▪ 28g fat ▪ 7g saturated fat ▪ **30g protein** ▪ **14g carbs** ▪ **7g sugar** ▪ 0g sugar alcohol ▪ 5g fiber ▪ 10g net carbs ▪ 127mg cholesterol ▪ 287mg sodium

BUFFALO CHICKEN ZUCCHINI BOATS

YIELDS 4 SERVINGS (2 FILLED ZUCCHINI BOATS PER SERVING)

Spice things up with these zucchini "boats." Bursting with flavor, they are sure to become a favorite. Tender, cheesy chicken is tossed in a spicy cream sauce and topped with crisp bacon.

INGREDIENTS

12 ounces boneless skinless chicken breasts

4 medium zucchini

4 slices raw bacon, chopped

2 tablespoons butter

2 ounces full-fat cream cheese

¼ cup plain whole-milk Greek yogurt

¼ cup hot sauce

¼ cup chopped celery

½ cup shredded full-fat cheddar cheese, divided

3 tablespoons canned black beans, rinsed and drained (optional)

2 tablespoons chopped fresh cilantro

DIRECTIONS

Preheat the oven to 375°F.

Place the chicken breasts in a medium pot, season with salt, pepper, and a few springs of fresh herbs, and then cover with water. Bring them to a boil over high heat. Reduce the heat to medium and cook for 15 to 20 minutes, until the chicken is cooked through. Remove the chicken breasts from the water, allow to them cool, then shred.

Slice the zucchini lengthwise. Scoop out and discard the seeds. Place the zucchini boats side by side in a 9 x 13-inch baking dish.

Place the chopped bacon in a medium pot over medium heat. Cook for 5 to 7 minutes, stirring occasionally, until crisp. Remove the bacon to a plate lined with a paper towel and set aside, reserving the bacon grease in the pot.

Add the butter to the bacon grease and melt over medium heat. Add the cream cheese, yogurt, and hot sauce. Stir for 1 to 2 minutes, until combined.

Remove the sauce from the heat. Add to the sauce the shredded chicken, celery, half the cheddar, and the black beans (if using). Season with salt and pepper to taste. Toss to coat.

Divide the chicken mixture evenly among the 8 scooped-out zucchini boats. Sprinkle each boat with the remaining cheddar.

Bake for 20 to 22 minutes, until the zucchini is just tender and the cheese is melted.

Garnish with the bacon bits and cilantro. Serve warm.

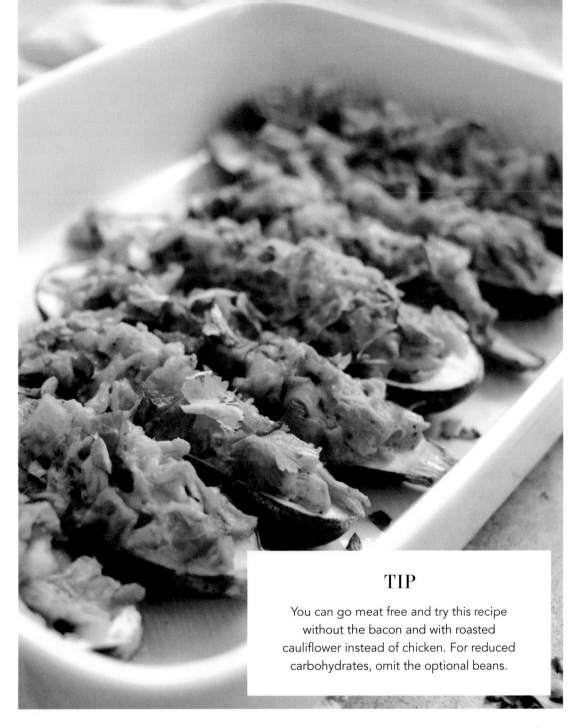

TIP

You can go meat free and try this recipe without the bacon and with roasted cauliflower instead of chicken. For reduced carbohydrates, omit the optional beans.

Nutrition information per serving (without beans): 282 calories ▪ 17g fat ▪ 9g saturated fat ▪ **26g protein** ▪ **7g carbs** ▪ **5g sugar** ▪ 0g sugar alcohol ▪ 2g fiber ▪ 5g net carbs ▪ 89mg cholesterol ▪ 277mg sodium

Nutrition information per serving (with beans): 293 calories ▪ 17g fat ▪ 9g saturated fat ▪ **27g protein** ▪ **9g carbs** ▪ **6g sugar** ▪ 0g sugar alcohol ▪ 3g fiber ▪ 6g net carbs ▪ 89mg cholesterol ▪ 308mg sodium

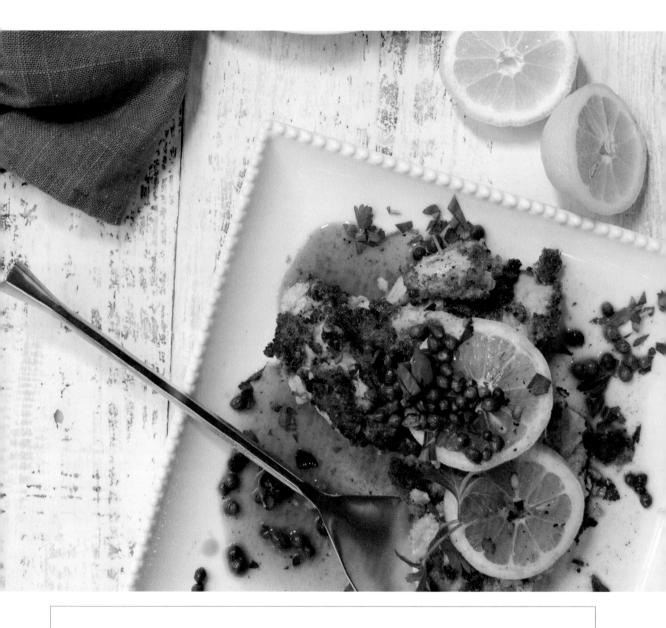

TIP

These breaded chicken breasts are great to make ahead. Once they have been pan fried, allow them to cool and then pack them in an airtight container. You can store them in the refrigerator for up to 5 days. For a versatile freezer stash meal, freeze the fully cooked cutlets on a baking sheet and then throw them all in a resealable bag. When you're ready to eat, reheat them in a 350°F oven until warmed through, make the sauce, and enjoy!

ALMOND FLOUR CHICKEN PICCATA

YIELDS 4 SERVINGS

Enjoy this comforting Italian classic with a low-carb twist. Thinly pounded chicken is encrusted in crispy almond flour breading and then smothered in a tart, buttery sauce.

INGREDIENTS

⅔ cup almond flour

¼ cup shredded Parmesan cheese

4 small-to-medium boneless skinless chicken breasts

1 egg

2 tablespoons whole buttermilk

2 tablespoons olive oil

2 tablespoons chopped parsley, divided

For the sauce

1 tablespoon butter

2 cloves garlic, minced

½ cup chicken broth

¼ cup lemon juice

3 tablespoons capers

Nutrition information per serving:
453 calories ▪ 28g fat ▪ 6g saturated fat
▪ **44g protein ▪ 7g carbs ▪ 2g sugar**
▪ 0g sugar alcohol ▪ 2g fiber ▪ 5g net carbs
▪ 157mg cholesterol ▪ 422mg sodium

DIRECTIONS

Combine the almond flour and Parmesan cheese with salt and pepper to taste in a shallow bowl and set aside.

Pat chicken dry and then season it with salt and pepper to taste. Place the chicken breasts in a resealable bag. Press out the air and seal the bag. Pound the chicken breasts until they are about ½ inch thick.

Whisk the egg, buttermilk, and 1 tablespoon of water in a small bowl until combined. Add the mixture to the bag with the chicken. Reseal it, and shake to coat the chicken breasts.

Heat the olive oil over medium-high heat in a large sauté pan.

Remove the chicken from the bag, allowing the excess egg mixture to drip away. Place the chicken breasts in the almond flour mixture and press to coat both sides. Shake away any excess and transfer the chicken to the hot pan.

Cook for 2 to 3 minutes per side, until cooked through and golden. Remove the chicken from the pan and keep it warm.

Melt the butter in the same sauté pan. Add the garlic and cook for 30 seconds, until fragrant.

Add the chicken broth, lemon juice, and salt and pepper to taste. Bring the mixture to a boil and then reduce the heat and cook for 2 to 3 minutes, until slightly thickened. Use a wooden spoon to scrape up any browned bits.

Remove the sauce from the heat. Add the capers and 1 tablespoon of the parsley; stir to combine.

Place one chicken breast on each of 4 plates, top with the sauce, and garnish with the remaining parsley.

SEARED STEAK WITH GORGONZOLA CREAM SAUCE

YIELDS 4 SERVINGS

Smother perfectly seared steak in an indulgent cream sauce
made with Greek yogurt and Gorgonzola cheese.

INGREDIENTS

1 tablespoon butter, divided

1 pound ribeye beef steak

1 tablespoon minced garlic

2 tablespoons lemon juice

2 tablespoons heavy cream

2 tablespoons plain whole-milk Greek yogurt

2 tablespoons Gorgonzola cheese

2 tablespoons sliced basil leaves

DIRECTIONS

Preheat the oven to 400°F.

Melt ½ tablespoon of the butter in a skillet over medium-high heat.

Pat the steak dry and then sprinkle it with salt and pepper to taste.

Add the steak to the melted butter and sear it for 5 to 8 minutes per side, until cooked to the desired doneness (about 6 minutes per side for medium rare).

Remove the steak from the pan and allow it to rest for 5 to 10 minutes. Tent it with foil to keep it warm.

Melt the remaining ½ tablespoon of butter in the same sauté pan over medium heat.

Add the garlic and cook for 1 minute, until fragrant.

Add the lemon juice to the pan and scrape up any browned bits with a wooden spoon.

Add the heavy cream, yogurt, and Gorgonzola cheese. Stir to combine. Simmer the sauce on low for 3 to 4 minutes, until thickened.

Slice the steak into thin strips, dividing equally between 4 plates and topping each with 2 tablespoons of the cream sauce. Garnish with the sliced basil leaves.

Note: This recipe can be made up to 4 days ahead; store the steak and cream sauce separately in the refrigerator.

Nutrition information per serving: 390 calories ▪ 39g fat ▪ 17g saturated fat ▪ **22g protein** ▪ **3g carbs** ▪ **1g sugar** ▪ 0g sugar alcohol ▪ 0g fiber ▪ 3g net carbs ▪ 104mg cholesterol ▪ 157mg sodium

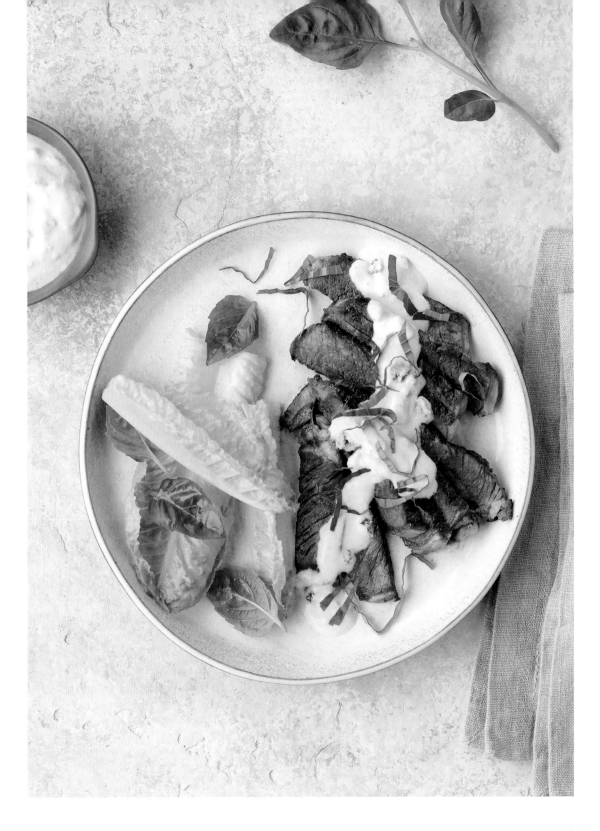

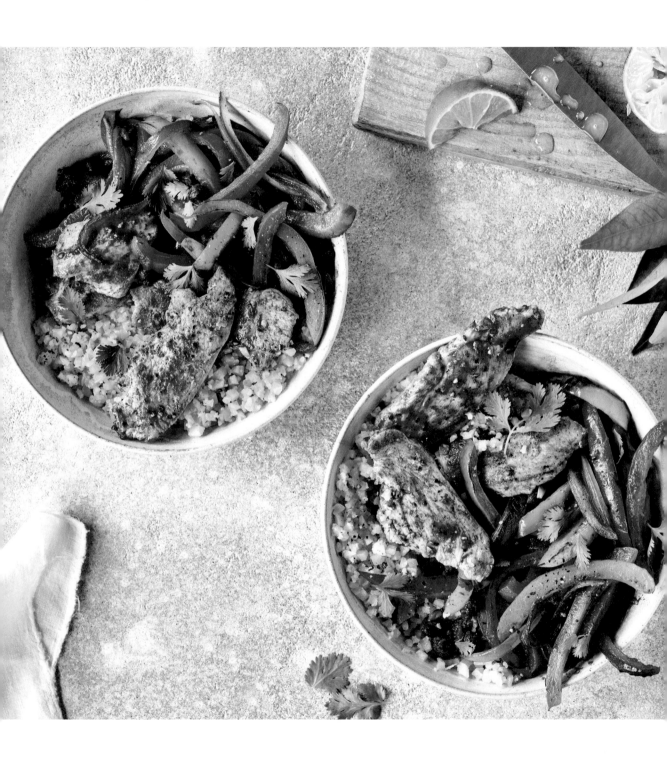

CHICKEN FAJITA BOWL

YIELDS 4 SERVINGS

Enjoy a fiesta in a bowl! Juicy pieces of chicken are coated in a flavorful fajita sauce and tossed with perfectly sautéed veggies and black beans. Serve over cauliflower rice and top it all with Monterey Jack cheese.

INGREDIENTS

1 tablespoon olive oil

1 pound boneless skinless chicken breasts

1 teaspoon paprika

¼ cup sliced onions

1 medium bell pepper, sliced

2 tablespoons tomato paste

2 tablespoons lime juice

1 teaspoon chipotle chili powder

¼ cup chicken broth

½ cup canned black beans, rinsed and drained

1½ cup cooked cauliflower rice

½ cup Monterey Jack cheese

2 tablespoons chopped cilantro

DIRECTIONS

Heat the olive oil over medium-high heat in a large skillet.

Pat the chicken dry. Dice it into ½-inch pieces and season it with paprika and salt and pepper to taste. Place it in the hot skillet and brown it for 3 to 4 minutes per side. Remove the chicken and set it aside, reserving the grease in the pan.

Reduce the heat to medium. Add the onion and bell pepper and cook for 3 to 4 minutes, until the onion is translucent.

Whisk together the tomato paste, lime juice, chipotle chili powder, chicken broth, and salt and pepper to taste in a small bowl.

Add this mixture along with the cooked chicken and the black beans to the veggies in the pan and cook for 3 to 4 minutes, until the sauce is slightly thickened.

Divide cauliflower rice into 4 bowls; then top with mixture from the pan. Garnish with the cheese and cilantro.

Note: This dish may be stored in an airtight container in the refrigerator for 3 to 4 days. For long-term storage, freeze individual portions. Defrost them overnight in the refrigerator and then reheat them over medium heat until heated through, about 5 to 6 minutes.

Nutrition information per serving: 354 calories ▪ 13g fat ▪ 5g saturated fat ▪ **43g protein** ▪ **14g carbs** ▪ **4g sugar** ▪ 0g sugar alcohol ▪ 5g fiber ▪ 9g net carbs ▪ 109mg cholesterol ▪ 408mg sodium

PORTOBELLO SHAKSHUKA

YIELDS 3 SERVINGS

This classic African dish is loaded with meaty portobello mushrooms in a savory tomato sauce. Top it with perfectly poached eggs and creamy feta cheese for a satisfying breakfast, lunch, or dinner.

INGREDIENTS

2 tablespoons olive oil

¼ cup chopped onion

8 ounces portobello mushrooms, cleaned and chopped

2 tablespoons minced garlic

2 teaspoons ground cumin

¼ cup harissa paste

¾ cup diced tomatoes

½ cup chicken broth

2 tablespoons lemon juice

2 cups chopped kale

6 eggs

2 ounces crumbled feta cheese

¼ cup chopped parsley

DIRECTIONS

Heat the olive oil over medium heat in a large saucepan or Dutch oven.

Add the onion and sauté for 3 to 4 minutes, until translucent. Add the mushrooms and cook for 5 to 6 minutes, until browned. Add the garlic and cook for 1 minute, until fragrant.

Add the cumin and harissa paste and stir to combine.

Add the tomatoes, chicken broth, lemon juice, and kale. Bring to a boil. Reduce the heat to medium and simmer for about 10 minutes, until the liquid is reduced by half.

Make 6 divots in this mixture and crack an egg into each divot. Cover the pot and cook for 8 to 12 minutes, until the eggs are cooked to the desired doneness.

Divide into 3 equal portions and serve the finished shakshuka garnished with the crumbled feta and parsley.

Note: You can make most of this recipe ahead of time: Follow the steps to make the shakshuka but do not add the eggs. This mixture may be stored in the refrigerator for 4 to 5 days. Cook the eggs with the shakshuka upon reheating.

Nutrition information per serving: 293 calories ▪ 20g fat ▪ 5g saturated fat ▪ **16g protein** ▪ **11g carbs** ▪ **4g sugar** ▪ 0g sugar alcohol ▪ 2g fiber ▪ 8g net carbs ▪ 373mg cholesterol ▪ 285mg sodium

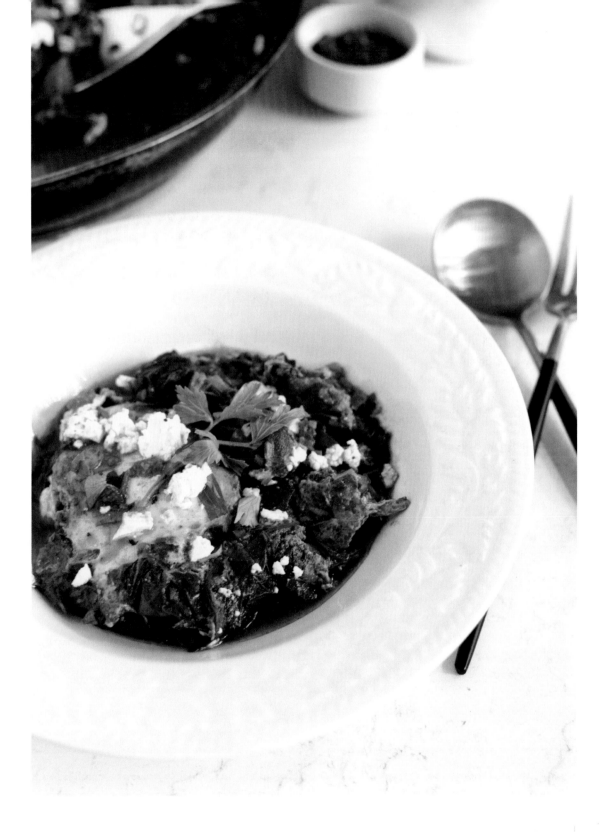

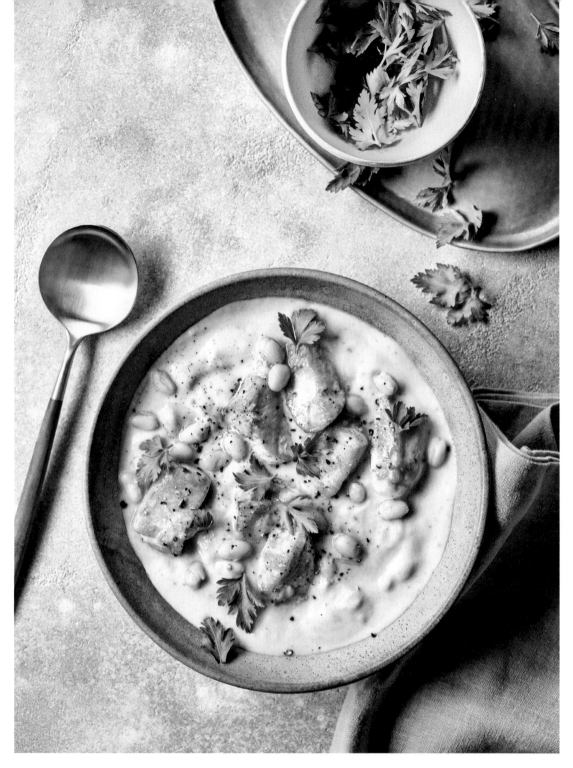

Nutrition information per serving: 302 calories ▪ 13g fat ▪ 4g saturated fat ▪ **38g protein** ▪ **7g carbs** ▪ **1g sugar** ▪ 0g sugar alcohol ▪ 2g fiber ▪ 5g net carbs ▪ 107mg cholesterol ▪ 293mg sodium

CREAMY CAULIFLOWER & CHICKEN

YIELDS 4 SERVINGS

This recipe's creamy Alfredo-like sauce is made with cauliflower
and white beans to give it an incredibly creamy texture.

INGREDIENTS

1 tablespoon olive oil

1 pound boneless skinless
chicken breasts

1 tablespoon butter

¼ cup diced onion

1 teaspoon minced garlic

1 cup cauliflower rice

¼ cup chicken broth

2 tablespoons grated
Parmesan cheese

½ teaspoon celery seeds

¼ cup canned white beans,
rinsed and drained

2 tablespoons chopped parsley

DIRECTIONS

Heat the olive oil over medium-high heat in a
large saucepan.

Pat the chicken dry. Dice it into ½-inch pieces and season
it with salt and pepper to taste. Add the chicken to the hot
pan and cook for 6 to 8 minutes, until cooked through.

Remove the chicken and set aside, reserving the grease
in the pan.

Reduce the heat to medium. Add the butter to melt.

Add the onions and cook for 3 to 4 minutes, until translucent. Add the garlic and cook for 1 minute, until fragrant.

Add the cauliflower rice and chicken broth. Bring the mixture to a boil and then reduce the heat and simmer for 4 to
5 minutes, until soft.

Transfer the cauliflower mixture to a food processor. Add
the Parmesan, celery seeds, and salt and pepper to taste.
Process for 1 to 2 minutes, until completely smooth.

Return the mixture to the pan over medium heat. Add the
cooked chicken and white beans and toss to coat. Heat for
2 to 3 minutes, until the chicken and beans are warmed.

Divide mixture into 4 portions and serve garnished
with parsley.

Note: This meal may be stored in an airtight container in the
refrigerator for 3 to 4 days. For long-term storage, freeze
individual portions. Defrost them overnight in the refrigerator
and reheat them over medium heat for 5 to 6 minutes until
heated through, or for 2 to 3 minutes in the microwave.

PROSCIUTTO & GOUDA PIZZA

YIELDS 6 SLICES (1 SLICE PER SERVING)

Indulge in a crispy almond flour pizza loaded with savory prosciutto and creamy Gouda cheese.

INGREDIENTS

1 tablespoon unflavored gelatin powder

2 cups almond flour

½ teaspoon sea salt

2 tablespoons melted butter

¼ cup grated Parmesan cheese

1 teaspoon baking powder

1 teaspoon dried thyme

1 teaspoon dried rosemary

½ teaspoon dried oregano

¼ cup crushed tomatoes

¼ cup basil leaves

½ cup shredded Gouda cheese

½ cup shredded whole-milk mozzarella cheese

1 ounce chopped prosciutto

DIRECTIONS

Preheat the oven to 350°F. Grease a baking sheet very lightly with olive oil and set aside.

Bring ¼ cup of water to a boil in a small pot. Pour it into a small heatproof bowl. Sprinkle the gelatin over the top. Set the mixture aside for at least 5 minutes.

Pulse the almond flour, salt, melted butter, Parmesan cheese, baking powder, thyme, rosemary, and oregano in a food processor until combined. Whisk the gelatin into the water to dissolve it and add this mixture to the food processor. Pulse for 1 minute, until a dough forms.

Turn the dough out onto a large sheet of parchment paper. Cover the dough with another large sheet of parchment paper.

Roll the dough out to a circle 8 inches in diameter and about ½ inch thick.

Top the dough with the crushed tomatoes, basil leaves, shredded Gouda, shredded mozzarella, and chopped prosciutto.

Transfer to the oven and bake for 12 to 15 minutes, until the crust is crispy and the cheese is bubbling.

Cut the pizza into 6 slices. Serve warm or store in an airtight container in the refrigerator for 3 to 4 days.

Nutrition information per serving: 349 calories ▪ 29g fat ▪ 8g saturated fat ▪ **16g protein** ▪ **10g carbs** ▪ **3g sugar** ▪ 0g sugar alcohol ▪ 5g fiber ▪ 5g net carbs ▪ 35mg cholesterol ▪ 615mg sodium

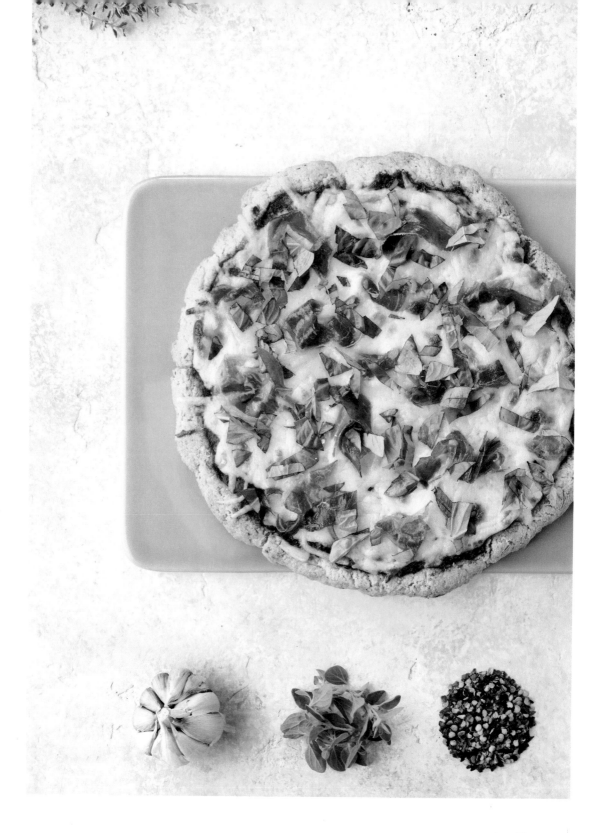

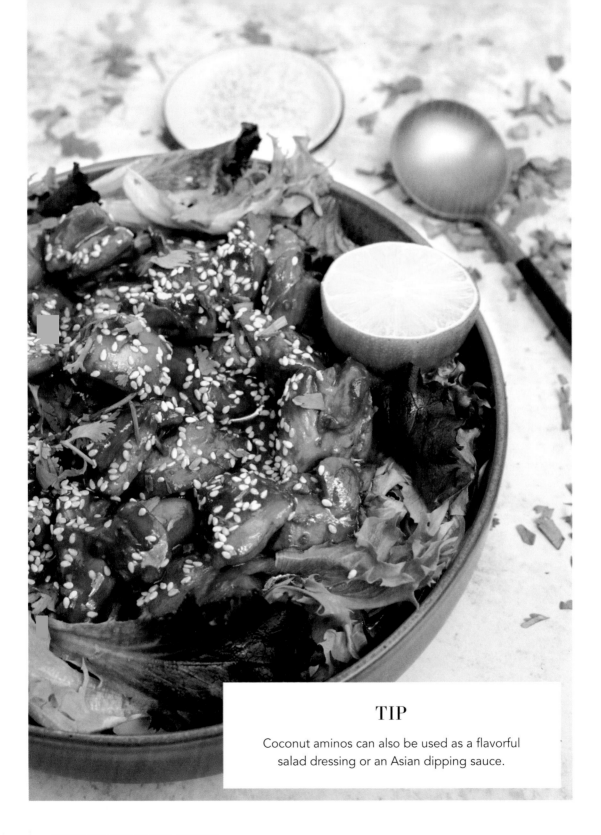

STICKY SESAME CHICKEN

YIELDS 4 SERVINGS

Skip the take-out and make a better version of this classic Asian dish. Juicy chicken thighs get a thick coating of sauce bursting with fresh garlic and ginger. This recipe uses coconut aminos, a soy sauce substitute made from fermented coconut palm sap that is soy, wheat, and gluten free. If you can't find coconut aminos, substitute tamari or soy sauce.

INGREDIENTS

1 pound boneless skinless chicken thighs

2 tablespoons olive oil

2 teaspoons tapioca flour

2 tablespoons sesame seeds

¼ cup chopped fresh cilantro

4 lime wedges

For the marinade

¼ cup coconut aminos

1 teaspoon erythritol brown sugar replacement

1 tablespoon minced fresh garlic

1 tablespoon minced fresh gingerroot

2 teaspoons sesame oil

3 tablespoons rice wine vinegar

DIRECTIONS

Pat the chicken dry. Dice into ½-inch pieces and season it with salt and pepper to taste.

In a large mixing bowl, whisk together the coconut aminos, erythritol brown sugar, garlic, ginger, sesame oil, rice wine vinegar, and salt and pepper to taste. Add the chicken and toss to coat. Cover and transfer to the refrigerator for 30 minutes to marinate.

Heat the olive oil over medium-high heat in a large sauté pan.

Remove the chicken from the marinade, allowing the excess to drip away. Reserve the marinade. Place the chicken in the hot pan and cook for 3 to 4 minutes per side.

Add the tapioca flour to the marinade and whisk to combine. Add the marinade to the pan with the chicken and cook for 4 to 5 minutes, until the sauce thickens.

Evenly divide among 4 bowls and serve the chicken garnished with sesame seeds, cilantro, and lime wedges. Stored in an airtight container in the refrigerator, this dish is good for 3 to 4 days.

Nutrition information per serving: 331 calories ▪ 18g fat ▪ 4g saturated fat ▪ **32g protein** ▪ **8g carbs** ▪ **5g sugar** ▪ 0g sugar alcohol ▪ 1g fiber ▪ 7g net carbs ▪ 145mg cholesterol ▪ 392mg sodium

BEEF & VEGETABLE STEW

YIELDS 4 SERVINGS

Enjoy the classic comfort of a thick, savory beef stew. This hearty stew is loaded with tender beef, delicate pearl onions, savory white beans, and juicy portobello mushrooms. For a lower-carb version, try it without the beans.

INGREDIENTS

3 tablespoons butter, divided

1 pound diced beef

½ cup pearl onions or chopped onions

¼ cup chopped celery (about ½ stalk)

½ cup chopped carrots (2 medium carrots)

8 ounces portobello mushrooms, cleaned and chopped

1 cup diced turnips (1½ small turnips)

1 teaspoon gelatin powder

2 teaspoons minced garlic

Juice of 1 lemon

2 tablespoons tomato paste

2 cups beef broth

¼ cup canned white beans, rinsed and drained (optional)

2 tablespoons chopped parsley

DIRECTIONS

Melt 2 tablespoons of the butter over medium-high heat in a large stockpot or Dutch oven.

Pat the beef dry and season it with salt and pepper to taste. Add the beef to the pot and brown it for 4 to 5 minutes on each side. Remove the beef and set aside.

Add the remaining 1 tablespoon of the butter to the pot and melt.

Add the onions, celery, and carrots to the pot. Cook for 4 to 5 minutes, stirring occasionally.

Add the mushrooms and turnips. Cook for an additional 5 to 7 minutes, stirring occasionally.

Meanwhile, pour ¼ cup of water into a small bowl and sprinkle the gelatin over the top. Set the mixture aside to soften for at least 5 minutes.

Add the garlic to the pot and cook for 1 minute, until golden.

Add the lemon juice, tomato paste, and beef broth and stir to combine, scraping up any browned bits with a wooden spoon.

Add the beef and beans (if using) to the pot and bring the stew to a boil. Once it is boiling, reduce the heat to medium-low.

Whisk the gelatin into the water and blend to dissolve it; then add the mixture to the stew. Simmer the stew for 15 to 20 minutes, until the vegetables are tender and the broth is slightly thickened.

When you are ready to serve, ladle the stew evenly into 4 bowls and garnish with the parsley.

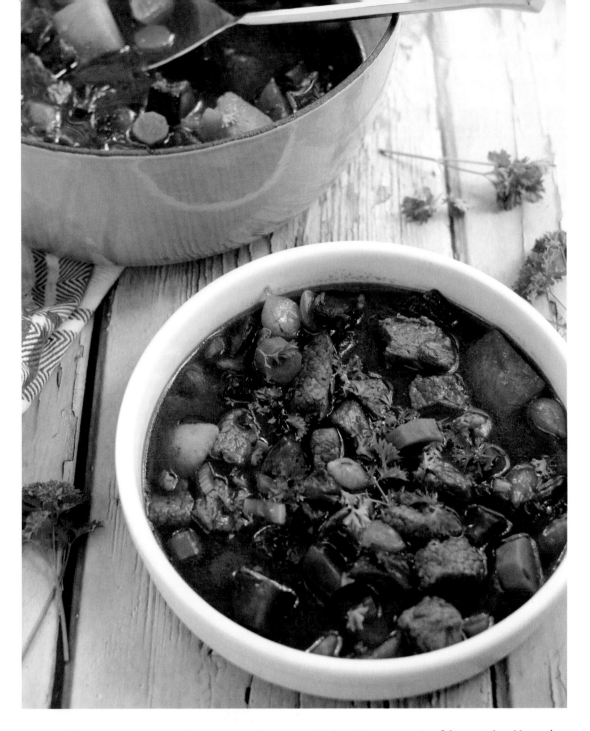

Nutrition information per serving (without beans): 418 calories ▪ 27g fat ▪ 12g saturated fat ▪ **34g protein** ▪ **11g carbs** ▪ **5g sugar** ▪ 1g sugar alcohol ▪ 2g fiber ▪ 8g net carbs ▪ 117mg cholesterol ▪ 171mg sodium

Nutrition information per serving (with beans): 463 calories ▪ 27g fat ▪ 12g saturated fat ▪ **35g protein** ▪ **14g carbs** ▪ **5g sugar** ▪ 1g sugar alcohol ▪ 3g fiber ▪ 10g net carbs ▪ 117mg cholesterol ▪ 171mg sodium

STUFFED CHICKEN BREAST

WITH ZUCCHINI FETTUCCINE

YIELDS 4 SERVINGS

These succulent chicken breasts are full of aromatic flavors and can be served either hot or cold. Freeze a few portions to reheat for a quick midweek dinner. Bound to become a family favorite, this recipe is also perfect for special occasions.

INGREDIENTS

For the chicken

2 tablespoons olive oil

2 shallots, finely chopped

1 teaspoon minced garlic

2 tablespoons sun-dried tomatoes

2 cups cremini mushrooms, thinly sliced

4 pieces (about 4 ounces each) thin-sliced boneless skinless chicken breasts

4 tablespoons cream cheese

½ cup chicken stock or water (more as necessary)

For the filling

2 tablespoons shredded Parmesan cheese

1 tablespoon capers, chopped

3 tablespoons fresh chopped Italian parsley

3 tablespoons pine nuts

For the fettuccine

1 tablespoon olive oil

2 medium zucchini or yellow squash, spiralized, sliced, or peeled into ribbons with a vegetable peeler, or sliced into thin rounds

1 garlic clove, finely chopped

½ cup cherry tomatoes, cut in half

2 tablespoons fresh chopped basil leaves

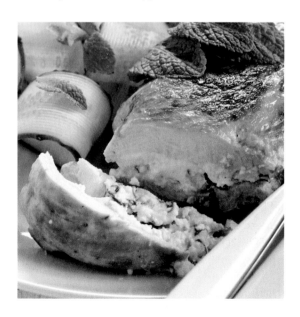

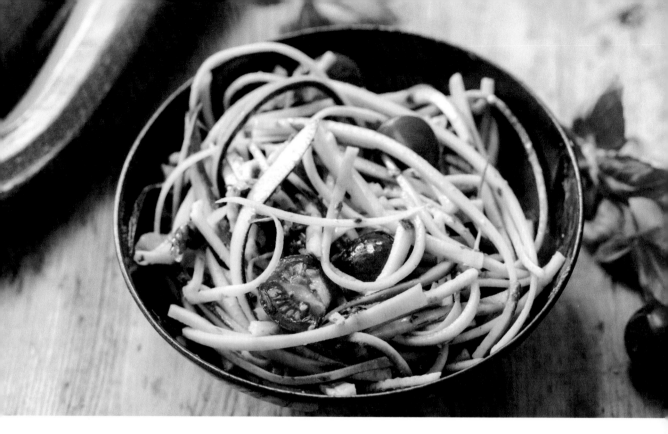

DIRECTIONS

Preheat the oven to 400°F. Lightly grease a 9 x 13-inch baking dish with olive oil and set it aside.

Heat the oil in a large skillet and sauté the shallots, garlic, and sun-dried tomatoes for 2 to 3 minutes. Add the mushrooms. Cook until the mushrooms are tender and all liquid has evaporated, about 4 to 5 minutes.

Transfer the mixture to a large bowl and stir in the Parmesan cheese, capers, parsley, and pine nuts to create a filling for the chicken.

Place the chicken breasts between 2 sheets of plastic food wrap and gently flatten them to about ½ inch, using a meat mallet. Season with salt and pepper to taste.

Spread each chicken fillet with 1 tablespoon of the cream cheese and spoon ¼ of the filling on top.

Roll up the breasts, tucking in the ends, and secure them with kitchen twine or wooden toothpicks.

Arrange the stuffed chicken, seam side down, onto the greased baking dish. Add the chicken stock and bake for about 20 to 25 minutes, or until the chicken is cooked through and golden. Transfer the chicken to a plate and tent with aluminum foil to keep warm; set aside.

To make the fettuccine, heat the olive oil in a large skillet over medium heat, adding the spiralized or otherwise precut zucchini and the garlic and tomatoes. Cook, tossing often, for 2 to 3 minutes, or until the zucchini pieces are just tender. Stir in the basil and remove the mixture from the heat. Salt and pepper to taste.

Slice the stuffed chicken breasts evenly into 4 slices and serve alongside the zucchini fettuccine.

Nutrition information per serving: 370 calories ▪ 18g fat ▪ 6g saturated fat ▪ **40g protein** ▪ **11g carbs** ▪ **7g sugar** ▪ 0g sugar alcohol ▪ 3g fiber ▪ 8g net carbs ▪ 112mg cholesterol ▪ 276mg sodium

COD

WITH ALMOND-BASIL RELISH

YIELDS 4 SERVINGS (1 FILLET PER SERVING)

This is an appetizing, no-fuss, and heart-healthy midweek meal that will be at the table in less than 15 minutes. Add a generous dollop of the almond and basil relish for a layer of Italian flavors, and serve with a side of steamed or roasted asparagus or broccolini.

INGREDIENTS

For the relish

½ cup almond-stuffed green olives, sliced (or substitute ¼ cup pitted green olives and ¼ cup blanched almonds)

2 tablespoons capers, chopped

1 tablespoon olive oil

2 tablespoons chopped roasted red peppers

4 tablespoons chopped fresh basil leaves

2 tablespoons lemon juice, or to taste

¼ teaspoon crushed red pepper (optional)

For the cod

4 (about 5 ounces each) skinless cod or haddock fillets

2 tablespoons olive oil

1 tablespoon unsalted butter or ghee

2 tablespoons chopped fresh Italian parsley

DIRECTIONS

Combine all the relish ingredients in a bowl and mix well. Season with salt and pepper to taste and refrigerate until needed.

Season the cod with salt and pepper to taste. Heat the oil and butter in a large skillet over medium-high heat and cook for about 4 minutes per side, or until golden.

Transfer the fish to a serving plate and serve topped with the relish and sprinkled with the parsley.

TIP

This relish can be made in advance without the basil and kept in the refrigerator for up to 2 days. Use it as a tasty addition to salads, wraps, and sandwiches.

Nutrition information per serving: 244 calories ▪ 14g fat ▪ 3g saturated fat ▪ **26g protein** ▪ **2g carbs** ▪ **1g sugar** ▪ 0g sugar alcohol ▪ 2g fiber ▪ 1g net carbs ▪ 73mg cholesterol ▪ 562mg sodium

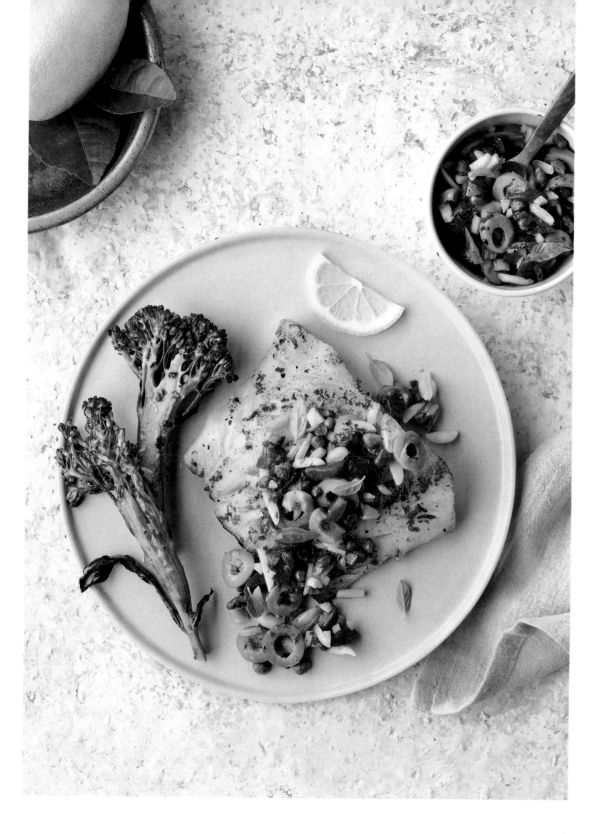

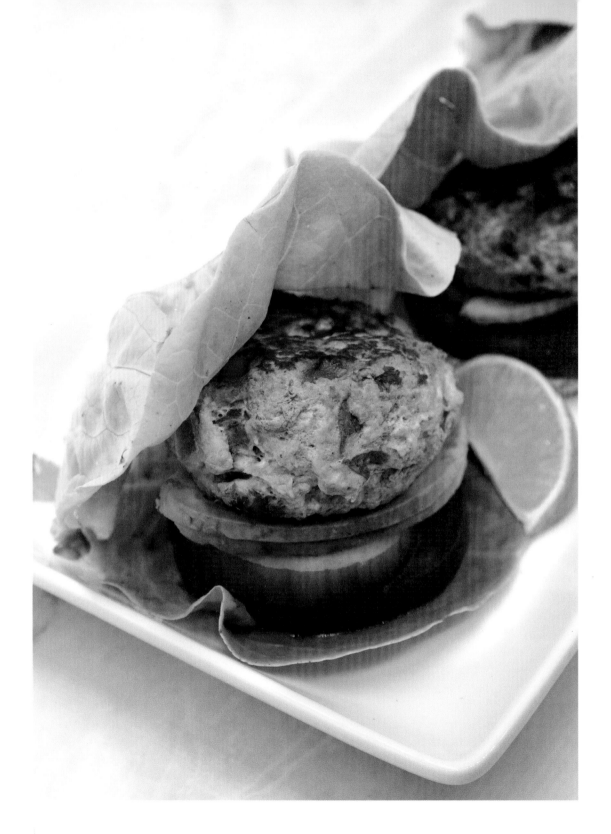

CILANTRO-LIME TURKEY BURGERS

YIELDS 4 SERVINGS (1 BURGER PER SERVING)

Fresh cilantro and lime juice make these turkey burgers extra flavorful. Serve with grilled veggies or a salad for a quick and easy meal. These are great for lunch or dinner.

INGREDIENTS

1 pound ground turkey, at least 93 percent lean

½ red onion, diced

⅓ cup fresh cilantro, chopped

Juice of half a lime

1 teaspoon garlic powder

½ teaspoon sea salt

½ teaspoon ground black pepper

1 teaspoon olive oil

8 leaves butter lettuce

¼ cup thinly sliced red onion

4 tomato slices, ¼ inch thick

DIRECTIONS

Place the ground turkey, onion, cilantro, lime juice, garlic powder, salt, and pepper in a large bowl and mix by hand until combined. Form into 4 patties.

Heat the olive oil in a large skillet over medium-high heat. Add the burgers and cook for 4 to 5 minutes on each side until cooked through, or until an instant-read thermometer inserted into the center of the patties reaches 165°F.

Transfer the burgers to a plate and let them rest. Serve them on butter lettuce wraps topped with red onion and tomato.

Nutrition information per serving: 183 calories ▪ 10g fat ▪ 2g saturated fat ▪ **22g protein** ▪ **1g carbs** ▪ **0g sugar** ▪ 0g sugar alcohol ▪ 0g fiber ▪ 1g net carbs ▪ 0mg cholesterol ▪ 290mg sodium

CHICKEN SHEPHERD'S PIE
WITH CAULIFLOWER

YIELDS 4 SERVINGS

Mashed potatoes are swapped for cauliflower in this version of a classic comfort dish. It is easy to prepare, and you can portion the pie into ramekins to freeze and have on hand for a quick meal.

INGREDIENTS

For the filling

2 tablespoons avocado oil

1 medium yellow onion, finely chopped

1 celery stick, finely chopped

1 one-inch piece fresh gingerroot, grated

2 garlic cloves, minced

1 teaspoon ground turmeric

1 pound lean ground chicken

½ cup halved cherry tomatoes (or ½ cup diced tomatoes)

½ teaspoon dried thyme

½ teaspoon dried marjoram

1 small dried bay leaf

2 cups packed baby kale

For the topping

2 cups finely chopped cauliflower florets

2 tablespoons ghee or butter

¼ cup heavy cream

½ teaspoon turmeric (optional)

½ cup shredded full-fat cheddar cheese

DIRECTIONS

Preheat the oven to 425°F.

Heat the oil in a large, deep skillet over medium heat. Add the onion and celery and cook until soft. Stir in the ginger, garlic, and turmeric and cook, stirring, for 30 seconds, until fragrant.

Add the chicken and turn up the heat to medium-high. Cook, stirring occasionally, until golden brown, about 5 to 6 minutes. Add the tomatoes, thyme, marjoram, and bay leaf, reduce the heat to medium-low, and simmer for about 15 to 20 minutes, until thickened. Stir in the baby kale and turn off the heat.

Meanwhile, steam the cauliflower florets for about 8 to 10 minutes, until soft. Transfer the cauliflower to a large saucepan and mash it with the ghee, heavy cream, turmeric (if using), and cheddar over medium heat, until creamy. If you prefer a smoother mash, blitz the mixture in a food processor. Season with salt and pepper to taste and set it aside.

Transfer the filling to a large pie dish or divide it among 4 individual pie dishes or ramekins. Top it with the mashed cauliflower, ruffling it with a fork.

Bake for about 15 minutes, or until bubbling and golden.

Note: To prepare this dish ahead, cover the baked pie with aluminum foil and keep it in the freezer for up to 2 months. Reheat from frozen, covered with the foil, at 375°F.

Nutrition information per serving: 417 calories ▪ 32g fat ▪ 14g saturated fat ▪ **25g protein** ▪ **9g carbs** ▪ **3g sugar** ▪ 0g sugar alcohol ▪ 2g fiber ▪ 7g net carbs ▪ 145mg cholesterol ▪ 184mg sodium

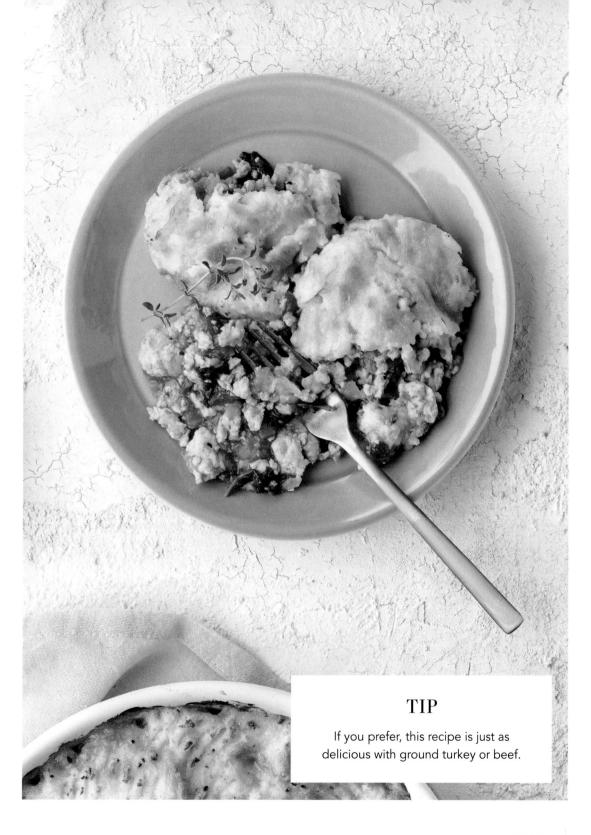

TIP

If you prefer, this recipe is just as delicious with ground turkey or beef.

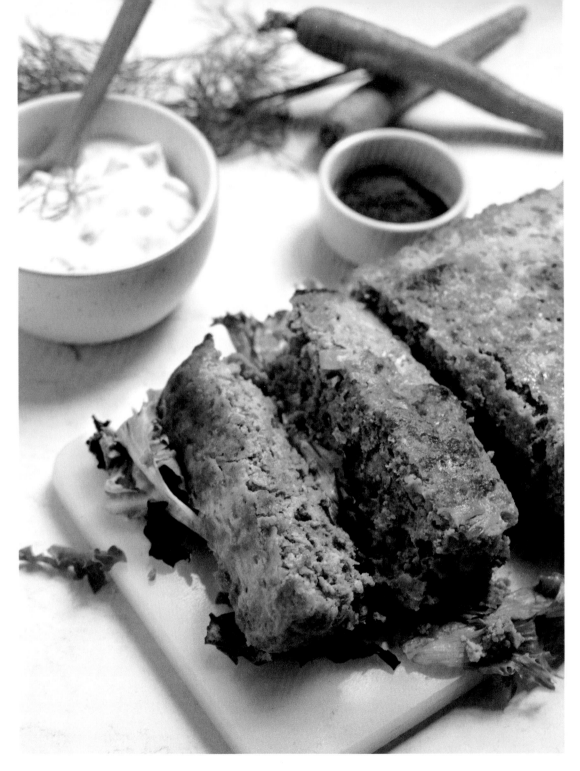

Nutrition information per serving: 296 calories ▪ 21g fat ▪ 9g saturated fat ▪ **18g protein** ▪ **9g carbs** ▪ **3g sugar**
▪ 0g sugar alcohol ▪ 2g fiber ▪ 7g net carbs ▪ 102mg cholesterol ▪ 326mg sodium

SPICED LAMB LOAF

YIELDS 8 SERVINGS (1 SLICE PER SERVING)

Sneak a few servings of vegetables into this sweet and savory lamb meatloaf, served with a creamy tzatziki sauce. This dish is great served warm for dinner, or in cold slices for lunch or a snack.

INGREDIENTS

1 cup chopped zucchini

½ cup chopped carrots (approximately 2 medium carrots)

½ cup chopped onions

½ cup diced tomatoes

1 pound ground lamb

1 tablespoon minced garlic

1 cup grated Parmesan cheese

⅓ cup almond flour

2 eggs

2 tablespoons tomato paste

2 teaspoons ground cumin

¼ teaspoon ground allspice

1 tablespoon lemon juice

For the tzatziki sauce

½ cup plain whole-milk Greek yogurt

2 tablespoons lemon juice

1 teaspoon minced garlic

1 tablespoon chopped dill

¼ cup small-diced cucumber

DIRECTIONS

Preheat the oven to 400°F.

Grease a loaf pan with olive oil and set aside. Put the zucchini, carrots, onions, and tomatoes in a food processor and pulse until softly textured and well combined. Transfer the vegetables to a colander and let drain for about 10 to 15 minutes, occasionally pressing with a clean towel to squeeze out any excess water.

Place the vegetables in a large mixing bowl. With a rubber spatula or similar tool, mix in the lamb, garlic, Parmesan, almond flour, eggs, tomato paste, cumin, allspice, lemon juice, and salt and pepper to taste.

When the mixture is uniform throughout, transfer it into the prepared loaf pan and smooth it into an even layer. Place the loaf pan inside a larger baking dish and fill the dish with enough water to come halfway up the sides of the loaf pan.

Bake for 60 to 70 minutes, until the loaf is golden and cooked through.

In a small mixing bowl, whisk together the yogurt, lemon juice, garlic, dill, and salt and pepper to taste. Add the cucumbers and stir to combine. Transfer the mixture to the refrigerator until you are ready to serve.

Carefully pour the excess oil from the loaf pan. Allow the loaf to cool for 10 to 15 minutes before removing from pan. Slice the loaf into 8 even slices and serve with the tzatziki on the side.

Note: The lamb loaf may be stored in the refrigerator for 3 to 4 days. To freeze, place individual slices on a baking sheet lined with parchment paper. Once they are frozen, they may be stored together in a large freezer-safe bag.

BLACKENED SALMON
WITH MANGO QUINOA

YIELDS 6 SERVINGS

This recipe sounds fancy, but you can whip it up in under 30 minutes.

INGREDIENTS

For the mango quinoa

1 tablespoon unsalted butter

⅓ cup pine nuts

1 cup quinoa, rinsed

1 cup full-fat coconut milk

¾ cup diced mango

½ teaspoon sea salt

For the salmon

3 tablespoons ground paprika

2 teaspoons ground cayenne pepper

1 tablespoon garlic powder

1 tablespoon onion powder

2 teaspoons sea salt

1½ teaspoons ground black pepper

¾ teaspoon dried oregano

½ cup unsalted butter, melted

6 (4 ounces each) wild Atlantic salmon fillets, skinless

DIRECTIONS

Turn on your oven's broiler. Line a baking sheet with parchment paper and set it aside.

Heat the butter in a medium saucepan over medium-high heat. When the butter is hot, add the pine nuts and stir constantly until they start to brown, about 4 minutes.

Add the quinoa and cook, stirring constantly, for another minute. Add the coconut milk, 1 cup of water, mango, and salt. Stir to combine.

Bring the quinoa to a boil, cover it, and reduce the heat to low. Simmer for 20 minutes, or until the liquid is absorbed and the quinoa is tender.

While the quinoa is cooking, prepare the salmon. Combine the paprika, cayenne, garlic powder, onion powder, salt, pepper, and oregano in a small bowl.

Brush both sides of the salmon with the melted butter, reserving a bit to drizzle in the next step. Generously rub the spice mixture onto both sides of the salmon.

Arrange the coated salmon on the prepared baking sheet and drizzle any remaining butter on top of the fillets.

Place the fillets in the preheated oven and broil for 5 minutes. Flip the salmon over and broil for another 5 minutes.

Change the oven setting to bake at 350°F and cook the salmon for another 10 minutes, or until the fish flakes easily with a fork. Remove the salmon from the oven and set it aside.

Fluff the quinoa with a fork and transfer as 6 equal individual portions to plates. Top each quinoa serving with a salmon fillet and serve.

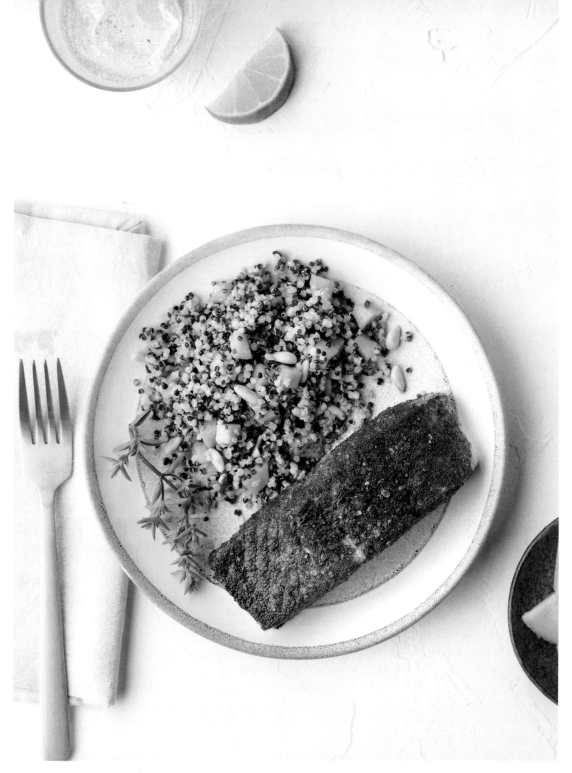

Nutrition information per serving: 412 calories ■ 24g fat ■ 11g saturated fat ■ **22g protein** ■ **26g carbs** ■ **3g sugar** ■ 0g sugar alcohol ■ 3g fiber ■ 23g net carbs ■ 67mg cholesterol ■ 65mg sodium

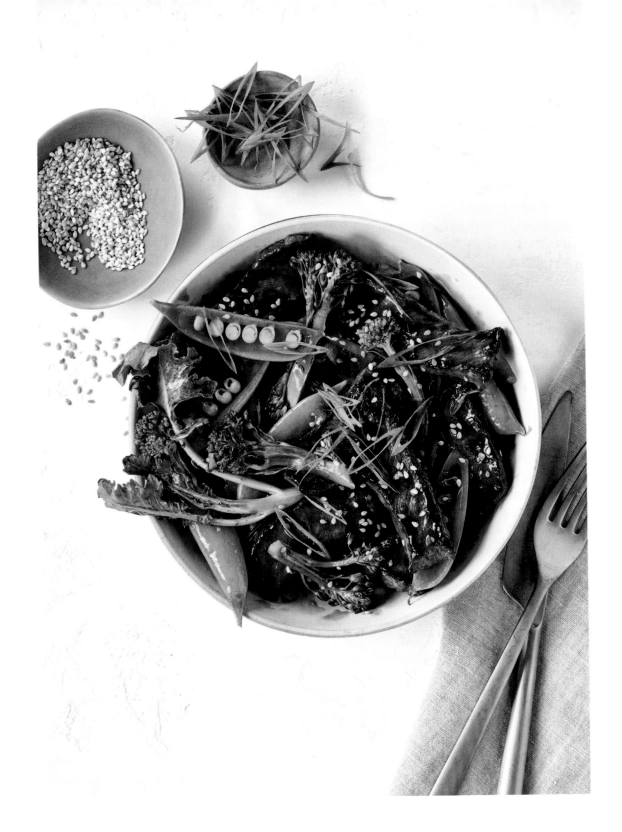

SESAME-GLAZED BEEF & VEGGIE BOWL

YIELDS 4 SERVINGS

Skip the take-out. Coat savory steak, crisp broccoli, and sweet sugar snap peas in a thick and creamy sesame glaze.

INGREDIENTS

1 tablespoon olive oil

1 pound beef steak

¼ cup diced onion

2 cups broccoli florets

½ cup sugar snap peas

¼ cup reduced-sodium tamari sauce

1 tablespoon toasted sesame oil

1 tablespoon minced garlic

½ cup beef broth

1 teaspoon tapioca flour

¼ cup chopped scallions

1 tablespoon sesame seeds

DIRECTIONS

In a large skillet, heat the olive oil over medium-high heat.

Pat the beef dry and season it with salt and pepper to taste. Add it to the hot pan and brown it for 3 to 4 minutes per side.

Remove the beef and set aside, reserving the grease in the skillet.

Reduce the heat to medium. Add the onion to the skillet and cook for 3 to 4 minutes, until translucent. Add the broccoli florets and cook for another 3 to 4 minutes, until brown. Add the sugar snap peas and cook for 1 to 2 minutes.

Meanwhile, in a small mixing bowl whisk together the tamari sauce, toasted sesame oil, minced garlic, beef broth, and tapioca flour until dissolved. Add the sauce to the skillet, stirring to coat the vegetables. Bring the mixture to a boil and then reduce the heat to medium-low.

Cut the steak into small pieces, about 1 inch square, and add it back to the pan, simmering for 5 to 7 minutes, until the beef is cooked to desired doneness.

Divide vegetables and steak mixture into 4 individual bowls. Garnish with the scallions and sesame seeds and serve.

Note: You can make this dish ahead or store leftovers in an airtight container in the refrigerator 3 to 4 days. For long-term storage, freeze individual portions. Defrost overnight in the refrigerator before reheating.

Nutrition information per serving: 402 calories ▪ 26g fat ▪ 8g saturated fat ▪ **35g protein** ▪ **7g carbs** ▪ **2g sugar** ▪ 0g sugar alcohol ▪ 2g fiber ▪ 5g net carbs ▪ 90mg cholesterol ▪ 839mg sodium

FISH TACOS
WITH CREAMY AVOCADO SAUCE

YIELDS 4 SERVINGS

Creamy avocado sauce complements a bold spice rub in these fish tacos.

INGREDIENTS

2 teaspoons chili powder
1 tablespoon lime juice
1 tablespoon avocado oil
½ teaspoon ground cumin
½ teaspoon garlic powder
½ teaspoon onion powder
½ teaspoon sea salt
1 pound cod
4 keto-friendly tortillas
2 cups shredded cabbage
¼ cup cilantro, chopped

For the sauce

1 avocado, pitted and peeled
Juice of 1 lime
⅓ cup chopped cilantro

DIRECTIONS

Stir together the chili powder, lime juice, avocado oil, cumin, garlic powder, onion powder, and salt in a small bowl.

Slice the fish into four small fillets and coat them with the spice rub.

Heat a large skillet over medium-high heat and pan fry the fillets for 2 to 3 minutes per side, until cooked through.

To make the sauce, place the avocado, lime juice, ⅓ cup cilantro, and salt and pepper to taste in a food processor and pulse until smooth. Add water as needed to adjust the consistency.

Serve the fish on 4 keto-friendly tortillas along with the cabbage and cilantro. Drizzle the sauce over the top of each.

Nutrition information per serving: 270 calories ▪ 13g fat ▪ 2.6g saturated fat ▪ **21.5g protein** ▪ **16g carbs** ▪ **0g sugar** ▪ 0g sugar alcohol ▪ 4g fiber ▪ 12g net carbs ▪ 49mg cholesterol ▪ 475mg sodium

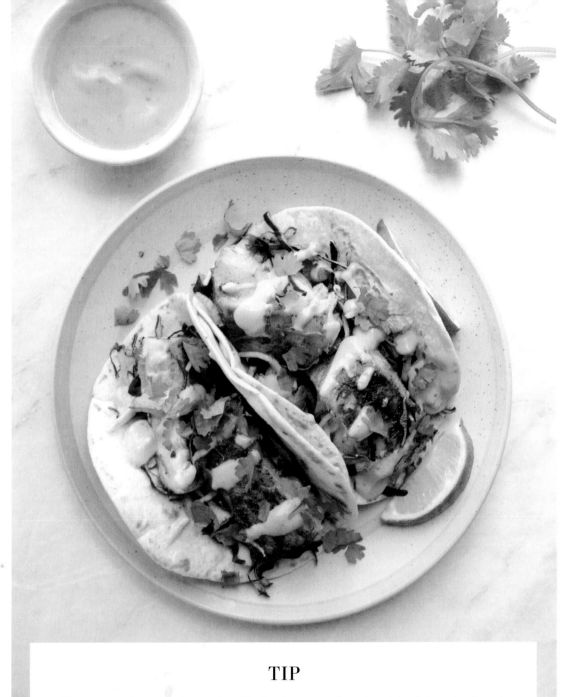

TIP

These tacos can also be made with tilapia or your favorite white fish and enjoyed over lettuce wraps or any keto-friendly tortillas. There are several keto-friendly tortillas available in most grocery stores, including almond flour and cassava flour tortillas, coconut wraps, and other low-carb tortilla wrap options.

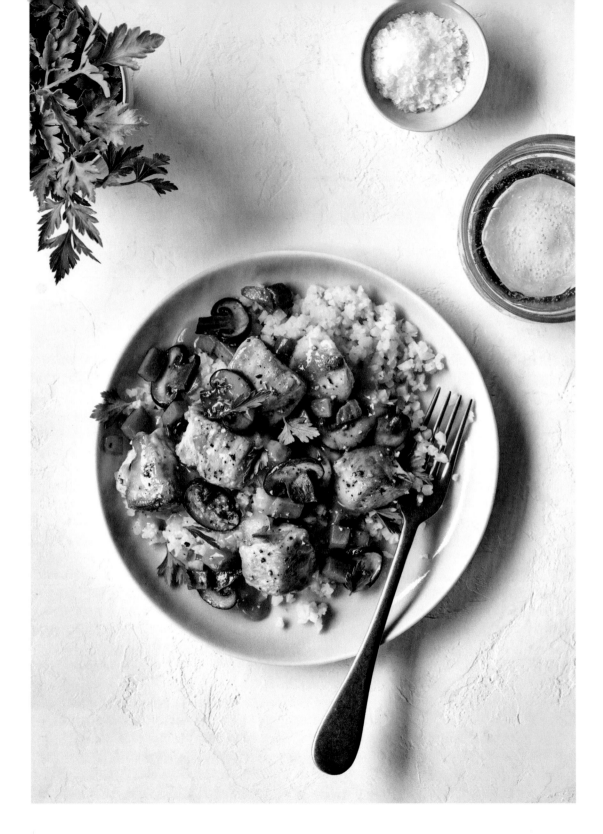

HOME-STYLE CHICKEN & "RICE"

YIELDS 4 SERVINGS

This downhome favorite is comfort in a bowl. Tender pieces of chicken and savory mushrooms are cooked in a creamy sauce and served over cauliflower rice.

INGREDIENTS

1 tablespoon olive oil

1 pound boneless skinless chicken breasts

½ tablespoon butter

¼ cup diced onion

¼ cup diced carrot (approximately 1 medium carrot)

1 cup sliced mushrooms

1 tablespoon tapioca flour

¼ cup heavy cream

½ cup chicken broth

1 teaspoon garlic powder

½ teaspoon paprika

1½ cups cooked cauliflower rice

2 tablespoons chopped fresh parsley

TIP

If you are using this recipe for Phase II, try serving it over ½ cup brown rice or quinoa.

DIRECTIONS

Heat the olive oil over medium-high heat in a large saucepan.

Pat the chicken dry. Dice it into ½-inch pieces and season it with salt and pepper to taste. Place the chicken in the hot pan and cook it for 3 to 4 minutes, until brown. Remove the chicken and set it aside, reserving the grease in the pan.

Reduce the heat to medium. Add the butter to melt.

Add the onion, carrot, and mushrooms. Cook for 3 to 4 minutes, until the onions are soft and the mushrooms are browned.

Sprinkle the vegetables with tapioca flour and stir for 1 minute to incorporate.

Add the heavy cream, chicken broth, garlic powder, and paprika to the mixture. Bring it to a light boil.

Return the chicken to the pan, reduce the heat to low, and simmer for 5 to 7 minutes, until the chicken is cooked through and the sauce is thickened. Evenly distribute the cauliflower rice into 4 individual bowls; then add the cooked chicken and veggies. Garnish with parsley and serve.

Note: If you are preparing this dish in advance, store it in an airtight container in the refrigerator for 3 to 4 days. For long-term storage, freeze individual portions and defrost them overnight in the refrigerator before reheating. Make the cauliflower rice fresh when you are ready to serve.

Nutrition information per serving: 331 calories ▪ 16g fat ▪ 6g saturated fat ▪ **38g protein** ▪ **7g carbs** ▪ **3g sugar** ▪ 0g sugar alcohol ▪ 2g fiber ▪ 5g net carbs ▪ 117mg cholesterol ▪ 248mg sodium

MINI TACO SALADS

WITH CILANTRO-LIME YOGURT DIP

YIELDS 6 SERVINGS (2 MINI TACO SALADS PER SERVING)

Who doesn't love tacos? These small salads will allow you to enjoy taco Tuesday while living your best South Beach Diet keto-friendly lifestyle! Make a double batch of the taco meat and serve it over a bed of lettuce for a quick next-day lunch option, or take it to go in a "salad jar."

INGREDIENTS

12 slices Colby Jack cheese
1 tablespoon avocado oil
1 clove garlic, minced
¼ small onion, chopped
1 pound ground turkey breast
½ cup packed spinach, chopped
½ teaspoon onion powder
½ teaspoon garlic powder
½ teaspoon smoked paprika
½ teaspoon chili powder
½ teaspoon ground cumin
½ teaspoon sea salt
½ teaspoon ground black pepper
24 cherry tomatoes, sliced in half
1 avocado, pitted and diced
¾ cup chopped fresh cilantro

DIRECTIONS

Preheat the oven to 400°F. Line two 9 x 13-inch baking sheets with parchment paper.

Evenly place 6 cheese slices on each baking sheet. Ensure adequate spacing between each cheese slice (approximately 2 inches) to avoid the slices melting together.

Bake for 5 to 6 minutes, or until the edges of the cheese slices are golden brown and bubbling. Watch the cheese closely to avoid overcooking.

Remove the cheese slices from the oven, allowing them to cool slightly (30 to 60 seconds). Blot any excess oil from the cheese slices with a paper towel, and allow the slices to cool for 1 to 2 minutes longer

Remove a cheese slice from the baking sheet with a spatula and mold it into the first of 12 cups of a muffin tin to make a small, bowl-shaped cheese shell. Use the back end of a spoon to help shape the cheese into a cup, if necessary.

TIP

To turn this recipe into a quick, make-ahead salad for lunch, chop half an avocado into cubes and place the cubes at the bottom of a mason jar or other airtight container. Add a squeeze of lime juice to the avocado to prevent browning. Add ½ cup sliced cherry tomatoes, ½ cup cooked turkey meat mixture, one cheese shell, shredded (or ¼ cup shredded cheese), and then top with the lettuce of your choice plus some cilantro. Store the salad in the airtight container overnight, and add Cilantro-Lime Yogurt Dip (recipe follows) immediately prior to eating.

Repeat with the remaining cheese slices and let them cool completely in the muffin tin while you make the taco meat filling.

Heat a large skillet over medium-high heat.

Add the avocado oil to the skillet.

Add the garlic and onion and sauté for 2 to 3 minutes.

Place the ground turkey in the skillet, breaking it up with a spoon or spatula as it cooks. Cook, stirring occasionally, for 6 to 7 minutes, or until the turkey is no longer pink in color.

Add the chopped spinach to the skillet and cook for another 2 to 3 minutes.

Mix together the onion powder, garlic powder, smoked paprika, chili powder, cumin, salt, and pepper in a small bowl.

Add the seasoning mixture to the skillet along with 1 tablespoon of water.

Stir the turkey mixture until the seasoning is well combined and cook for another minute before removing it from the heat.

Add ¼ cup of the cooked turkey mixture to each of the 12 cheese shells. Garnish the cups with the cherry tomatoes, avocado, and cilantro and serve with Cilantro-Lime Yogurt Dip (recipe follows).

Nutrition information per serving: 297 calories ▪ 19g fat ▪ 9g saturated fat ▪ **27g protein** ▪ **6g carbs** ▪ **2g sugar** ▪ 0g sugar alcohol ▪ 3g fiber ▪ 3g net carbs ▪ 13mg cholesterol ▪ 566mg sodium

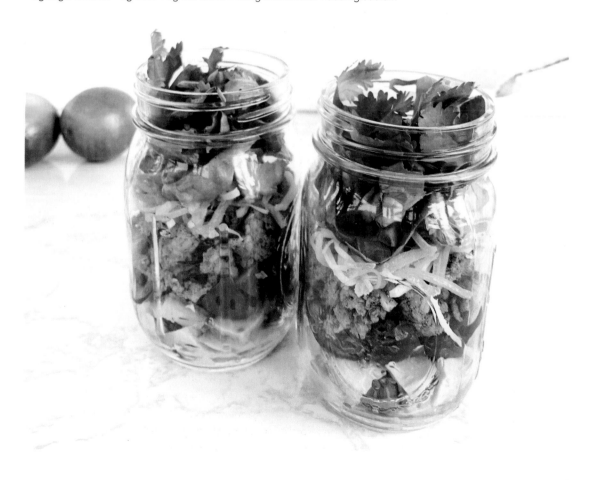

CILANTRO-LIME YOGURT DIP

YIELDS 1 CUP (2 TABLESPOONS PER SERVING)

This creamy, tangy dip makes the perfect accompaniment to our Mini Taco Salads (page 234). But don't limit yourself to just tacos! Try this as a creamy dip for fresh vegetables or add a dollop to soups for a flavorful twist.

INGREDIENTS

1 cup plain whole-milk Greek yogurt

Juice of 1 lime (about 2 tablespoons)

1 to 2 tablespoons chopped fresh cilantro

¼ teaspoon sea salt

¼ teaspoon ground black pepper

DIRECTIONS

Combine the yogurt, lime juice, cilantro, salt, and pepper in a small bowl. Stir until they are well mixed.

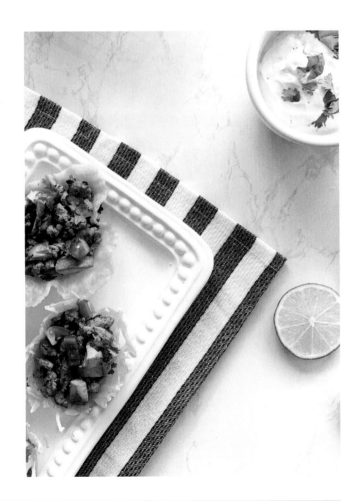

Nutrition information per serving: 28 calories ▪ 1g fat ▪ 1g saturated fat ▪ **3g protein** ▪ **1g carbs** ▪ **1g sugar** ▪ 0g sugar alcohol ▪ 0g fiber ▪ 1g net carbs ▪ 4mg cholesterol ▪ 83mg sodium

KALE CAESAR SALAD

WITH CREAMY CASHEW DRESSING

YIELDS 2 SERVINGS

A thick, creamy, dairy-free Caesar dressing coats crunchy romaine and baby kale for an easy, plant-based lunch. Nutritional yeast adds protein and a cheesy flavor to the dressing, so don't skip it!

INGREDIENTS

4 cups chopped romaine lettuce

2 cups baby kale

½ cup raw cashews

2 tablespoons fresh lemon juice

1 tablespoon extra virgin olive oil

1 tablespoon capers

1 tablespoon apple cider vinegar

2 tablespoons nutritional yeast

1 garlic clove

½ teaspoon Dijon mustard

¼ teaspoon ground black pepper

DIRECTIONS

Mix the romaine and kale together in a large bowl.

Place all the remaining ingredients into the bowl of a food processor or a small blender and process/blend on high until completely smooth. Taste and add salt, a pinch at a time, if you feel it necessary. Since capers are already quite salty, you may not need any.

Drizzle the dressing over the lettuce mixture and toss well to combine. Distribute evenly between two smaller bowls. Serve immediately.

TIP

Serve this salad as is for a meatless meal, or for a heartier meal, top it with grilled chicken or steak.

Nutrition information per serving: 329 calories ▪ 24g fat ▪ 4g saturated fat ▪ **14g protein** ▪ **21g carbs** ▪ **3g sugar** ▪ 0g sugar alcohol ▪ 7g fiber ▪ 15g net carbs ▪ 0mg cholesterol ▪ 198mg sodium

HEIRLOOM TOMATO LASAGNA

YIELDS 6 SERVINGS

A lasagna with a twist—this is an amazingly vibrant plant-based dish that
is bursting with the colors and flavors of the Mediterranean. It can be assembled
in advance and refrigerated until you are ready to cook.

INGREDIENTS

2 medium zucchini or yellow squash,
sliced lengthwise ¼ inch thick

3 tablespoons olive oil

1 medium onion, chopped

3 cups cremini mushrooms, sliced

1 tablespoon lemon juice

½ small red bell pepper, chopped

2 cloves garlic, chopped

½ cup canned chopped artichoke
hearts, rinsed

2 tablespoons fresh basil leaves,
shredded

1 tablespoon fresh oregano leaves,
chopped

3 large heirloom tomatoes (or any vine
ripe tomatoes), sliced ½ inch thick,
divided

1 cup whole-milk ricotta cheese

¼ cup grated Parmesan cheese

DIRECTIONS

Preheat the oven to 375°F. Lightly grease a 9-inch square
baking dish and set it aside.

Place the sliced zucchini in a colander and sprinkle it lightly
with salt; set it aside.

Heat the olive oil in a large skillet over medium heat. Add
the onion and sauté it until softened, about 3 to 4 minutes.
Stir in the mushrooms, lemon juice, red bell pepper, and
garlic. Cook for 5 to 6 minutes, until the vegetables are tender and the liquid has evaporated.

Stir in the artichoke hearts, basil, and oregano and season
with salt and pepper to taste. Turn off the heat.

Pat dry the zucchini slices with paper towels.

Cover the bottom of the prepared dish with slightly over-
lapping tomato slices, using half the slices. Layer the zucchini, mushroom mixture, ricotta cheese, and most of the
Parmesan, retaining a small amount for the topping. Finish
off the dish with the remaining tomatoes. Brush the top of
the tomatoes with a little olive oil, sprinkle them with salt
and pepper, and scatter the remaining Parmesan on top.

Bake for 18 to 20 minutes, or until the tomatoes begin
to brown. Let the lasagna cool slightly in the baking dish
before slicing into 6 evenly cut pieces and serving.

Nutrition information per serving: 211 calories ▪ 14g fat ▪ 5g saturated fat ▪ **10g protein** ▪ **14g carbs** ▪ **6g sugar**
▪ 0g sugar alcohol ▪ 3g fiber ▪ 10g net carbs ▪ 23mg cholesterol ▪ 183mg sodium

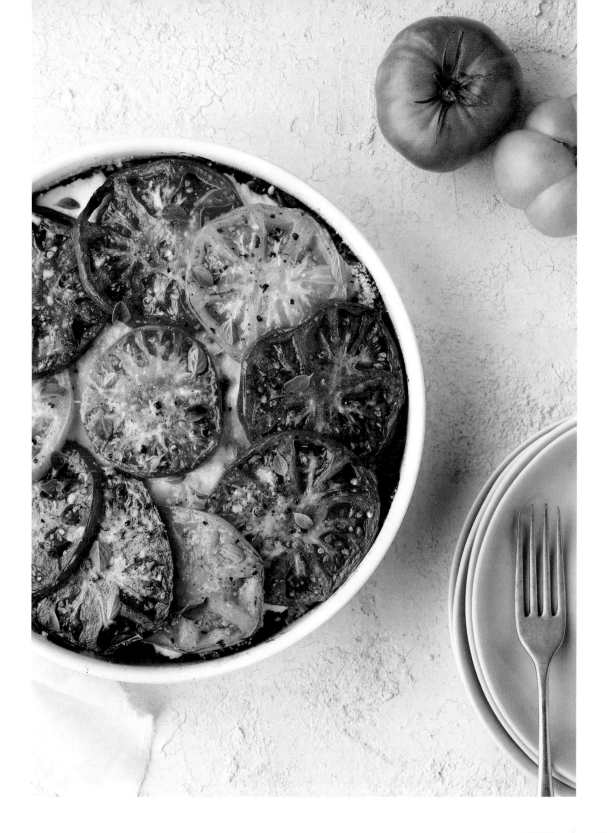

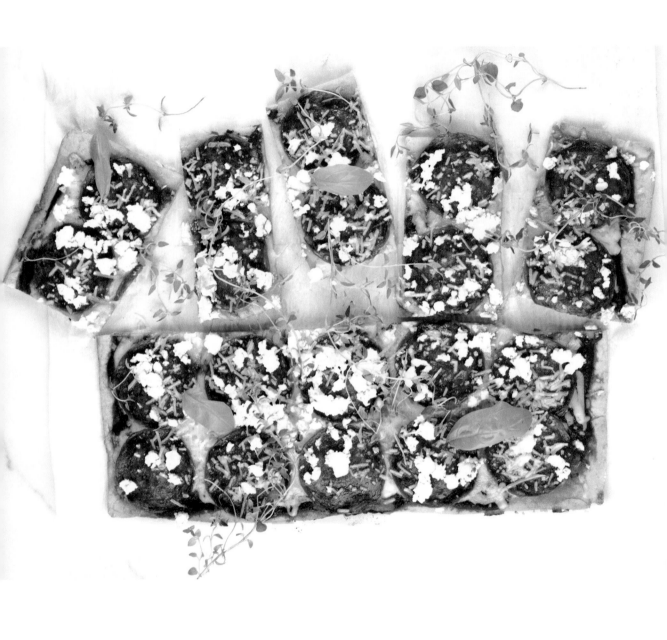

Nutrition information per serving: 346.8 calories ▪ 28.5g fat ▪ 10.9g saturated fat ▪ **17.2g protein** ▪ **7.4g carbs** ▪ **2.2g sugar** ▪ 0g sugar alcohol ▪ 2.6g fiber ▪ 4.8g net carbs ▪ 75mg cholesterol ▪ 532.8mg sodium

PEPPERONI & GOAT CHEESE PIZZA

YIELDS 8 SLICES (1 SLICE PER SERVING)

Who says pizza is off limits when you're eating low carb? Once you try this version of your favorite comfort food, you won't even want to go back to delivery.

INGREDIENTS

For the crust

1½ cups shredded whole-milk mozzarella cheese

2 ounces full-fat cream cheese

1½ cups almond flour

1 large egg

1 teaspoon minced garlic

For the toppings

½ cup pizza sauce (no sugar added)

1 cup whole-milk mozzarella cheese

32 thin slices of pepperoni (2 to 3 ounces)

½ cup crumbled goat cheese

2 tablespoons grated Parmesan cheese

DIRECTIONS

Place an oven rack at the bottom of the oven and preheat it to 425°F. Take out a baking sheet and cut two pieces of parchment paper the same size. Set these aside.

Combine the 1½ cups mozzarella and cream cheese in a saucepan over low heat and stir until melted and smooth. Remove from the heat and allow the mixture to cool slightly. Transfer it to a food processor.

Add the almond flour and egg to the cheese mixture and pulse until a dough forms, about 2 minutes.

Remove the dough from the food processor and transfer it to a piece of parchment paper. Cover the dough with the other piece of parchment paper and use a rolling pin to roll the dough into a rectangle about the size of your baking sheet, approximately ¼ inch thick.

Remove the top piece of parchment paper and transfer the dough along with the bottom piece of parchment paper to a baking sheet.

Use a fork to poke holes all over the dough. Spread the minced garlic evenly on top.

Place the baking sheet in the preheated oven. Bake for 9 minutes or until the dough starts to turn golden. Remove it from the oven.

For the topping, spread the pizza sauce evenly over the dough. Sprinkle 1 cup mozzarella evenly on top, followed by the pepperoni and crumbled goat cheese. Sprinkle the Parmesan over the other toppings.

Bake for 10 to 15 more minutes or until the cheese melts and starts to bubble. Remove the pizza from the oven and allow it to cool before slicing and serving. Cut the pizza into 8 slices.

MOROCCAN LENTIL STEW

YIELDS 6 SERVINGS

Lentils are high in fiber and a good source of plant-based protein. Make sure you're using green lentils for this recipe, which remain firm, instead of red lentils, which disintegrate when you cook them for too long.

INGREDIENTS

1½ teaspoons ground cumin

1 teaspoon curry powder

1 teaspoon sea salt

½ teaspoon ground black pepper

½ teaspoon ground cinnamon

½ teaspoon ground turmeric

¼ teaspoon ground coriander

¼ teaspoon ground ginger

¼ teaspoon ground cloves

¼ teaspoon ground nutmeg

¾ pound boneless skinless chicken thighs

3 tablespoons coconut oil

½ cup finely diced sweet onion

1 clove garlic, minced

6 cups vegetable broth (no sugar added)

½ cup chopped tomatoes

2 medium zucchini, diced

½ cup chopped celery

1 cup dried green lentils

4 cups chopped spinach

½ cup plain whole-milk Greek yogurt

1 medium avocado, pitted and sliced

Fresh chopped cilantro (optional)

DIRECTIONS

Combine cumin, curry powder, salt, pepper, cinnamon, turmeric, coriander, ginger, cloves, and nutmeg in a small bowl and mix well. Set the bowl aside.

Pat the chicken dry and dice it into bite-size pieces. Season it with salt and pepper on all sides.

Heat the coconut oil in a large stockpot over medium heat. When the oil is hot, add the onion and cook for 5 minutes, or until softened and translucent, stirring occasionally. Add the garlic and cook for another 2 minutes.

Add the chicken and cook it for 3 minutes, stirring to brown it on all sides. Sprinkle the prepared spice mixture over the chicken and cook for another 3 minutes.

Pour in the vegetable broth and add the tomatoes, zucchini, celery, and lentils.

Bring the mixture to a boil and then reduce the heat to medium-low. Stir in the spinach and cook until wilted, about 2 minutes.

Reduce the heat to low and simmer the stew uncovered for 20 minutes, or until the vegetables and lentils are tender and the chicken is cooked through.

Distribute the stew evenly into 6 bowls and top each with a dollop of yogurt and the avocado slices. Add a sprinkle of the cilantro, if desired.

Note: This stew may be stored in an airtight container for 4 to 5 days in the refrigerator, or you may freeze individual portions in resealable bags. (For maximum freezer storage, lay resealable bags flat to freeze.) Reheat the portions from frozen on the stovetop over medium heat for 8 to 10 minutes, until warmed through.

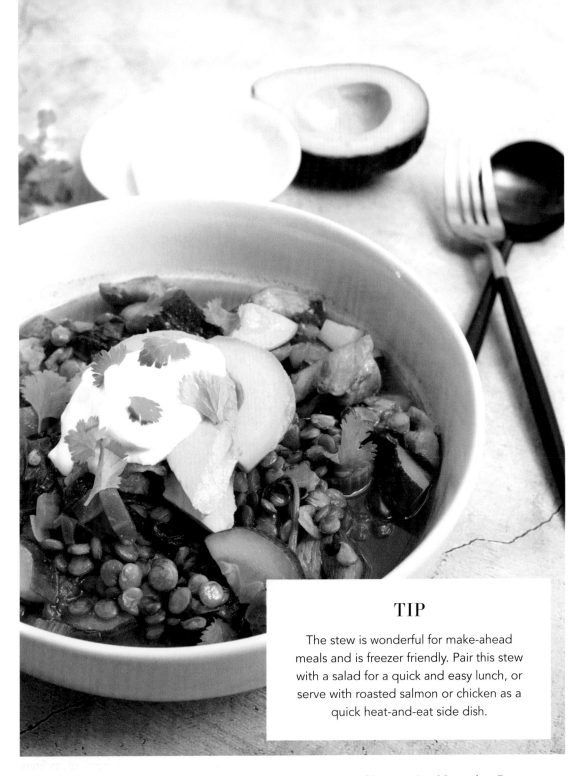

Nutrition information per serving: 347 calories ▪ 16g fat ▪ 9g saturated fat ▪ **23g protein** ▪ **30g carbs** ▪ **5g sugar**
▪ 0g sugar alcohol ▪ 7g fiber ▪ 23g net carbs ▪ 56mg cholesterol ▪ 623mg sodium

SPICE-RUBBED SALMON
WITH CREAMY DILL DRESSING

YIELDS 4 SERVINGS

Rub juicy salmon fillets with this spiced Dijon glaze and they will bake to perfection.
Cool things down with a creamy dill dressing made with crumbled feta and Greek yogurt.

INGREDIENTS

1 pound salmon fillets

1 tablespoon olive oil

1 teaspoon Dijon mustard

½ teaspoon ground cumin

½ teaspoon paprika

½ teaspoon ground coriander

½ cup plain whole-milk Greek yogurt

2 ounces crumbled feta cheese

2 tablespoons lemon juice

2 tablespoons chopped chives

¼ cup chopped fresh dill

DIRECTIONS

Preheat the oven to 375°F. Grease a sheet pan with olive oil and set it aside.

Pat the salmon dry. Rub it with olive oil and place the fillets skin side down on the prepared baking sheet. Brush the salmon with the Dijon mustard.

Combine the cumin, paprika, and coriander in a small bowl.

Sprinkle the salmon with the spice mix and salt and pepper to taste.

Transfer the salmon to the oven and bake it for 15 to 18 minutes, until the salmon is cooked through.

Meanwhile, whisk together the yogurt, feta cheese, lemon juice, chives, and half the dill in a bowl.

Divide the salmon into 4 equal portions and serve warm, drizzled with the creamy dill dressing and garnished with the remaining dill. The salmon and dressing may be kept for 3 to 4 days in the refrigerator, stored separately in airtight containers.

Nutrition information per serving: 221 calories ▪ 12g fat ▪ 4g saturated fat ▪ **27g protein** ▪ **3g carbs** ▪ **2g sugar** ▪ 0g sugar alcohol ▪ 0g fiber ▪ 2g net carbs ▪ 18mg cholesterol ▪ 263mg sodium

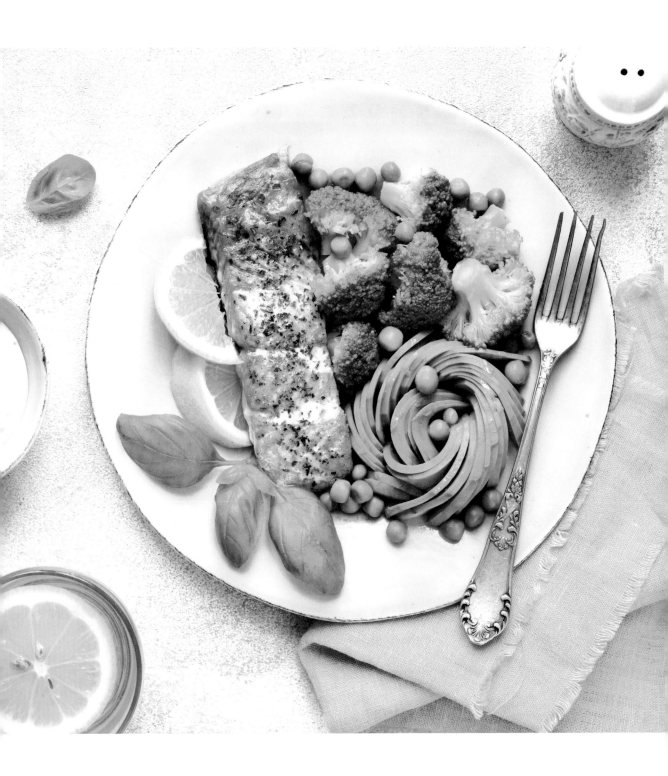

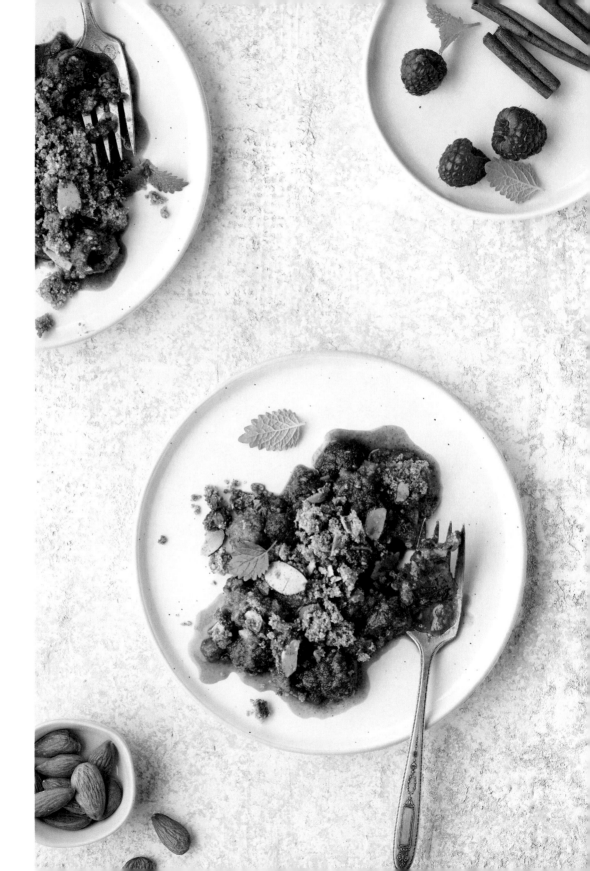

SIDES, SNACKS & SWEETS

PARMESAN ROASTED BRUSSELS SPROUTS

YIELDS 4 SERVINGS

Take your brussels sprouts game to the next level by roasting them in a blend of crushed pork rinds and Parmesan cheese.

INGREDIENTS

1 pound brussels sprouts
2 tablespoons olive oil
⅓ cup crushed pork rinds
⅓ cup grated Parmesan cheese

DIRECTIONS

Preheat the oven to 400°F.

Trim the brussels sprouts and cut them in half. Toss them with olive oil in a large bowl.

Add the pork rinds, Parmesan, and salt and pepper to taste. Toss to coat.

Arrange the mixture in a single layer on a baking sheet and roast for 15 to 18 minutes, until golden and tender. Divide into 4 equal portions and serve.

Note: This dish can be made ahead and stored in an airtight container in the refrigerator for 3 to 4 days.

TIP

If you don't eat pork, crispy turkey bacon broken into bits is a great alternative.

Nutrition information per serving: 165 calories ▪ 11g fat ▪ 3g saturated fat ▪ **9g protein** ▪ **11g carbs** ▪ **2g sugar** ▪ 0g sugar alcohol ▪ 4g fiber ▪ 7g net carbs ▪ 11mg cholesterol ▪ 251mg sodium

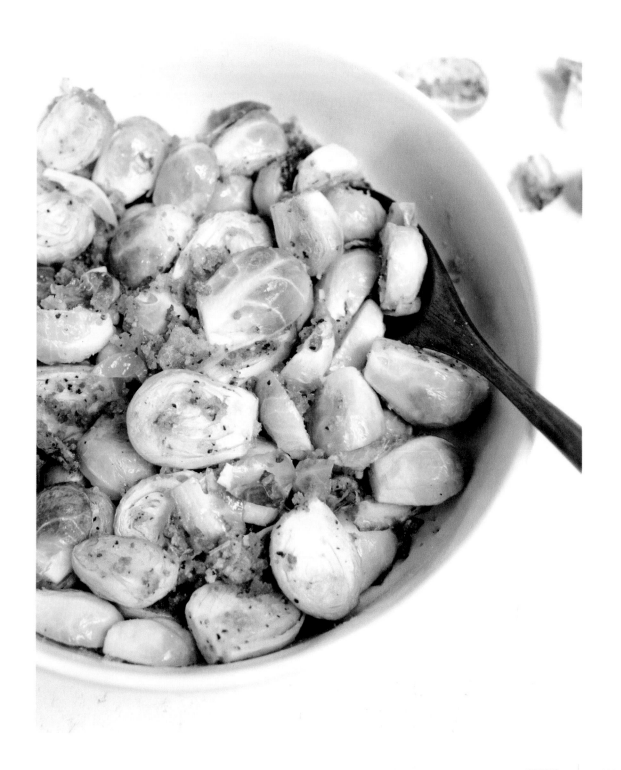

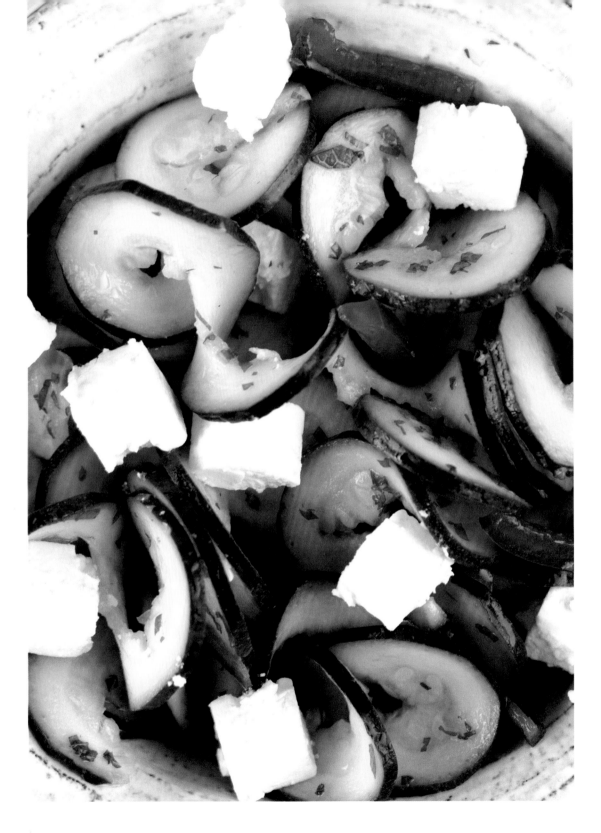

ZUCCHINI FETA SALAD

YIELDS 4 SERVINGS

This fresh salad can be enjoyed on its own as a starter or a light lunch.

INGREDIENTS

½ small cucumber, peeled, deseeded, and diced

1 shallot, diced

2 tablespoons fresh chopped mint leaves

3 tablespoons extra virgin olive oil, divided

1 to 2 tablespoons apple cider vinegar (or to taste)

2 to 3 tablespoons plain whole-milk Greek yogurt or sour cream (optional)

2 medium zucchini, thinly sliced or shaved

1 small (about 4 ounce) red bell pepper, deseeded and cut into thin strips

⅓ cup crumbled (or cut into small cubes) feta cheese

DIRECTIONS

Put the cucumber, shallot, mint leaves, olive oil, apple cider vinegar, and yogurt (if using) into a blender and pulse until smooth. Season with salt and pepper to taste.

Combine the zucchini, bell pepper, and feta cheese in a salad bowl, drizzle with the dressing, and toss lightly before dividing into 4 portions. Refrigerate the salad until you are ready to serve.

TIP

Sprinkle a handful of chopped toasted walnuts over the salad for an extra layer of crunchiness.

Nutrition information per serving: 168 calories ▪ 14g fat ▪ 4g saturated fat ▪ **4g protein** ▪ **6g carbs** ▪ **5g sugar** ▪ 0g sugar alcohol ▪ 2g fiber ▪ 6g net carbs ▪ 16mg cholesterol ▪ 179mg sodium

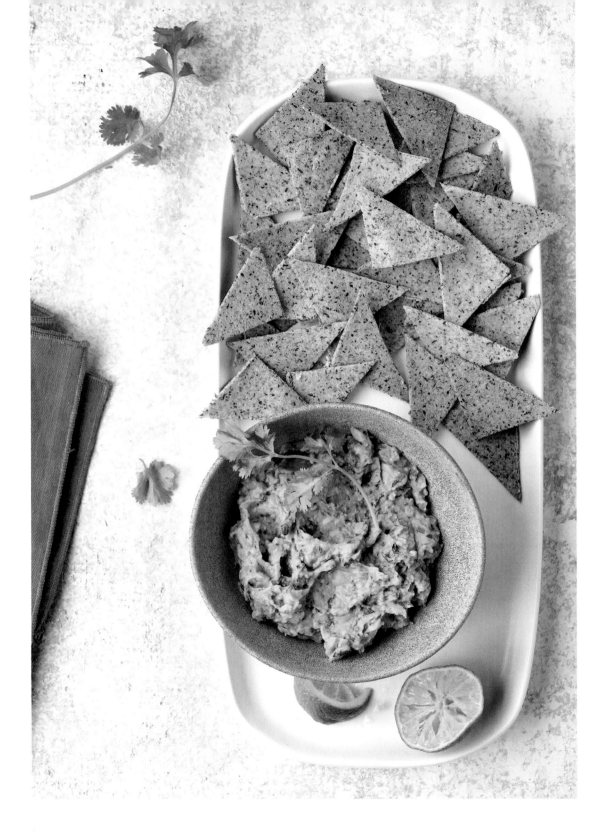

ALMOND FLOUR TORTILLA CHIPS

WITH HOMEMADE GUACAMOLE

YIELDS: 4 SERVINGS

These low-carb tortilla chips are made with almond flour and flaxseeds for a crispy, crunchy chip that's perfect for scooping up freshly made guacamole!

INGREDIENTS

¾ cup almond flour

¼ cup ground flaxseeds

1 large egg white

¼ teaspoon sea salt

¼ teaspoon baking powder

Olive oil

For the guacamole

2 large ripe avocados, pitted

Juice from 1 lime

¼ cup roughly chopped fresh cilantro

½ teaspoon sea salt

¼ teaspoon garlic powder

DIRECTIONS

Preheat the oven to 350°F. Cut 2 pieces of parchment paper to the size of a baking sheet and set them aside.

Place the almond flour, flaxseeds, egg white, salt, and baking powder into the bowl of a food processor and pulse until a dough forms.

Turn the dough out onto one of the pieces of parchment paper and then top it with the second piece of parchment paper. Use a rolling pin to roll the dough out into a large oval, about the same length and width as the parchment. The dough should be very thin.

Slide the parchment-covered dough onto a baking sheet and then carefully remove the top piece of parchment paper. Using a pizza cutter, cut the dough into 2-inch squares. Then cut each square diagonally into 2 triangles.

Spray the top of the dough with the olive oil and bake for 12 to 15 minutes, or until the chips are golden.

Meanwhile, scoop out the ripe avocado and place it in a large bowl. Add the lime juice, cilantro, salt, and garlic powder. Mash with a fork to combine. Taste and add more salt, if needed.

Serve immediately, or divide the chips and guacamole into 4 separate containers for a pre-portioned snack to enjoy throughout the week.

Nutrition information per serving: 222 calories ▪ 18g fat ▪ 2g saturated fat ▪ 5g protein ▪ 12g carbs ▪ 1g sugar ▪ 0g sugar alcohol ▪ 8g fiber ▪ 3g net carbs ▪ 0mg cholesterol ▪ 310mg sodium

GARLIC & PARMESAN MASHED CAULIFLOWER

YIELDS 4 SERVINGS

Mashed cauliflower is the perfect lower-carb alternative to mashed potatoes.
While cauliflower is often bland, when mashed with lots of garlic and
Parmesan cheese it becomes a flavorful and indulgent addition to any meal.

INGREDIENTS

1 large head of cauliflower
4 tablespoons butter
1 teaspoon sea salt
½ teaspoon garlic powder
¼ teaspoon ground black pepper
½ cup grated Parmesan cheese

DIRECTIONS

Bring a large pot of water to a boil.

Cut the cauliflower in half, discard the core, and break it
into large florets. Cook the cauliflower in boiling water for
10 to 12 minutes, or until soft.

Drain the cauliflower and place it back in the pot over low
heat. Add the butter, salt, garlic, pepper, and Parmesan
to the pot and use a potato masher to mash until smooth.
Taste and add more salt, if needed. Divide the prepared
cauliflower into 4 portions and serve.

Nutrition information per serving: 199 calories ▪ 15g fat ▪ 9g saturated fat ▪ **9g protein** ▪ **12g carbs** ▪ **3g sugar**
▪ 0g sugar alcohol ▪ 5g fiber ▪ 6g net carbs ▪ 9mg cholesterol ▪ 540mg sodium

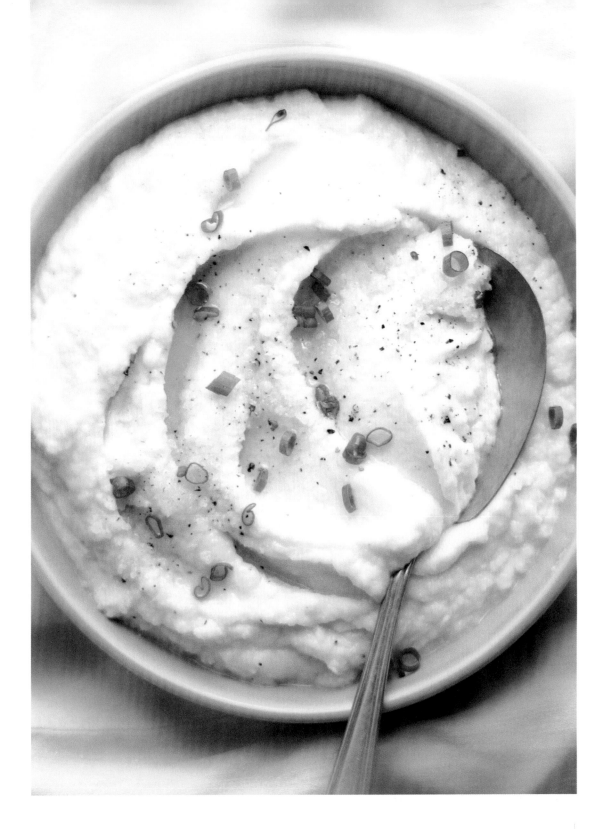

HERBED SEED CRACKERS

YIELDS 48 CRACKERS (8 CRACKERS PER SERVING)

Snack on healthy fats and fiber with these crunchy crackers. They're a great low-carb option for your favorite dips or terrific on their own. Best of all, they're easy to make!

INGREDIENTS

¼ cup pumpkin seeds

2 tablespoons sunflower seeds

2 tablespoons sesame seeds

2 tablespoons ground flaxseeds

2 tablespoons hemp seeds

¼ cup chia seeds

1 teaspoon dried thyme

1 teaspoon dried basil

1 teaspoon dried rosemary

1 teaspoon poppy seeds

½ teaspoon coarse sea salt

DIRECTIONS

Place 2 oven racks in the center of the oven and preheat it to 200°F. Line 2 baking sheets with parchment paper and set aside.

Combine all the ingredients, along with pepper to taste, in a small mixing bowl. Add ¾ cup water and stir to combine. Set the mixture aside to soak for 15 minutes, until thick and uniform.

After soaking, stir the mixture to combine. Divide evenly between the prepared baking sheets and press the mixture into even ⅛-inch-thick layers.

Bake for 1 hour, until golden and crisp on top.

Remove the baking sheets from the oven, keeping the oven on. Carefully lift the parchment paper and cracker dough from the baking sheets and flip them over, back onto the hot baking sheets. Slowly peel the parchment away to expose the bottom of the cracker dough. Return the baking sheets to the oven for another 30 minutes.

Cool the cracker dough for 30 minutes and then break or cut it into crackers that are approximately 2 by 2 inches (about 24 crackers per sheet).

Note: These crackers may be stored in an airtight container at room temperature for 4 to 5 days. For long-term storage, lay the crackers on a baking sheet in a single layer, with the crackers not touching, to freeze before storing them in a freezer-safe bag.

Nutrition information per serving: 129 calories ▪ 10g fat ▪ 1g saturated fat ▪ **5g protein** ▪ **6g carbs** ▪ **0g sugar** ▪ 0g sugar alcohol ▪ 4g fiber ▪ 2g net carbs ▪ 0mg cholesterol ▪ 135mg sodium

RADICCHIO & MUSHROOM GRATIN

YIELDS 6 SERVINGS

This flavorful, creamy side dish is also great as a meal on its own. Cooking radicchio mellows out its bitter taste and enhances its flavor. When mixed with the sweet taste of caramelized onions and the earthiness of mushrooms, the result is delicious.

INGREDIENTS

½ cup full-fat sour cream

1 cup whole milk

⅓ cup soft goat cheese

¼ teaspoon nutmeg

2 tablespoons olive oil

1 large red onion, thinly sliced

2 garlic cloves, chopped

2 sprigs fresh thyme or fresh oregano

2 tablespoons balsamic vinegar

10 ounces red radicchio, thinly sliced

2 tablespoons butter

2 cups white mushrooms, sliced

6 to 7 broccolini stems, cut into 1½-inch pieces

6 to 7 young asparagus spears, cut into 1½-inch pieces

½ cup shredded full-fat cheddar cheese

DIRECTIONS

Preheat the oven to 400°F. Lightly grease a 9-inch square baking dish (alternatively, use 6 ramekins) and set aside.

Whisk together the sour cream, milk, goat cheese, and nutmeg, and season with salt and pepper to taste; set aside.

Heat the olive oil in a large, heavy-bottomed skillet. Add the onion, and cook for about 10 minutes, stirring occasionally until the onions are tender and begin to caramelize. Add the garlic, thyme, balsamic vinegar, and radicchio and cook, stirring occasionally, for about 5 minutes, until the radicchio softens.

Add the butter and mushrooms and continue cooking for 5 minutes. Stir in the broccolini and asparagus.

Stir the sour cream and milk mixture into the skillet and adjust the seasoning to taste.

Transfer the mixture to the prepared dish and sprinkle with the cheddar. Bake for 12 to 15 minutes, or until bubbly and the cheese is melted.

Carefully remove the dish from the oven and let it cool for 5 minutes before portioning the contents into 6 servings.

Note: The gratin can be made ahead and frozen in the baking dish (covered with plastic food wrap) for up to 2 weeks. Thaw it in the refrigerator and bake it as directed above.

Nutrition information per serving: 257 calories ▪ 20g fat ▪ 10g saturated fat ▪ **10g protein** ▪ **11g carbs** ▪ **6g sugar** ▪ 0g sugar alcohol ▪ 2g fiber ▪ 9g net carbs ▪ 42mg cholesterol ▪ 171mg sodium

TIP

Endive or watercress may be substituted for the radicchio.

KETO CLOUD BREAD 2 WAYS

YIELDS 12 CLOUD BREADS (2 CLOUD BREADS PER SERVING)

You don't have to give up bread to eat a Keto-Friendly South Beach Diet! This perfectly named bread is light as air. It's great for everything from morning toast to sandwich bread.

INGREDIENTS

For the bread

6 room-temperature eggs, whites and yolks separated

¼ teaspoon cream of tartar

3 tablespoons room-temperature cream cheese

3 tablespoons room-temperature plain whole-milk Greek yogurt

⅛ teaspoon sea salt

For garlic Parmesan topping

1 tablespoon grated Parmesan cheese

1 teaspoon garlic powder

For everything bagel topping

1 teaspoon white sesame seeds

½ teaspoon dried onion powder

¼ teaspoon black sesame seeds

⅛ teaspoon garlic powder

⅛ teaspoon poppy seeds

⅛ teaspoon sea salt

DIRECTIONS

Place 2 oven racks in the center of the oven and preheat it to 300°F. Line 2 baking sheets with parchment paper and set aside.

Beat the egg whites in a large mixing bowl with an electric mixer on medium, until frothy. Add the cream of tartar and continue to beat, slowly increasing the mixer speed until stiff peaks form.

In a separate, large mixing bowl, beat together the egg yolks, cream cheese, yogurt, and salt with an electric mixer on medium, until completely smooth.

Add half the prepared egg whites to the cream cheese mixture and fold gently to combine. Slowly fold in the other half of the egg whites to incorporate.

Scoop the mixture onto the prepared baking sheets, 6 scoops per sheet, to form 12 rounded cloud breads. Combine the ingredients for each topping, and sprinkle one baking sheet with Parmesan topping and the other with everything bagel topping.

Bake for 30 to 35 minutes, until golden. Cool completely before serving.

Note: Baked cloud bread can be stored in the refrigerator, separated by parchment paper or paper towels, for 4 to 5 days. For long-term storage, lay individual bread on a baking sheet lined with parchment paper and place it in the freezer. Once the bread is frozen, store it in freezer-safe bags. Thaw it in the refrigerator overnight.

Nutrition information per serving: 109 calories ▪ 8g fat ▪ 3g saturated fat ▪ **7g protein** ▪ **1g carbs** ▪ **1g sugar** ▪ 0g sugar alcohol ▪ 0g fiber ▪ 1g net carbs ▪ 195mg cholesterol ▪ 136mg sodium

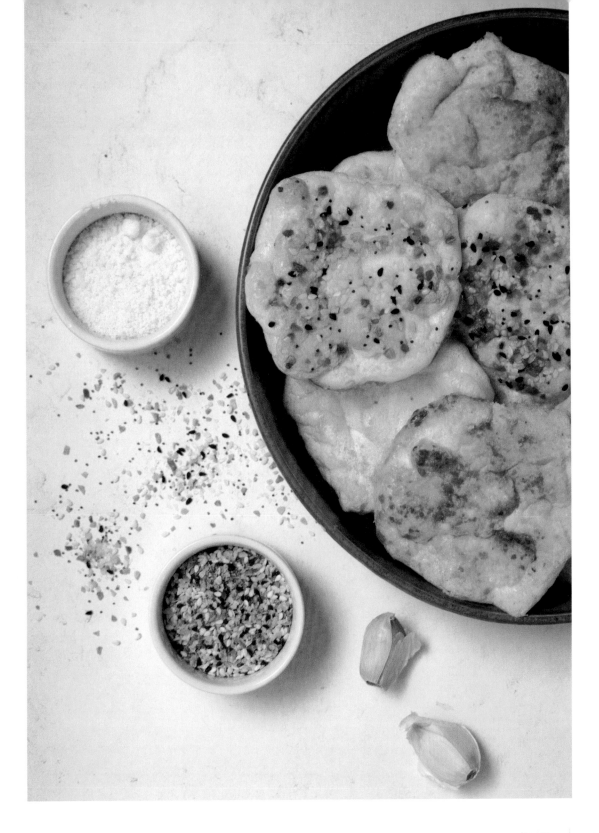

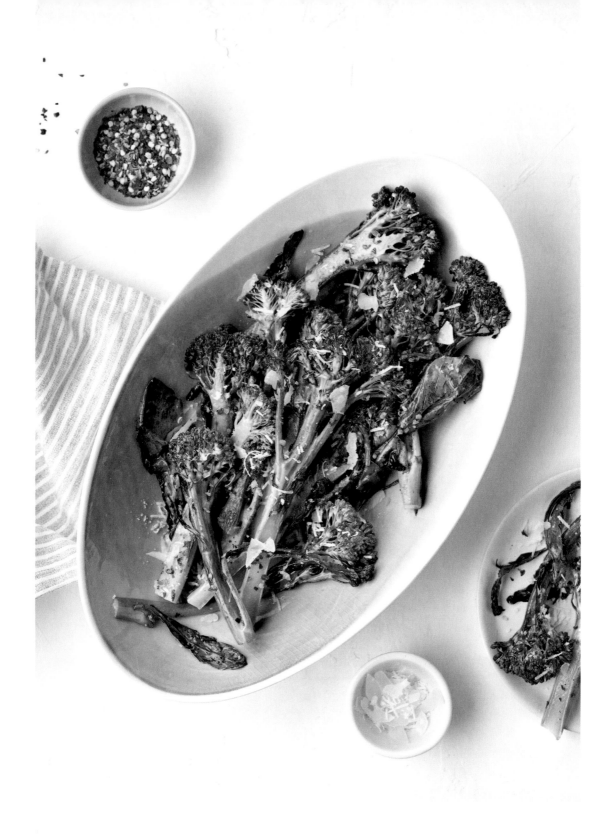

PARMESAN ROASTED BROCCOLI RABE

YIELDS 4 SERVINGS

Broccoli rabe is a lower-carb alternative to broccoli, and is a great way to add more green vegetables to a keto-friendly diet. When roasted and tossed with Parmesan cheese, it becomes the perfect side dish for roast chicken, burgers, and salmon.

INGREDIENTS

1 pound broccoli rabe
1 tablespoon olive oil
½ teaspoon sea salt
¼ teaspoon garlic powder
¼ teaspoon chili flakes
¼ cup grated Parmesan cheese

DIRECTIONS

Preheat the oven to 400°F.

Trim the broccoli rabe to remove 1 to 2 inches of tough stem at the bottom. Cut the larger florets in half lengthwise. Place the broccoli rabe on a baking sheet and drizzle it with the olive oil, tossing to combine. Sprinkle the salt, garlic, and chili flakes on top.

Bake for 20 minutes, or until the broccoli rabe is tender. Remove it from the oven and toss it with the Parmesan cheese in a large bowl. Divide the prepared broccoli rabe into 4 portions and serve.

Nutrition information per serving: 77 calories ▪ 5g fat ▪ 1g saturated fat ▪ **5g protein** ▪ **4g carbs** ▪ **0g sugar** ▪ 0g sugar alcohol ▪ 4g fiber ▪ 0g net carbs ▪ 5mg cholesterol ▪ 437mg sodium

SAVORY PESTO YOGURT BOWLS

YIELDS 1 SERVING

Yogurt isn't just for breakfast! Try it as an Italian-inspired snack topped with store-bought pesto, cherry tomatoes, and avocado for a cold, creamy, savory yogurt bowl full of fresh flavors. Most store-bought pestos are naturally South Beach Diet keto friendly; just check the label to be sure there isn't any added sugar.

INGREDIENTS

½ cup plain whole-milk Greek yogurt

1 tablespoon basil pesto

4 cherry tomatoes, halved

¼ avocado, pitted and diced

DIRECTIONS

Spread the yogurt into the bottom of a bowl.

Top with the pesto, tomatoes, avocado, and a pinch each of salt and pepper, to taste.

Serve immediately.

Nutrition information per serving: 193 calories ▪ 12g fat ▪ 4g saturated fat ▪ **13g protein** ▪ **12g carbs** ▪ **5g sugar** ▪ 0g sugar alcohol ▪ 4g fiber ▪ 7g net carbs ▪ 25mg cholesterol ▪ 59mg sodium

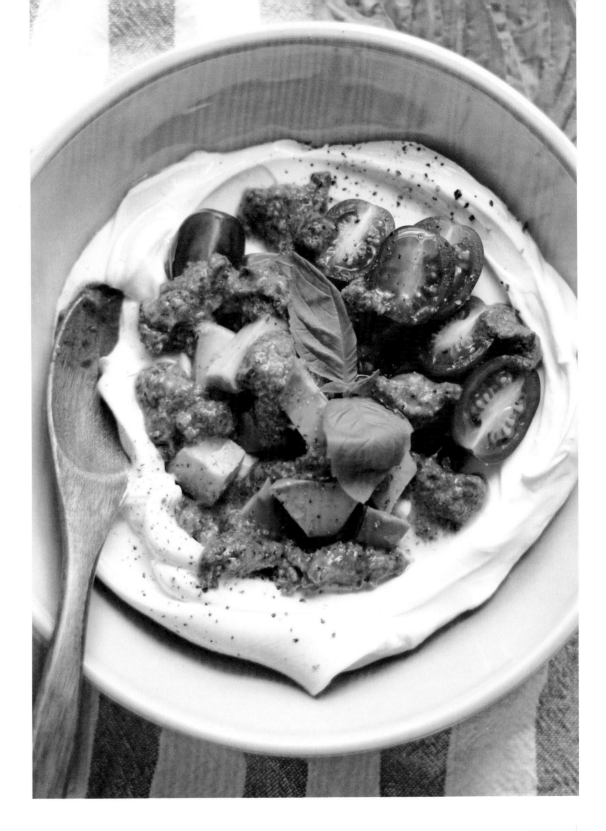

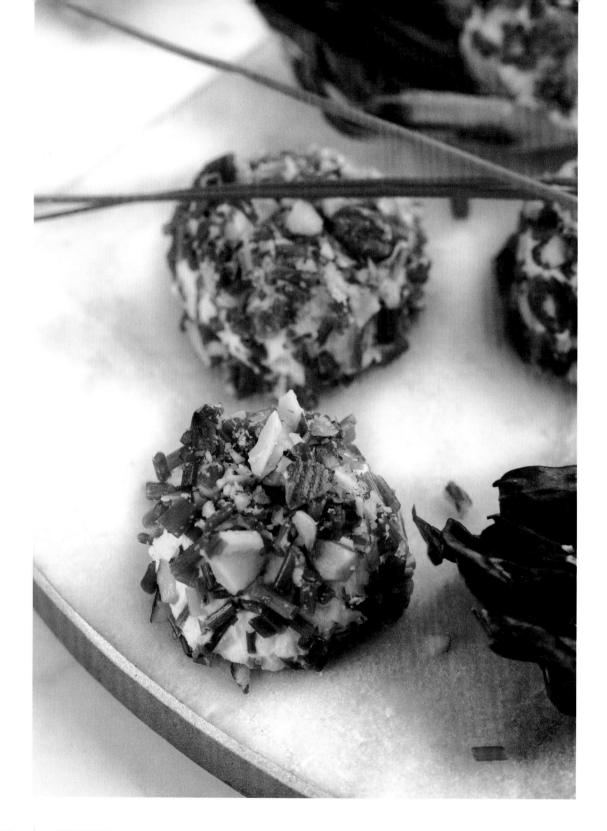

SMOKY GOAT CHEESE & ALMOND BALLS

YIELDS 24 BALLS (1 BALL PER SERVING)

Delight your guests by serving these colorful, bite-size goat cheese balls at your next dinner party, or make one large cheese ball for an informal gathering. They work as a savory snack, either on their own or with keto-friendly chips, and can be made up to a day ahead.

INGREDIENTS

One 8-ounce package cream cheese

One 10.5-ounce package soft goat cheese

1 ripe avocado, mashed

1 tablespoon lemon juice

⅓ cup shredded Parmesan or full-fat sharp cheddar cheese

3 tablespoons unsalted butter, softened at room temperature

¼ teaspoon smoked paprika

¼ teaspoon garlic and/or onion powder

¼ teaspoon ground cumin

For the garnish

⅓ cup smoked almonds, chopped

3 tablespoons fresh chopped chives

1 teaspoon fresh chopped thyme

DIRECTIONS

Whisk together all of the cheese ball ingredients until thoroughly combined. Add salt and pepper to taste. Refrigerate the mixture for about 30 minutes.

Line a flat serving platter with parchment paper and set it aside.

Mix together the garnish of smoked almonds, chives, and thyme in a small bowl.

Scoop out 1 rounded tablespoon of the cheese ball mixture and roll it into the almond garnish. Arrange the balls on the prepared platter and refrigerate until firm.

Nutrition information per serving: 105 calories ▪ 10g fat ▪ 5g saturated fat ▪ **4g protein** ▪ **2g carbs** ▪ **0g sugar** ▪ 0g sugar alcohol ▪ 0g fiber ▪ 1g net carbs ▪ 23mg cholesterol ▪ 129mg sodium

SPICY PARMESAN CRISPS

YIELDS 10 CRISPS (5 CRISPS PER SERVING)

Ready in less than 10 minutes, these Parmesan crisps are the best accompaniment for keto dips or can be served on their own as a snack at any time of the day.

INGREDIENTS

1 cup shredded Parmesan cheese

1 small serrano pepper, thinly sliced

2 sweet mini peppers, thinly sliced

½ teaspoon Italian seasoning

¼ teaspoon chili flakes

For the toppings (optional)

¼ cup shredded full-fat sharp cheddar cheese

½ tablespoon hemp seeds

½ teaspoon smoked paprika

½ teaspoon onion powder

DIRECTIONS

Preheat the oven to 400°F. Line a large baking sheet with parchment paper or a large silicon baking mat.

Place a heaping tablespoon of Parmesan on the prepared baking sheet and spread it into a 3-inch circle. This is most easily done using a 3-inch egg ring or cookie cutter as a guide. Repeat until all the cheese has been used; you should have enough for 10 circles.

Carefully portion the sliced serrano pepper and sweet peppers on top of the cheese circles and sprinkle each circle with the Italian seasoning and chili pepper flakes. Additional toppings may be added or substituted.

Bake for about 5 to 7 minutes, or until the edges begin to brown.

Let the crisps cool slightly for a minute or two on the baking sheet before serving. Store them in an airtight container for up to 2 days.

TIP

Turn these crisps into colorful mini taco shells by draping them while still warm over the handle of a wooden spoon suspended between 2 cans.

Nutrition information per serving: 61 calories ▪ 4g fat ▪ 3g saturated fat ▪ **5g protein** ▪ **1g carbs** ▪ **0g sugar** ▪ 0g sugar alcohol ▪ 0g fiber ▪ 1g net carbs ▪ 10mg cholesterol ▪ 204mg sodium

SWEET & SALTY TRAIL MIX

YIELDS 2 CUPS (APPROXIMATELY ⅓ CUP PER SERVING)

Homemade trail mix with freshly roasted nuts and sugar-free chocolate
makes for a fun snack to take with you on the go! See the note below
for variations, including maple cinnamon and chocolate coconut.

INGREDIENTS

1 cup raw cashews

1 cup raw pecans

Olive oil spray

¼ teaspoon sea salt

¼ cup roughly chopped sugar-free
chocolate

DIRECTIONS

Preheat the oven to 350°F.

Place the nuts in a small bowl, spray them with olive oil,
and sprinkle them with salt. Toss them to combine and then
place the nuts on a baking sheet.

Roast the nuts for 8 to 10 minutes, or until they are golden
brown. Let them cool completely in the pan.

In a large bowl, mix together the roasted and cooled nuts
with the chocolate and store in an airtight container or
divide into 6 resealable bags for a pre-portioned snack to
enjoy throughout the week.

TIP

Any nuts, seeds, and unsweetened chocolate can be used interchangeably in
this recipe to yield a custom trail mix blend. To make maple cinnamon trail mix,
omit the salt and olive oil and instead roast the nuts with ½ teaspoon cinnamon
and 1 tablespoon sugar-free maple syrup. To make coconut trail mix, replace
1 cup of nuts with 1 cup of shredded unsweetened coconut.

Nutrition information per serving: 184 calories ▪ 15g fat ▪ 3g saturated fat ▪ **4g protein** ▪ **9g carbs** ▪ **2g sugar**
▪ 6g sugar alcohol ▪ 3g fiber ▪ 0g net carbs ▪ 0mg cholesterol ▪ 102mg sodium

CHEESY GARLIC CAULIFLOWER BREADSTICKS

YIELDS 12 BREADSTICKS (2 BREADSTICKS PER SERVING)

Indulge in a take-out classic without the guilt. These crispy breadsticks are dripping with melted cheese and bursting with savory garlic and Italian seasoning.

INGREDIENTS

2 cups cauliflower rice

¾ cup shredded whole-milk mozzarella cheese, divided

6 tablespoons grated Parmesan cheese, divided

1 large egg

3 teaspoons minced garlic

2 tablespoons olive oil

2 teaspoons dried minced onion

½ teaspoon dried thyme

½ teaspoon dried rosemary

¼ teaspoon dried oregano

DIRECTIONS

Place oven racks on the top and middle rungs of the oven and preheat it to 450°F. Line a baking sheet with parchment paper and set it aside.

Press the cauliflower rice between 2 clean towels to remove the excess liquid. Transfer it to a large mixing bowl.

Add ½ cup of the mozzarella, 4 tablespoons of the Parmesan, the egg, and the minced garlic. Season with salt and pepper to taste. Stir to combine into a dough that holds its shape when pinched together.

Transfer the dough to the prepared baking sheet. Press it into an oval about ¼ inch thick.

Transfer the baking sheet to the lower of the 2 oven racks and bake for 12 to 15 minutes, until the bottom is crisp and golden.

Meanwhile, whisk together in a small bowl the olive oil, minced onion, thyme, rosemary, and oregano. Season with salt and pepper to taste and set the mixture aside.

Remove the baking sheet from the oven. Increase the heat to broil.

Nutrition information per serving: 135 calories ▪ 11g fat ▪ 4g saturated fat ▪ **7g protein** ▪ **4g carbs** ▪ **1g sugar** ▪ 0g sugar alcohol ▪ 1g fiber ▪ 3g net carbs ▪ 49mg cholesterol ▪ 233mg sodium

Brush the olive oil mixture all over the bread and then sprinkle it with the remaining mozzarella and Parmesan. Return it to the top rack of the oven and broil for 1 to 2 minutes, until the cheese is bubbly and golden. Keep a close eye on the bread to prevent burning.

Allow the bread to cool for 5 minutes. Cut it into 12 slices and enjoy it warm.

Note: These breadsticks keep very well in the refrigerator or freezer. To store them in the refrigerator, allow them to cool on a wire rack and then store them in an airtight container for up to 5 days. To store them in the freezer, cool them completely on a wire rack and then transfer the individual pieces to a baking sheet placed in the freezer. Once they are frozen, toss them all in a bag and store them in the freezer.

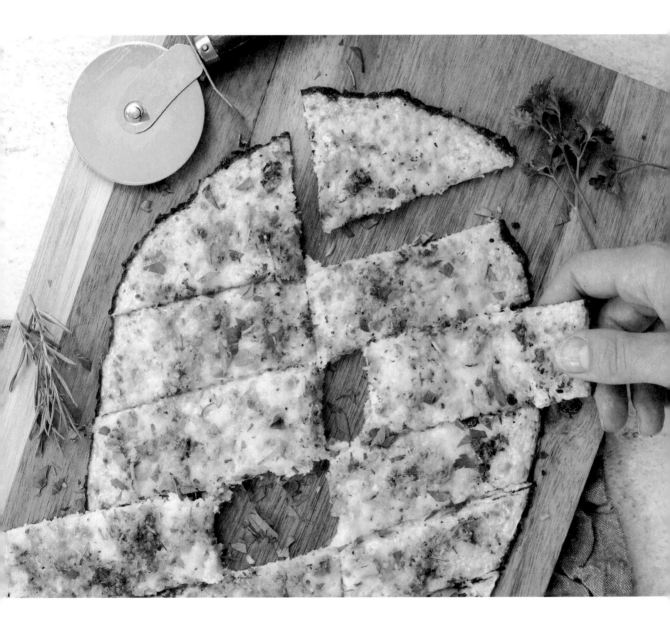

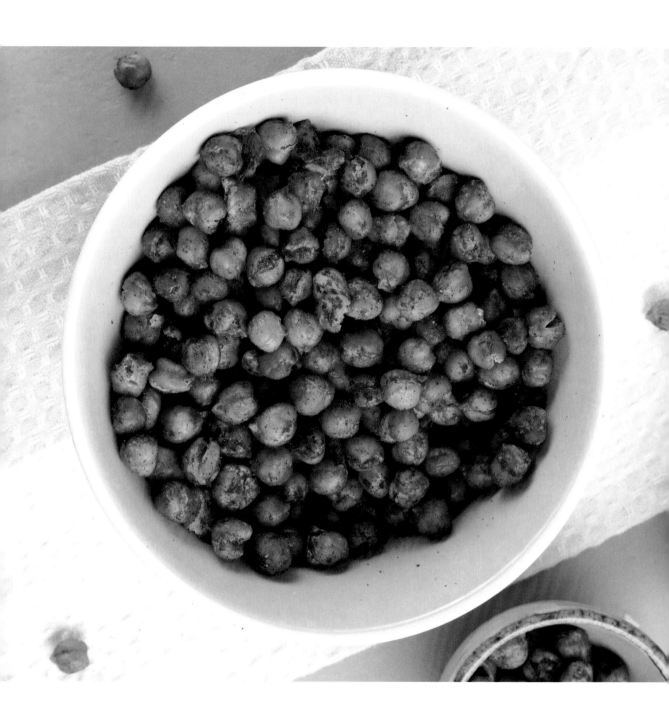

CINNAMON ROASTED CHICKPEAS

YIELDS 2 CUPS (¼ CUP PER SERVING)

Chickpeas might not be the first thing you think of now when you're looking for a sweet snack, but you will after you try this easy-to-make recipe that satisfies your sweet tooth while also providing protein and fiber.

INGREDIENTS

Two 15-ounce cans chickpeas, rinsed and drained

2 tablespoons coconut oil, melted

2 tablespoons ground cinnamon

½ teaspoon ground nutmeg

¼ cup granulated erythritol sweetener

DIRECTIONS

Preheat the oven to 400°F. Line a baking sheet with parchment paper and set it aside.

Place the chickpeas in a bowl and pour the oil on top. Toss to coat. Sprinkle the cinnamon, nutmeg, and erythritol on top and toss again to coat evenly.

Spread out the chickpeas on the prepared baking sheet.

Bake for 45 minutes, or until the chickpeas turn crunchy and golden brown.

Remove the chickpeas from the oven and allow them to cool before eating. You can divide the chickpeas into 8 separate containers for a pre-portioned snack to enjoy throughout the week.

Nutrition information per serving: 139 calories ▪ 4g fat ▪ 3g saturated fat ▪ **5g protein** ▪ **25g carbs** ▪ **1g sugar** ▪ 6g sugar alcohol ▪ 5g fiber ▪ 14g net carbs ▪ 0mg cholesterol ▪ 333mg sodium

SALTED TAHINI DARK CHOCOLATE FUDGE CUPS

YIELDS 12 CUPS (1 CUP PER SERVING)

Creamy tahini is combined with rich, dark chocolate in these decadent fudge cups. They make a great sweet treat for a guilt-free indulgence.

INGREDIENTS

½ cup tahini

2 bars sugar-free dark chocolate

¼ cup coconut oil

½ teaspoon vanilla extract

Coarse sea salt for topping

DIRECTIONS

Line a 12-cup muffin tin with silicone cups or paper cupcake liners.

Microwave the tahini, dark chocolate, and coconut oil together in 30-second increments, until the chocolate is melted.

Stir in the vanilla extract and pour the mixture into the prepared muffin tin. Sprinkle with salt and freeze for at least 2 hours.

Nutrition information per serving: 155 calories ▪ 15g fat ▪ 8g saturated fat ▪ **2g protein** ▪ **8g carbs** ▪ **0g sugar** ▪ 2g sugar alcohol ▪ 3g fiber ▪ 3g net carbs ▪ 0mg cholesterol ▪ 3mg sodium

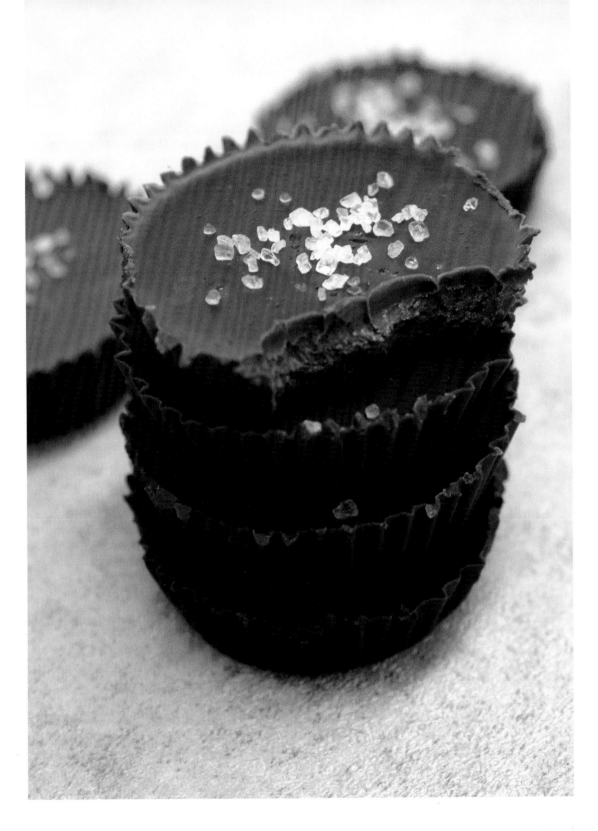

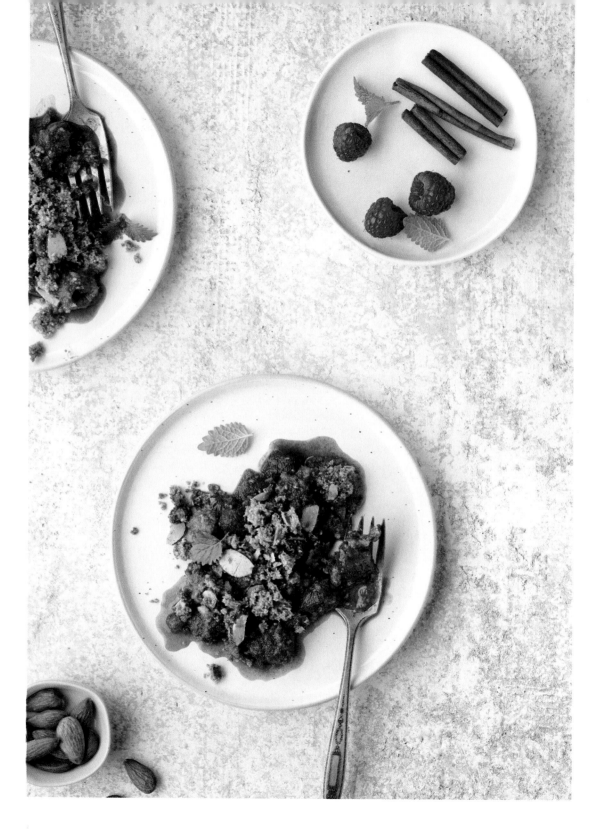

WARM RASPBERRY CRISP

YIELDS 8 SERVINGS (1 SQUARE PER SERVING)

Raspberries are naturally lower in net carbs than other fruit, so they're a great South Beach Diet keto-friendly choice for a warm fruit crisp. Topped with a crumbly almond flour and coconut topping and baked until bubbling, this dessert is just calling for a scoop of sugar-free ice cream!

INGREDIENTS

3 cups fresh raspberries
⅓ cup granulated erythritol sweetener
1 teaspoon vanilla extract

For the topping

⅔ cup almond flour
¼ cup sliced almonds
¼ cup shredded unsweetened coconut
¼ cup granulated erythritol sweetener
1 teaspoon cinnamon
4 tablespoons melted butter or coconut oil

DIRECTIONS

Preheat the oven to 350°F.

Mix the raspberries, erythritol, and vanilla in an 8-inch square baking dish. Spread evenly in the dish.

To make the topping, stir together all remaining ingredients in a bowl and then use your hands to crumble it over the berries.

Bake for 20 to 25 minutes, or until golden and bubbling. Allow the crisp to cool in the pan for 15 minutes. Cut into 8 squares and serve.

Nutrition information per serving: 163 calories ▪ 44g fat ▪ 8.7g saturated fat ▪ **2g protein** ▪ **22g carbs** ▪ **3g sugar** ▪ 13g sugar alcohol ▪ 5g fiber ▪ 4g net carbs ▪ 15mg cholesterol ▪ 46mg sodium

CHOCOLATE FREEZER FUDGE

YIELDS 16 SQUARES (1 SQUARE PER SERVING)

This super-creamy freezer fudge can be made with 6 basic
ingredients and lots of options for customization.

INGREDIENTS

1 cup almond butter

5 tablespoons coconut oil, melted

3 tablespoons cocoa powder

3 tablespoons granulated erythritol
sweetener

1 teaspoon vanilla extract

⅛ teaspoon sea salt

DIRECTIONS

Line a loaf pan with parchment paper and set it aside.

Whisk together all the ingredients and pour the mixture into
the prepared pan. Place the pan in the freezer for at least
30 minutes, or until set.

Use the parchment paper to lift the fudge out of the pan.
Cut it into 16 squares. Store the fudge in the freezer for a
firm texture, or the refrigerator for a softer texture.

TIP

Top with your favorite nuts, use peanut butter
instead of almond butter, or swap in other
extracts (such as almond or maple instead of
vanilla) for endless fudge flavor varieties!

Nutrition information per serving: 137 calories ▪ 13g fat ▪ 4g saturated fat ▪ **3g protein** ▪ **6g carbs** ▪ **1g sugar**
▪ 2g sugar alcohol ▪ 2g fiber ▪ 1g net carbs ▪ 0mg cholesterol ▪ 20mg sodium

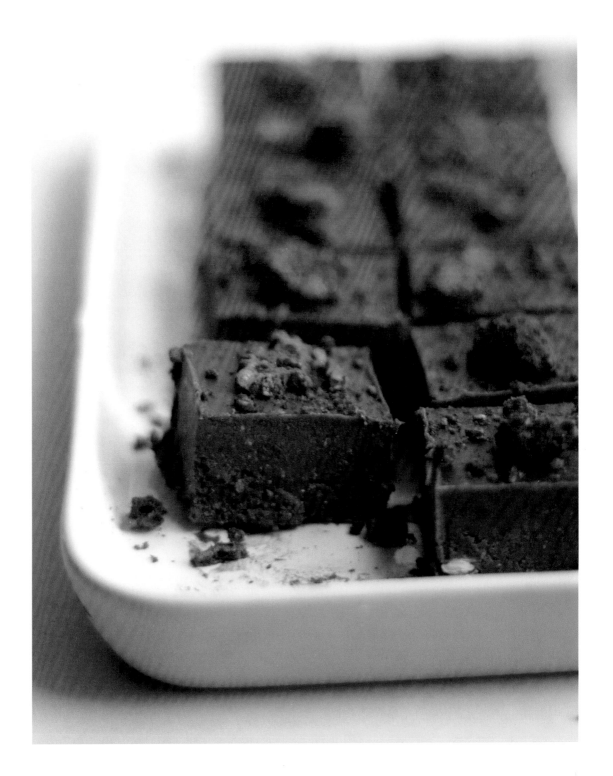

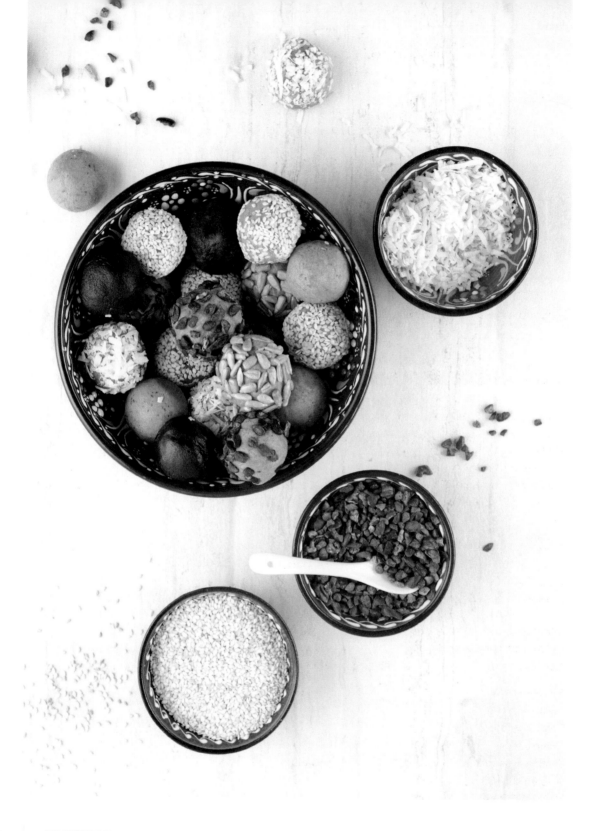

PEANUT BUTTER & TAHINI PROTEIN BITES

YIELDS 24 BALLS (1 BALL PER SERVING)

An energy-boosting snack at any time of day, these delicious
bites are also the perfect after-dinner treat.

INGREDIENTS

1 cup unsalted unsweetened
natural peanut butter

¼ cup tahini

1 tablespoon MCT oil

½ cup coconut flour (plus 1 to 2
tablespoons, if needed)

2 tablespoons ground flaxseeds

½ teaspoon cinnamon

2 scoops (about 4 tablespoons) keto-
friendly vanilla protein powder

2 scoops (about 4 tablespoons)
collagen peptides

2 tablespoons powdered erythritol
sweetener

¼ teaspoon Himalayan pink salt

Choose from among the following for an optional garnish:

Sesame seeds

Cacao nibs

Carob powder

Hemp seeds

Sunflower seeds

Toasted shredded
unsweetened coconut

DIRECTIONS

Line a flat serving platter or a baking sheet with parchment
paper and set it aside.

Mix together the peanut butter, tahini, and MCT oil in a
large bowl until smooth.

Add the coconut flour, flaxseeds, cinnamon, protein powder, collagen peptides, erythritol, and salt; stir thoroughly.

Scoop out a rounded tablespoon of the mixture and form
it into a ball; roll it onto the desired garnish, and place it on
the prepared baking sheet. Repeat until all the mixture has
been used (approximately 24 balls).

Place the balls in the freezer and let them chill for about 10
minutes, or until firm. The balls are best stored in an airtight
container in the freezer and can be kept for up to 2 months.

Nutrition information per serving: 108 calories ▪ 8g fat
▪ 2.1g saturated fat ▪ **6g protein** ▪ **6g carbs** ▪ **1g sugar**
▪ 1g sugar alcohol ▪ 2g fiber ▪ 3g net carbs ▪ 1mg cholesterol
▪ 40mg sodium

KETO BROWNIES

YIELDS 9 BROWNIES (1 BROWNIE PER SERVING)

Find your brownie nirvana with these chocolaty brownies
bursting with chocolate chips and a touch of spice.

INGREDIENTS

1 cup sugar-free chocolate chips, divided

⅔ cup butter, melted

½ cup powdered erythritol sweetener

2 eggs

1 teaspoon vanilla extract

2 tablespoons coconut flour

2 tablespoons cacao powder

1 teaspoon sea salt

DIRECTIONS

Preheat the oven to 350°F. Line an 8-inch square baking dish with parchment paper and set it aside.

In a double boiler, or in the microwave, melt ½ cup of the chocolate chips.

Whisk the butter and erythritol together in a large mixing bowl with an electric mixer until combined.

Add the eggs and vanilla extract. Beat for 1 minute to combine.

Add the melted chocolate and stir until it is incorporated.

Whisk together the coconut flour, cacao powder, and salt in a separate bowl.

Add the coconut flour mixture to the chocolate mixture. Stir until just combined. Do not overmix.

Fold in the remaining chocolate chips.

Transfer the batter to the prepared baking dish and smooth it into an even layer.

Bake for 25 to 30 minutes, until set.

Allow the brownies to cool in the pan for 30 minutes. Lift the parchment paper to remove the brownies from the baking dish. Slice them into 9 squares, and enjoy.

Note: Brownies may be stored in an airtight container in the refrigerator for 4 to 5 days. For long-term storage, freeze individual brownies on a baking sheet lined with parchment paper. Once they are frozen, they may be stored together in a large freezer-safe bag.

Nutrition information per serving: 231 calories ▪ 21g fat ▪ 13g saturated fat ▪ **3g protein** ▪ **34g carbs** ▪ **0g sugar** ▪ 29g sugar alcohol ▪ 3g fiber ▪ 2g net carbs ▪ 78mg cholesterol ▪ 282mg sodium

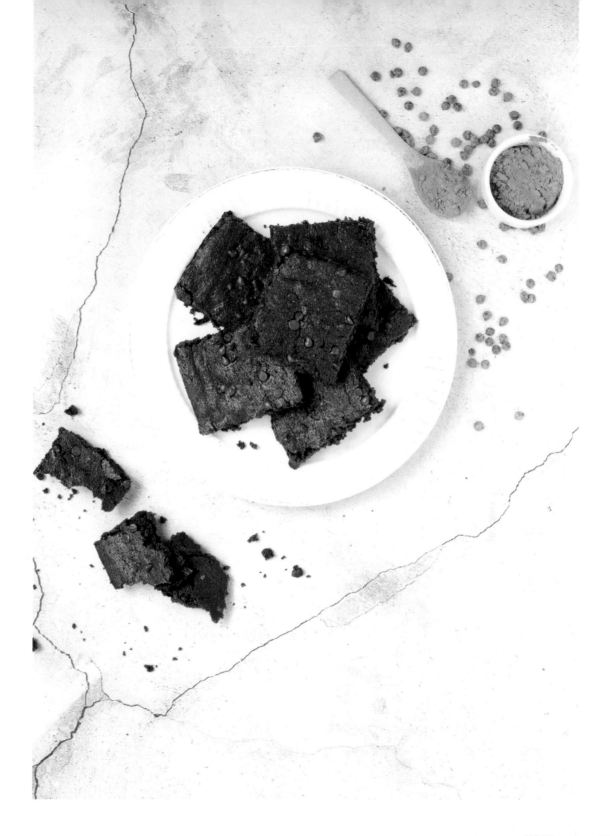

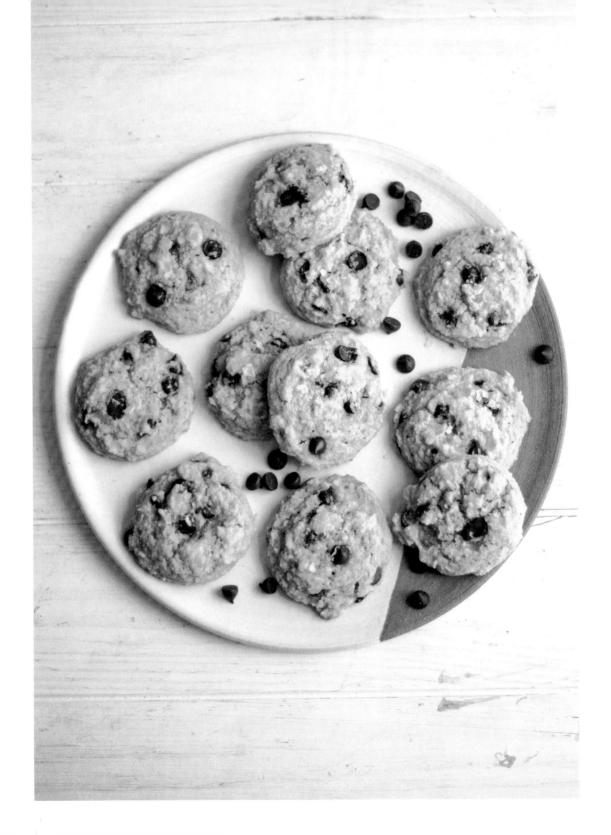

CHOCOLATE CHIP COOKIES

YIELDS 16 COOKIES (1 COOKIE PER SERVING)

These tender, soft baked cookies are made with almond flour for a South Beach Diet keto-friendly version of the classic. Be sure to buy sugar-free chocolate chips, or chop up a bar of sugar-free chocolate to make chocolate chunk cookies!

INGREDIENTS

⅓ cup coconut oil, melted

2 large eggs

½ cup granulated erythritol sweetener

2 teaspoons vanilla extract

1½ cups almond flour

1 teaspoon baking soda

½ teaspoon baking powder

¼ teaspoon sea salt

½ cup sugar-free chocolate chips

DIRECTIONS

Preheat the oven to 350°F. Line a baking sheet with parchment paper.

Whisk together the coconut oil, eggs, erythritol, and vanilla extract in a mixing bowl. Add the almond flour, baking soda, baking powder, salt, and chocolate chips. Stir well to fully combine.

Scoop the cookie dough by heaping tablespoons onto the prepared baking sheet, leaving at least 1 inch of space between each cookie until all the mixture has been used (approximately 16 cookies).

Bake for 8 to 10 minutes, or until the cookies are just barely cooked through. Since these cookies don't have sugar in them, they won't turn golden brown in the oven like traditional cookies do. Instead, keep an eye out for firm edges and still-soft centers to know when they're done.

Allow the cookies to cool for 10 minutes on the baking sheet before serving.

Nutrition information per serving: 93 calories ▪ 8g fat ▪ 5g saturated fat ▪ **2g protein** ▪ **11g carbs** ▪ **0g sugar** ▪ 10g sugar alcohol ▪ 1g fiber ▪ 0g net carbs ▪ 23mg cholesterol ▪ 45mg sodium

PEANUT BUTTER CUPS

YIELDS 6 CUPS (1 CUP PER SERVING)

This sugar-free take on the classic candy couldn't be easier to make and is filled with a thick layer of creamy peanut butter!

INGREDIENTS

⅓ cup cocoa powder

½ cup coconut oil, melted

2 tablespoons granulated erythritol sweetener

¼ teaspoon vanilla extract

6 tablespoons unsweetened natural peanut butter

Coarse sea salt, for topping (optional)

DIRECTIONS

Line a 6-count muffin tin with paper cupcake liners.

Whisk together the cocoa, coconut oil, erythritol, and vanilla extract in a small bowl. Scoop 1 rounded tablespoon of the cocoa mixture into the bottom of each muffin cup.

Place the muffin tin in the freezer and leave it for 5 minutes to allow the chocolate to solidify.

Scoop 1 tablespoon of the peanut butter into each muffin cup, spreading it into an even layer. Top with another tablespoon of the cocoa mixture.

Freeze the peanut butter cups for another 5 minutes. Top each with a pinch of coarse sea salt (if desired). Serve immediately or transfer to a container in the refrigerator to store for up to 1 week.

Nutrition information per serving: 262 calories ▪ 27g fat ▪ 18g saturated fat ▪ **5g protein** ▪ **14g carbs** ▪ **2g sugar** ▪ 4g sugar alcohol ▪ 2g fiber ▪ 7g net carbs ▪ 0mg cholesterol ▪ 74mg sodium

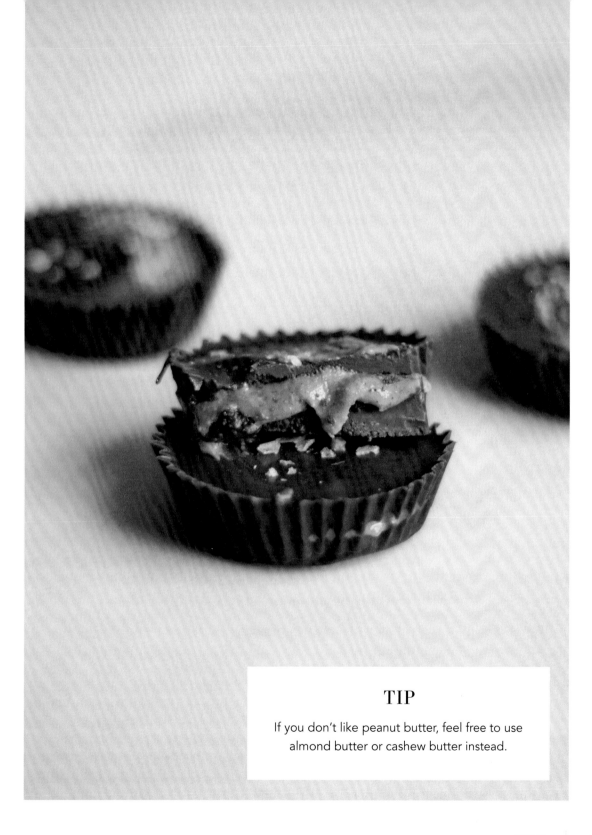

TIP

If you don't like peanut butter, feel free to use almond butter or cashew butter instead.

CHOCOLATE CHIP COOKIE DOUGH BITES

YIELDS 12 BALLS (1 BALL PER SERVING)

These cookie dough bites taste like eating cold, creamy cookie dough straight from the fridge! Cashew butter is used here for its neutral flavor, but this recipe is equally delicious made with almond butter or peanut butter.

INGREDIENTS

½ cup cashew butter

2 tablespoons coconut oil, melted

2 tablespoons granulated erythritol sweetener

½ teaspoon vanilla extract

¼ cup coconut flour

¼ teaspoon sea salt

2 tablespoons sugar-free chocolate chips

DIRECTIONS

Stir together the cashew butter, coconut oil, erythritol, and vanilla extract in a small bowl. Add all the remaining ingredients and stir well to combine.

Transfer the bowl to the refrigerator to chill for 15 to 20 minutes, or until firm.

Using a heaping tablespoon, portion the cookie dough into 12 balls.

Place the balls in a container with a lid and store them in the refrigerator for up to 1 week.

TIP

For a shortcut, try spreading the mixture into a parchment-lined loaf pan, chill it until firm, and instead of rolling it into balls, cut it into 12 squares.

Nutrition information per serving: 106 calories ▪ 8g fat ▪ 4g saturated fat ▪ **3g protein** ▪ **6g carbs** ▪ **0g sugar** ▪ 1g sugar alcohol ▪ 2g fiber ▪ 3g net carbs ▪ 0mg cholesterol ▪ 62mg sodium

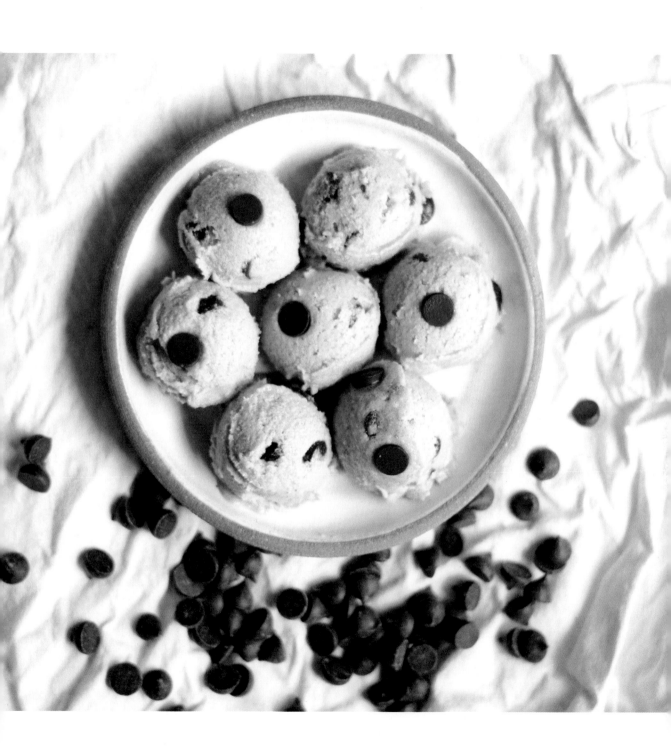

CONVERSION CHARTS

The recipes in this book use the standard United States method for measuring liquid and dry or solid ingredients (teaspoons, tablespoons, and cups). The following charts are provided to help cooks outside the U.S. successfully use these recipes. All equivalents are approximate.

STANDARD CUP	FINE POWDER (e.g., flour)	GRAIN (e.g., rice)	GRANULAR (e.g., sugar)	LIQUID SOLIDS (e.g., butter)	LIQUID (e.g., milk)
1	140 g	150 g	190 g	200 g	240 ml
¾	105 g	113 g	143 g	150 g	180 ml
⅔	93 g	100 g	125 g	133 g	160 ml
½	70 g	75 g	95 g	100 g	120 ml
⅓	47 g	50 g	63 g	67 g	80 ml
¼	35 g	38 g	48 g	50 g	60 ml
⅛	18 g	19 g	24 g	25 g	30 ml

USEFUL EQUIVALENTS FOR LIQUID INGREDIENTS BY VOLUME				
¼ tsp			1 ml	
½ tsp			2 ml	
1 tsp			5 ml	
3 tsp	1 tbsp		½ fl oz	15 ml
	2 tbsp	⅛ cup	1 fl oz	30 ml
	4 tbsp	¼ cup	2 fl oz	60 ml
	5 ⅓ tbsp	⅓ cup	3 fl oz	80 ml
	8 tbsp	½ cup	4 fl oz	120 ml
	10 ⅔ tbsp	⅔ cup	5 fl oz	160 ml
	12 tbsp	¾ cup	6 fl oz	180 ml
	16 tbsp	1 cup	8 fl oz	240 ml
	1 pt	2 cups	16 fl oz	480 ml
	1 qt	4 cups	32 fl oz	960 ml
			33 fl oz	1000 ml 1 l

USEFUL EQUIVALENTS FOR DRY INGREDIENTS BY WEIGHT		
(To convert ounces to grams, multiply the number of ounces by 30.)		
1 oz	$\frac{1}{16}$ lb	30 g
4 oz	$\frac{1}{4}$ lb	120 g
8 oz	$\frac{1}{2}$ lb	240 g
12 oz	$\frac{3}{4}$ lb	360 g
16 oz	1 lb	480 g

USEFUL EQUIVALENTS FOR COOKING/OVEN TEMPERATURES			
Process	Fahrenheit	Celsius	Gas Mark
Freeze Water	32° F	0° C	
Room Temperature	68° F	20° C	
Boil Water	212° F	100° C	
Bake	325° F	160° C	3
	350° F	180° C	4
	375° F	190° C	5
	400° F	200° C	6
	425° F	220° C	7
	450° F	230° C	8
Broil			Grill

USEFUL EQUIVALENTS FOR LENGTH				
(To convert inches to centimeters, multiply the number of inches by 2.5.)				
1 in			2.5 cm	
6 in	1/2 ft		15 cm	
12 in	1 ft		30 cm	
36 in	3 ft	1 yd	90 cm	
40 in			100 cm	1 m

REFERENCES

CHAPTER 1

Avena, N. M., P. Rada, and B. G. H. Hoebel. Evidence for sugar addiction: Behavioral and neurochemical effects of intermittent, excessive sugar intake. *Neuroscience and Biobehavioral Reviews* 32, no. 1 (May 18, 2007): 20–39. https://doi.org/10.1016/j.neubiorev.2007.04.019

Davey, C. G., M. Yu, and N. B. Allen. The emergence of depression in adolescence: Development of the prefrontal cortex and the representation of reward. *Neuroscience and Biobehavioral Reviews* 32, no. 1 (May 16, 2007): 1–19. https://doi.org/10.1016/j.neubiorev.2007.04.016

Lenoir, M., F. Serre, L. Cantin, and S. H. Ahmed. Intense sweetness surpasses cocaine reward. *PLoS ONE* 2, no. 8 (August 1, 2007): e98. https://doi.org/10.1371/journal.pone.0000698

Page, K. A., O. Chan, G. W. Cline, S. Naik, R. T. Constable, and R. S. Sherwin. Effects of fructose vs glucose on regional cerebral blood flow in brain regions involved with appetite and reward pathways. *JAMA* 309, no. 17 (January 2, 2013): 63–70. https://www.ncbi.nlm.nih.gov/pubmed/23280226

Wiss, D. A., N. Avena, and P. Rada. Sugar addiction: From evolution to revolution. *Frontiers in Psychiatry* 9 (November 7, 2018): 1–16. https://doi.org/10.3389/fpsyt.2018.00545

CHAPTER 2

Aude, Y. W., A. S. Agatston, F. Lopez-Jimenez, E. H. Lieberman, M. Almon, M. Hansen, G. Rojas et al. The National Cholesterol Education Program Diet vs a diet lower in carbohydrates and higher in protein and monounsaturated fat: A randomized trial. *Archives of Internal Medicine* 164, no. 19 (October 25, 2004): 2141–46. https://doi.org/10.1001/archinte.164.19.2141

Avena, N. M. et al. Evidence for sugar addiction: Behavioral and neurochemical effects of intermittent, excessive sugar intake.

Cefalu, W. T., M. P. Petersen, and R. E. Ratner. The alarming and rising costs of diabetes and prediabetes: A call for action! *Diabetes Care* 37 (December 2014): 3137–38. https://doi.org/10.2337/dc14-2329

Dall, T. M., W. Yang, P. Halder, B. Pang, M. Massoudi, N. Wintfeld, A. P. Semilla, J. Franz, and P. F. Hogan. The economic burden of elevated blood glucose levels in 2012: Diagnosed and undiagnosed diabetes, gestational diabetes. *Diabetes Care* 37 (December 2014): 3172–79. https://doi.org/10.2337/dc14-1036

Davey, Yu, and Allen. The emergence of depression in adolescence: Development of the prefrontal cortex and the representation of reward.

Hallberg, S., A. L. McKenzie, P. T. Williams, S. D. Phinney, and J. S. Volek. Effectiveness and safety of a novel care model for the management of type 2 diabetes at 1 year: An open-label, non-randomized, controlled study. *Diabetes Therapy* 9, no. 2 (April 2018): 583–612. https://www.ncbi.nlm.nih.gov/pubmed/29417495

Hollar, D., S. E. Messiah, G. Lopez-Mitnik, T. L. Hollar, M. Almon, and A. S. Agatston. Healthier options for public schoolchildren program improves weight and blood pressure in 6- to 13-year-olds. *Journal of the Academy of Nutrition and Dietetics* 110, no. 2 (February 2010): 261–67. https://doi.org/10.1016/j.jada.2009.10.029

Page, K. A. et al. Effects of fructose vs glucose on regional cerebral blood flow in brain regions involved with appetite and reward pathways.

Saslow, L. R., J. Daubenmier, J. T. Moskowitz, S. Kim, E. J. Murphy, S. D. Phinney, R. Ploutz-Snyder et al. Twelve-month outcomes of a randomized trial of a moderate-carbohydrate versus very low-carbohydrate diet in overweight adults with Type 2 diabetes mellitus or prediabetes. *Nutrition and Diabetes* 7, article 304 (December 21, 2017): 1–6. https://doi.org/10.1038/s41387-017-0006-9

Shai, I., D. Schwarzfuchs, Y. Henkin, D. R. Shahar, S. Witkow, I. Greenberg, R. Golan et al. Weight loss with a low-carbohydrate, Mediterranean, or low-fat diet. *New England Journal of Medicine* 359, no. 3 (July 17, 2008): 229–41. https://www.nejm.org/doi/full/10.1056/NEJMoa0708681

Wiss, D. A. et al. Sugar addiction: From evolution to revolution.

CHAPTER 3

Ayashi, T. O. H. Patterns of insulin concentration during the OGTT predict the risk of type 2 diabetes in Japanese Americans. *Diabetes Care* 36, no. 5 (October 2013): 1229–35. https://doi.org/10.2337/dc12-0246

Bancks, M. P., A. O. Odegaard, J. S. Pankow, W. Koh, J. Yuan, and M. D. Gross. Glycated hemoglobin and all-cause and cause-specific mortality in Singaporean Chinese without diagnosed diabetes: The Singapore Chinese Health Study. *Diabetes Care* 37, no. 12 (December 2014): 3180–87. https://doi.org/10.2337/dc14-0390

Borg, R., J. C. Kuenen, B. Carstensen, H. Zheng, D. M. Nathan, and R. J. Heine. Real-life glycaemic profiles in non-diabetic individuals with low fasting glucose and normal HbA1c: The A1C-Derived Average Glucose (ADAG) study. *Diabetologica* 53, no. 8 (August 2010): 1608–11. https://doi.org/10.1007/s00125-010-1741-9

Chang, A. M., and J. B. Halter. Aging and insulin secretion. *American Journal of Physiology Endocrinology and Metabolism* 284, no. 4 (January 2003): 7–12. https://www.ncbi.nlm.nih.gov/pubmed/12485807

England, T. N. Prevention of type 2 diabetes mellitus by changes in lifestyle among subjects with impaired glucose tolerance. *New England Journal of Medicine* 344, no. 18 (May 3, 2001): 1343–50. https://www.ncbi.nlm.nih.gov/pubmed/11333990

Gyberg, V., D. De Bacquer, K. Kotseva, G. De Backer, O. Schnell, J. Sundvall, J. Tuomilehto, D. Wood, and L. Rydén. Disease management screening for dysglycaemia in patients with coronary artery disease as reflected by fasting glucose, oral glucose tolerance test, and HbA1c: a report from EUROASPIRE IV—a survey from the European Society of Cardiology. *European Heart Journal* 36, no. 19 (May 14, 2015): 1171–77. https://doi.org/10.1093/eurheartj/ehv008

Hall, H., D. Perelman, A. Breschi, P. Limcaoco, R. Kellogg, T. McLaughlin, and M. Snyder. Glucotypes reveal new patterns of glucose dysregulation. *PLoS Biology* 16, no. 7 (July 24, 2018): 1–23. https://www.ncbi.nlm.nih.gov/pubmed/30040822

Meigs, J. B., M. G. Larson, R. B. D'Agostino, D. Levy, M. E. Clouse, D. M. Nathan, P. W. Wilson, and C. J. O'Connell. Coronary artery calcification in Type 2 diabetes and insulin resistance: The Framingham Offspring Study. *Diabetes Care* 25, no. 8 (August 2002), 1313–19. https://www.ncbi.nlm.nih.gov/pubmed/12145227

Menke, A., S. Casagrande, L. Geiss, and C. C. Cowie. Prevalence of and trends in diabetes among adults in the United States, 1988–2012. *Journal of the American Medical Association* 314, no.10 (September 8, 2015): 1021–29. https://doi.org/10.1001/jama.2015.10029

Mensink, M., E. E. Blaak, M. A. van Baak, A. J. Wagenmakers, and W. H. Saris. Plasma free fatty acid uptake and oxidation are already diminished in subjects at high risk for developing Type 2 diabetes. *Diabetes* 50, no. 11 (November 2001): 2548–54. https://www.ncbi.nlm.nih.gov/pubmed/11679433

Nathan, D. M., M. B. Davidson, R. A. DeFronzo, R. J. Heine, R. R. Henry, R. Pratley, and B. Zinman. Impaired fasting glucose and impaired glucose tolerance: Implications for care. *Diabetes Care* 30, no. 3 (March 2007): 753–59. https://doi.org/10.2337/dc07-9920

Pratipanawatr, W., T. Pratipanawatr, K. Cusi, R. Berria, J. M. Adams, C. P. Jenkinson, K. Maezono, R. A. DeFronzo, and L. J. Mandarino. Skeletal muscle insulin resistance in normoglycemic subjects with a strong family history of type 2 diabetes is associated with decreased insulin-stimulated insulin receptor substrate-1 tyrosine phosphorylation. *Diabetes* 50, no. 11 (November 2001): 2572–78. https://www.ncbi.nlm.nih.gov/pubmed/11679436

Pyörälä, M., H. Miettinen, M. Laakso, and K. Pyörälä. Hyperinsulinemia predicts coronary heart disease risk in the 22-year rollow-up results of the Helsinki Policemen Study. *Circulation* 98, no. 5 (August 4, 1998): 398–404. https://www.ncbi.nlm.nih.gov/pubmed/9714089

Rasmussen-Torvik, L. J., M. Li, W. H. Kao, D. Couper, E. Boerwinkle, S. J. Bielinski, A. R. Folsom, and J. S. Pankow. Association of a fasting glucose genetic risk score with subclinical atherosclerosis: The Atherosclerosis Risk in Communities (ARIC) Study. *Diabetes* 60, no. 1 (January 2011): 331–35. https://doi.org/10.2337/db10-0839

Reaven, G. (2012). Insulin resistance and coronary heart disease in nondiabetic individuals. *Arteriosclerosis, Thrombosis, and Vascular Biology* 32 (August 1, 2012): 1754–59. https://doi.org/10.1161/ATVBAHA.111.241885

Retnakaran, R., Y. Qi, M. Sermer, P. W. Connelly, A. J. G. Hanley, and B. Zinman. An abnormal screening glucose challenge test in pregnancy predicts postpartum metabolic dysfunction, even when the antepartum oral glucose tolerance test is normal. *Clinical Endocrinology* 71, no. 2 (July 6, 2009): 208–14. https://doi.org/10.1111/j.1365-2265.2008.03460.x

Rigano, K. S., J. L. Gehring, B. D. Evans Hutzenbiler, A. V. Chen, O. L. Nelson, C. A. Vella, C. T. Robbins, and H. T. Jansen. Life in the fat lane: seasonal regulation of insulin sensitivity, food intake, and adipose biology in brown bears. *Journal of Comparative Physiology B* 187, no. 4 (May 2017): 649–76. https://doi.org/10.1007/s00360-016-1050-9

Soleimani, M. Insulin resistance and hypertension: New insights. *Kidney International* 87, no. 3 (March 2015): 497–99. https://doi.org/10.1038/ki.2014.392

Utzschneider, K. M., R. L. Prigeon, M. V. Faulenbach, J. Tong, D. B. Carr, E. J. Boyko, D. L. Leonetti et al. Oral disposition index predicts the development of future diabetes above and beyond fasting and 2-h glucose levels. *Diabetes Care* 32, no. 2 (February 2009): 335–41. https://doi.org/10.2337/dc08-1478

CHAPTER 4

Abdelmalek, M. F., and C. Day. Sugar sweetened beverages and fatty liver disease: Rising concern and call to action. Editorial. *Journal of Hepatology* 63, no. 2 (August 2015): 306–8. https://doi.org/10.1016/j. jhep.2015.05.021

Agatston, A. S., W. R. Janowitz, F. J. Hildner, N. R. Zusmer, M. Viamonte, and R. Detrano. Quantification of coronary artery calcium using ultrafast computed tomography. *Journal of the American College of Cardiology* 15, no. 4 (March 15, 1990): 827–32. https://doi.org/10.1016/0735-1097(90)90282-T

Bergeron, N., S. Chiu, P. T. Williams, S. M. King, and R. M. Krauss. Effects of red meat, white meat, and nonmeat protein sources on atherogenic lipoprotein measures in the context of low compared with high saturated fat intake: A randomized controlled trial. *American Journal of Clinical Nutrition* 110, no. 1 (June 4, 2019): 24–33. https://www.ncbi.nlm.nih.gov/pubmed/31161217

Blasbalg, T. L., J. R. Hibbeln, C. E. Ramsden, S. F. Majchrzak, and R. R. Rawlings. Changes in consumption of omega-3 and omega-6 fatty acids in the United States during the 20th century. *American Journal of Clinical Nutrition* 93, no. 5 (May 2011): 950–62. https://www.ncbi.nlm.nih.gov/pubmed/21367944

Cali, A. M, A. M. De Oliveira, H. Kim, S. Chen, M. Reyes-Mugica, S. Escalera, J. Dziura, S. E. Taksali et al. Glucose dysregulation and hepatic steatosis in obese adolescents: Is there a link? *Hepatology* 49, no. 6 (June 2009): 1896. https://doi.org/10.1002/hep.22858

Carrel, G., L. Eglie, C. Tran, P. Schneiter, V. Giusti, D. D'Alessio, and L. Tappy. Contributions of fat and protein to the incretin effect of a mixed meal. *American Journal of Clinical Nutrition* 94, no. 4 (October 2011): 997–1003. https://academic.oup.com/ajcn/article/94/4/997/4598165

Chazelas, E., B. Srour, E. Desmetz, E. Kesse-Guyot, C. Julia, V. Deschamps, N. Druesne-Pecollo et al. Sugary drink consumption and risk of cancer: Results from NutriNet-Santé prospective cohort. *British Medical Journal* 365 (July 10, 2019): 1–13. https://doi.org/10.1136/bmj.l2408

Cox, C. L., K. L. Stanhope, J. M. Schwarz,, J. L. Graham, B. Hatcher, S. C. Griffen, A. A. Bremer et al. Consumption of fructose-sweetened beverages for 10 weeks reduces net fat oxidation and energy expenditure in overweight/obese men and women. *European Journal of Clinical Nutrition* 66, no. 2 (September 28, 2011): 201–8. https://doi.org/10.1038/ejcn.2011.159

Cunnane, S. C., A. Courchesne-Loyer, C. Vandenberghe, V. St-Pierre, M. Fortier, M. Hennebelle, E. Croteau et al. Can ketones help rescue brain fuel supply in later life? Implications for cognitive health during aging and the treatment of Alzheimer's disease. *Frontiers in Molecular Neuroscience* 9 (July 8, 2016): 1–21. https://doi.org/10.3389/fnmol.2016.00053

DeFronzo, R. A. Insulin resistance, lipotoxicity, type 2 diabetes and atherosclerosis: The missing links. The Claude Bernard Lecture 2009. *Diaberologia* 53, no. 7 (July 2010): 1270–87. https://doi.org/10.1007/s00125-010-1684-1

DeFronzo, R. A., and M. A. Abdul-Ghani. Preservation of β-cell function: The key to diabetes prevention. *Journal of Clinical Endocrinology and Metabolism* 96, no. 8 (August 1, 2011): 2354–66. https://doi.org/10.1210/jc.2011-0246

DiNicolantonio, J. J. and J. H. O'Keefe. Importance of maintaining a low omega–6/omega–3 ratio for reducing inflammation. *Open Heart* 5, no. 2 (November 26, 2018). https://doi.org/10.1136/openhrt-2018-000946

DiNicolantonio, J. J., and J. H. O'Keefe. Omega-6 vegetable oils as a driver of coronary heart disease: the oxidized linoleic acid hypothesis. *Open Heart* 5, no. 2 (September 26, 2018): 1–6. https://doi.org/10.1136/openhrt-2018-000898

Dusilová, T. J. Kovář, M. Drobný, P. Šedivý, M. Dezortová, R. Poledne, K. Zemánková, and M. Hájek. Different acute effects of fructose and glucose administration on hepatic fat content. *American Journal of Clinical Nutrition* 109, no. 6 (June 2019): 1519–26. https://doi.org/10.1093/ajcn/nqy386

Eelderink, C., S. Rietsema, I. M. Y. van Vliet, L. C. Loef, T. Boer, M. Koehorst, I. M. Nolte et al. The effect of high compared with low dairy consumption on glucose metabolism, insulin sensitivity, and metabolic flexibility in overweight adults: a randomized crossover trial. *American Journal of Clinical Nutrition* 109, no. 6 (June 1, 2019): 1555–68. https://www.ncbi.nlm.nih.gov/pubmed/30997492

Fabbrini, E., F. Magkos, B. S. Mohammed, T. Pietka, N. A. Abumrad, B. W. Patterson, A. Okunade, and S. Klein. Intrahepatic fat, not visceral fat, is linked with metabolic complications of obesity. *Proceedings of the National Academy of Sciences of the United States of America* 106, no. 36 (September 8, 2009): 15430–35. https://www.ncbi.nlm.nih.gov/pubmed/19706383

Gunter, M. J., X. Xie, X. Xue, G. C. Kabat, T. E. Rohan, S. Wassertheil-Smoller, G. Y. F. Ho et al. Breast cancer risk in metabolically healthy but overweight postmenopausal women. *Cancer Research* 75, no. 2 (January 2015): 270–75. https://doi.org/10.1158/0008-5472.CAN-14-2317

Haffner, S. M., L. Mykka, A. Festa, J. P. Burke, and M. P. Stern. Insulin-resistant prediabetic subjects have more atherogenic risk factors than insulin-sensitive prediabetic subjects: Implications for preventing coronary heart disease during the prediabetic state. *Circulation* 101, no. 9 (March 7, 2000): 975–80. https://www.ncbi.nlm.nih.gov/pubmed/10704163

Hammarstedt, A., T. E. Graham, and B. B. Kahn. Adipose tissue dysregulation and reduced insulin sensitivity in non-obese individuals with enlarged abdominal adipose cells. *Diabetology& Metabolic Syndrome* 4, no. 1 (September 19, 2012): 1–9. https://www.ncbi.nlm.nih.gov/pubmed/22992414

Heni, M., J. Machann, H. Staiger, N. F. Schwenzer, A. Peter, F Schick, C. D. Claussen, N. Stefan, H. U. Häring, and A. Fritsche. Pancreatic fat is negatively associated with insulin secretion in individuals with impaired fasting glucose and/or impaired glucose tolerance: A nuclear magnetic resonance study. *Diabetes / Metabolism Research and Reviews* 26, no. 3 (March 2010): 200–205. https://www.ncbi.nlm.nih.gov/pubmed/20225188

Joshi, P. H., B. Patel, M. J. Blaha, J. D. Berry, R. Blankstein, M. J. Budoff, N. Wong, A. Agatston, R. S. Blumenthal, and K. Nasir. Coronary artery calcium predicts cardiovascular events in participants with a low lifetime risk of cardiovascular disease: The Multi-Ethnic Study of Atherosclerosis (MESA). *Atherosclerosis* 246 (March 2016): 367–73. https://doi.org/10.1016/j.atherosclerosis.2016.01.017

Juntunen, K. S., L. K. Niskanen, K. H. Liukkonen, K. S. Poutanen, J. J. Holst, and H. M. Mykkänen. Postprandial glucose, insulin, and incretin responses to grain products in healthy subjects. *American Journal of Clinical Nutrition* 75, no. 2 (February 2002): 254–62. https://www.ncbi.nlm.nih.gov/pubmed/11815315

Kaplan, H., R. C. Thompson, B. C. Trumble, L. S. Wann, A. H. Allam, B. Beheim, B. Frolich et al. Coronary atherosclerosis in indigenous South American Tsimane: A cross-sectional cohort study. *The Lancet* 389, no. 10080 (March 17, 2017): 1730–39. https://www.ncbi.nlm.nih.gov/pubmed/28320601

Li, N., J. Fu, D. P. Koonen, J. Albert, H. Snieder, and M. H. Hofker. Are hypertriglyceridemia and low HDL causal factors in the development of insulin resistance? *Atherosclerosis* 233, no. 1 (March 2014): 130–38. https://doi.org/10.1016/j.atherosclerosis.2013.12.013

Lim, J. S., M. Mietus-Snyder, A. Valente, J. Schwarz, and R. H. Lustig. The role of fructose in the pathogenesis of naFID and the metabolic syndrome. *Nature Reviews Gastroenterology & Hepatology* 7 (April 6, 2010): 251–64. https://doi.org/10.1038/nrgastro.2010.41

Ma, J., C. S. Fox, P. F. Jacques, E. K. Speliotes, U. Hoffmann, C. E. Smith, E. Saltzman, and N. M. McKeown. Sugar-sweetened beverage, diet soda, and fatty liver disease in the Framingham Heart Study cohorts. *Journal of Hepatology* 63, no. 2 (August 2015): 462–69. https://doi.org/10.1016/j.jhep.2015.03.032

Mathur, A., M. Marine, D. Lu, D. A. Swartz-Basile, R. Saxena, N. J. Zyromski, and H. A. Pitt. Nonalcoholic fatty pancreas disease. *HPB* 9, no. 4 (August 2007): 312–18. https://doi.org/10.1080/13651820701504157

McQuaid, S. E., L. Hodson, M. J. Neville, A. L. Dennis, J. Cheeseman, S. M. Humphreys, T. Ruge et al. Down-regulation of adipose tissue fatty acid trafficking. *Diabetes* 60, no. 1 (January 2011): 47–55. https://doi.org/10.2337/db10-0867

Meier, J. J., K. Hücking, J. J. Holst, C. F. Deacon, W. H. Schmiegel, and M. A. Nauck. Reduced insulinotropic effect of gastric inhibitory polypeptide in first-degree relatives of patients with type 2 diabetes. *Diabetes* 50 (November 2001): 2497–2504. https://diabetes.diabetesjournals.org/content/diabetes/50/11/2497.full.pdf

Miedema, M. D., Z. A. Dardari, K. Nasir, R. Blankstein, T. Knickelbine, S. Oberembt, and L. Shaw. Association of coronary artery calcium with long-term, cause-specific mortality among young adults. *JAMA Network Open* 2, no. 7 (July 19, 2019): 1–12. https://doi.org/10.1001/jamanetworkopen.2019.7440

Montero, Carlos. The issue is not food, nor nutrients, so much as processing. Invited commentary. *Public Health Nutrition* 12, no. 5 (May 2009): 729–31. https://doi.org/10.1017/S1368980009005291

Ong, K. L., R. L. McClelland, K. A. Rye, B. M. Y. Cheung. W. S. Post, D. Vaidya, M. H. Criqui, M. Cushman, P. J. Barter, and M. A. Allison. The relationship between insulin resistance and vascular calcification in coronary arteries, and the thoracic and abdominal aorta: The Multi-Ethnic Study of Atherosclerosis. *Atherosclerosis* 236, no. 2 (October 2014): 257–62. https://doi.org/10.1016/j.atherosclerosis.2014.07.015

Oni, E. T., A. S. Agatston, M. J. Blaha, J. Fialkow, R. Cury, A. Sposito, E. Erbel et al. A systematic review: Burden and severity of subclinical cardiovascular disease among those with nonalcoholic fatty liver; should we care? *Atherosclerosis* 230, no. 2 (October 2013): 258–67. https://doi.org/10.1016/j.atherosclerosis.2013.07.052

Ozturk, Y., and O. B. Soylu. Fatty liver in childhood. *World Journal of Hepatology* 6, no. 1 (January 27, 2014): 33–40. https://doi.org/10.4254/wjh.v6.i1.33

Patterson, E., R. Wall, G. F. Fitzgerald, R. P. Ross, and C. Stanton. Health implications of high dietary omega-6 polyunsaturated fatty acids. *Journal of Nutrition and Metabolism* 2012 (November 20, 2011). https://doi.org/10.1155/2012/539426

Pfeiffer, A. F. H., and F. Keyhani-Nejad. High glycemic index metabolic damage—a pivotal role of GIP and GLP-1. *Trends in Endocrinology & Metabolism* 29, no. 5 (May 1, 2018): 289–99. https://doi.org/10.1016/j.tem.2018.03.003

Samieri, C., C. Féart, L. Letenneur, J. F. Dartigues, K. Pérès, S. Auriacombe, E. Peuchant, C. Delcourt, and P. Barberger-Gateau. Low plasma eicosapentaenoic acid and depressive symptomatology are independent predictors of dementia risk. *American Journal of Clinical Nutrition* 88, no. 3 (September 2008): 714–21. https://www.ncbi.nlm.nih.gov/pubmed/18779288

Schauer, I. E., J. K. Snell-Bergeon, B. C. Bergman, D. M. Maahs, A. Kretowski, R. H. Eckel, and M. Rewers. Insulin resistance, defective insulin-mediated fatty acid suppression, and coronary artery calcification in subjects with and without type 1 diabetes. The CACTI Study. *Diabetes Care* 60, no. 11 (January 2011): 306–14. https://doi.org/10.2337/db10-0328

Schwarz, J., [?] foot, D. Dare, and K. Aghajanian. Hepatic de novo lipogenesis in normoinsulinemic and hyperinsulinemic subjects consuming high-fat , low-carbohydrate. *American Journal of Clinical Nutrition* 77, no. 1 (January 2003): 43–50. https://www.ncbi.nlm.nih.gov/pubmed/12499321

Siri-Tarino, P. W., Q. Sun, F. B. Hu, and R. M. Krauss. Saturated fat, carbohydrate, and cardiovascular disease. *American Journal of Clinical Nutrition* 91, no. 3 (March 2010): 502–9. https://academic.oup.com/ajcn/article/91/3/502/4597078

Smith, G. I., P. Atherton, D. N. Reeds, B. S. Mohammed, D. Rankin, D., M. J. Rennie, and B. Mittendorfer. Dietary omega-3 fatty acid supplementation increases the rate of muscle protein synthesis in older adults: a randomized controlled trial. *American Journal of Clinical Nutrition* 93, no. 2 (February 2011): 402–12. https://www.ncbi.nlm.nih.gov/pubmed/21159787

Srikanthan, P., C. J. Crandall, D. Miller-Martinez, T. E. Seeman, G. A. Greendale, N. Binkley, and A. S. Karlamangla. Insulin resistance and bone strength: Findings from the study of midlife in the United States. *Journal of Bone and Mineral Research* 29, no. 4 (August 26, 2013): 796–803. https://asbmr.onlinelibrary.wiley.com/doi/full/10.1002/jbmr.2083

Stanhope, K., J. M. Schwarz, and P. Havel. Adverse metabolic effects of dietary fructose: results from the recent epidemiological, clinical, and mechanistic studies. *Current Opinion in Lipidology* 24, no. 3 (June 2013): 198–206. https://doi.org/10.1097/MOL.0b013e3283613bca.

Sugeedha, J., U. K. Putcha, V. S. Mullapudi, S. Ghosh, A. Sakamuri, S. R. Kona, S. S. Vadakattu, C. Madakasira, and A. Ibrahim. Chronic consumption of fructose in combination with trans fatty acids but not with saturated fatty acids induces nonalcoholic steatohepatitis with fibrosis in rats. *European Journal of Nutrition* 57, no. 6 (September 2018): 2171–87. https://doi.org/10.1007/s00394-017-1492-1

Sung, K., J. Choi, H. Gwon, S. Choi, B. Kim, H. J. Kwag, and S. H. Kim. Relationship between insulin resistance and coronary artery calcium in young men and women. *PLoS ONE* 8, no. 1 (January 16, 2013): e53316. https://doi.org/10.1371/journal.pone.0053316

Takahashi, K., H. Nakamura, H. Sato, H. Matsuda, K. Takada, and T. Tsuji. Four plasma glucose and insulin responses to a 75g OGTT in healthy young Japanese women. *Journal of Diabetes Research* (January 30, 2018). https://www.ncbi.nlm.nih.gov/pubmed/29629377

Toth, P. P. Epicardial steatosis, insulin resistance, and coronary artery disease. *Heart Failure Clinics* 8, no. 4 (October 2012): 671–78. https://doi.org/10.1016/j.hfc.2012.06.013

Wilcox, G. Insulin and insulin resistance. *Clinical Biochemist Reviews* 26, no. 2 (May 2005): 19–39. https://www.ncbi.nlm.nih.gov/pmc/articles/PMC1204764/

Williams, R. Liver disease in the UK: Startling findings and urgent need for action. *Journal of Hepatology* 63, no. 2 (August 2015): 297–99. https://doi.org/10.1016/j.jhep.2015.04.022

Wong, N. D., M. G. Sciammarella, D. Polk, A. Gallagher, L. Miranda-Peats, B. Whitcomb, R. Hachamovitch et al. The metabolic syndrome, diabetes, and subclinical atherosclerosis assessed by coronary calcium. *Journal of the American College of Cardiology* 41, no. 9 (May 2003): 1547–53. https://doi.org/10.1016/S0735-1097(03)00193-1

Yamazoe, M., T. Hisamatsu, K. Miura, S. Kadowaki, M. Zaid, A. Kadota, S. Torii et al. Relationship of insulin resistance to prevalence and progression of coronary artery calcification. *Arteriosclerosis, Thrombosis, and Vascular Biology* 36, no. 8 (June 9, 2016): 1703–8. https://doi.org/10.1161/ATVBAHA.116.307612

CHAPTER 5

Akilen, R., N. Deljoomanesh, S. Hunschede, C. E. Smith, M. U. Arshad, R. Kubant, and G. H. Anderson. The effects of potatoes and other carbohydrate side dishes consumed with meat on food intake, glycemia and satiety response in children. *Nutrition & Diabetes* 6, no. 2 (February 15, 2016): e195-8. https://doi.org/10.1038/nutd.2016.1

Blanchet, C. M., Lucas, P. Julien, R. Morin, S. Gingras, and E. Dewailly. Fatty acid composition of wild and farmed Atlantic salmon *(Salmo salar)* and rainbow trout *(Oncorhynchus mykiss)*. *Lipids* 40, no. 5 (May 2005): 529–31. https://www.ncbi.nlm.nih.gov/pubmed/16094864

Blasbalg, T. L. et al. Changes in consumption of omega-3 and omega-6 fatty acids in the United States during the 20th century.

Boden, G., K. Sargrad, C. Homko, M. Mozzoli, and T. P. Stein. Effect of a low-carbohydrate diet on appetite, blood glucose levels, and insulin resistance in obese patients with type 2 diabetes. *Annals of Internal Medicine* 142, no. 6 (March 15, 2005): 403–12. https://www.ncbi.nlm.nih.gov/pubmed/15767618

Chen, Y., R. Feng, X. Yang, J. Dai, M. Huang, X. Ji, Y. Li et al. Yogurt improves insulin resistance and liver fat in obese women with nonalcoholic fatty liver disease and metabolic syndrome: a randomized controlled trial. *American Journal of Clinical Nutrition* 109, no. 6 (June 1, 2019): 1611–19. https://www.ncbi.nlm.nih.gov/pubmed/31136662

De Alzaa, F. C. Guillaume, and L. Ravetti (2018). Evaluation of chemical and physical changes in different commercial oils during heating. *ACTA Scientific Nutritional Health* 2, no. 6 (May 5, 2018): 2–11. https://actascientific.com/ASNH/pdf/ASNH-02-0083.pdf

DiNicolantonio, J. J., J. Liu, and J. H. O'Keefe. (2018). Magnesium for the prevention and treatment of cardiovascular disease. *Open Heart* 5, no. 2 (July 1, 2018): e000775. https://www.ncbi.nlm.nih.gov/pmc/articles/PMC6045762/

Douchi, T., T. Matsuo, H. Uto, T. Kuwahata, T. Oki, and Y. Nagata. Lean body mass and bone mineral density in physically exercising postmenopausal women. *Maturitas* 45, no. 3 (July 25, 2003): 185–90. https://doi.org/10.1016/S0378-5122(03)00143-9

Genuis, S. J., and R. A. Lobo. Gluten sensitivity presenting as a neuropsychiatric disorder. *Gastroenterology Research and Practice* 2014 (February 12, 2014): 2–7. https://doi.org/10.1155/2014/293206

Gunnerud, U. J., E. M. Östman, and I. M. E. Björck. Effects of whey proteins on glycaemia and insulinaemia to an oral glucose load in healthy adults; a dose-response study. *European Journal of Clinical Nutrition* 67 (May 1, 2013): 749–53. https://doi.org/10.1038/ejcn.2013.88

Hartwich, J., M. M. Malec, L. Partyka, P. Pérez-Martinez, C. Marin, J. López-Miranda, A. C. Tierney et al. The effect of the plasma n-3/n-6 polyunsaturated fatty acid ratio on the dietary LDL phenotype transformation—insights from the LIPGENE study. *Clinical Nutrition* 28, no. 5 (October 2009): 510–15. https://doi.org/10.1016/j.clnu.2009.04.016

Ho, K. Y., J. D. Veldhuls, M. L. Johnson, R. Furlanetto, W. S. Evans, K. G. Alberti, and M. O. Thomer. Fasting enhances growth hormone secretion and amplifies the complex rhythms of growth hormone secretion in man. *Journal of Clinical Investigation* 81, no. 4 (April 1988): 968–75. https://www.ncbi.nlm.nih.gov/pubmed/3127426

Key, T. J. (2011). Fruit and vegetables and cancer risk. *British Journal of Cancer* 104, no. 1 (January 4, 2011): 6–11. https://doi.org/10.1038/sj.bjc.6606032

Layman, D. K., P. Clifton, M. C. Gannon, R. M. Krauss, and F. Q. Nuttall. Protein in optimal health: Heart disease and type 2 diabetes. *American Journal of Clinical Nutrition* 87, no. 5 (May 2008): 1571S-75S. https://www.ncbi.nlm.nih.gov/pubmed/18469290

Phillips, S. M., and W. Martinson. Nutrient-rich, high-quality, protein-containing dairy foods in combination with exercise in aging persons to mitigate sarcopenia. *Nutrition Reviews* 77, no. 4 (April 2019): 216–29. https://doi.org/10.1093/nutrit/nuy062

Woo, S., J. Yang, M. Hsu, A.Yang, L. Zhang, R. P. Lee, I. Gilbuena et al. Effects of branched-chain amino acids on glucose metabolism in obese , prediabetic men and women: A randomized crossover study. *American Journal of Clinical Nutrition* 109, no. 6 (June 1, 2019): 1569–77. https://www.ncbi.nlm.nih.gov/pubmed/31005973

SUGGESTED READING

Agatston, Arthur. *The South Beach Diet Gluten Solution*. New York: Rodale, 2014.

Cummins, Ivor, and Jeffry Gerber. *Eat Rich, Live Long: Use the Power of Low-Carb and Keto for Weight Loss and Great Health*. Las Vegas: Victory Belt Publishing, 2018.

Fung, Jason. *The Obesity Code*. Vancouver: Greystone Books, 2016.

Hyman, Mark. *The Blood Sugar Solution: 10-Day Detox Diet*. New York: Little, Brown, 2014.

Ludwig, David S. *Always Hungry?: Conquer Cravings, Retrain Your Fat Cells, and Lose Weight Permanently*. New York: Grand Central Life & Style, 2016.

Lustig, Robert H. *The Hacking of the American Mind: The Science Behind the Corporate Takeover of Our Bodies and Brains*. New York: Avery, 2016.

Noakes, Tim. *The Lore of Nutrition*. Cape Town: Penguin Random House South Africa, 2018.

Phinney, Stephen D., and Jeff S. Volek. *The Art and Science of Low Carbohydrate Living: An Expert Guide to Making the Life-Saving Benefits of Carbohydrate Restriction Sustainable and Enjoyable*. Miami: Beyond Obesity, 2018.

Taubes, Gary. *Good Calories, Bad Calories: Fats, Carbs, and the Controversial Science of Diet and Health*. New York: Knopf, 2007.

Teicholz, Nina. *The Big Fat Surprise: Why Butter, Meat and Cheese Belong in a Healthy Diet*. New York: Simon & Schuster, 2014.

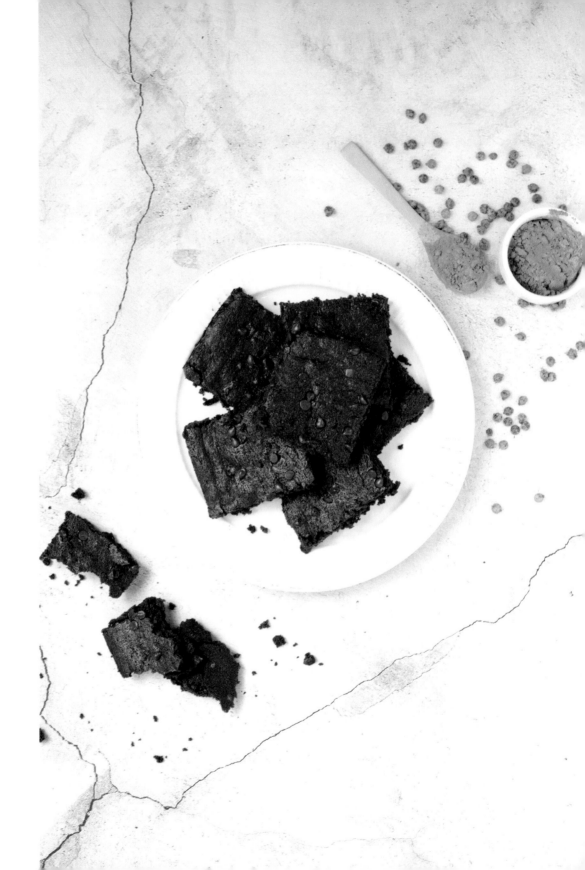

INDEX

Note: Page numbers in *italics* indicate recipe photos on pages separate from recipes.

A

addiction, to sugar, 3, 5–6, 7–8, 18, 42, 90

Agatston Calcium Score, 51–52

aging, 42, 71, 72

alcohol consumption, 3–4, 53, 91

almond butter

  about, 85

  Chocolate Chip Cookie Dough Bites variation, 286

  Chocolate Freezer Fudge, 276–277

  Deviled Egg Salad, 170–171

  Peanut Butter Cups tip, 285

almond flour

  about, 80, 89; keto-friendly tortillas tip, 231; pizza crusts, 210–*211*, 240–241

  Almond Flour Chicken Piccata, *200*–201

  Almond Flour Tortilla Chips, 177, *252*–253

almonds

  about, 85

  Cream of Broccoli Soup, *178*–179

  Grab-and-Go Nut & Berry Yogurt Bark, *152*–153

  Smoky Goat Cheese & Almond Balls, *264*–265

  Warm Raspberry Crisp, *274*–275

Alzheimer prevention, 53–54

American Plains Indians, 44

anchovies, 85

Arroyo, Juan, 8

arteriosclerosis, 16–17, 27, 41, 44, 50–52

artichokes

  about, 87

  Heirloom Tomato Lasagna, 238–*239*

  Spinach & Artichoke Quiche Cups, *144*–145

arugula, 150–*151*

Asian diet paradox, 44–45, 72

Asian dipping sauce tip, 212

asparagus, 257

atherogenic lipid profile, 50

athletic performance, 21–22, 54–55, 62

avocado oil, 65, 82

avocados

  about: storage tip, 234

  Cauliflower Tahini Rice Bowl, 192

  Fish Tacos with Creamy Avocado Sauce, 230–*231*

  Homemade Guacamole, *252*–253

  Mini Taco Salads with Cilantro-Lime Yogurt Dip, 234–*235*

  Moroccan Lentil Stew, 242–243

  Savory Pesto Yogurt Bowls, *262*–263

  Shrimp & Avocado Salad, 180–*181*

  Smoked Salmon Bowl, 142–*143*

  Smoky Goat Cheese & Almond Balls, *264*–265

  Warm Avocado with Egg, 150–*151*

B

bacon

  Buffalo Chicken Zucchini Boats, 198–*199*

  Cream of Broccoli Soup, *178*–179

  Egg Cups 3 Ways, 138–*139*

  Lemon-Rosemary Braised Chicken Breasts, *188*–189

  Parmesan Roasted Brussels Sprouts tip, 248

  Spinach & Artichoke Quiche Cups, *144*–145

  Warm Avocado with Egg tip, 151

basil pesto, *262*–263

beans and legumes. *See also specific beans and legumes*

  about, 63, 79, 89, 91

  Beef & Vegetable Stew, 214–*215*

  Buffalo Chicken Zucchini Boats, 198–*199*

  Chicken Fajita Bowl, 204–205

  Chockfull of Veggie Chili, *182*–183

  Cinnamon Roasted Chickpeas, *270*–271

  Creamy Cauliflower & Chicken, *208*–209

  Moroccan Lentil Stew, 242–243

  Pumpkin & Black Bean Chili, 176–*177*

  Thai Chickpea Curry, 186–*187*

beef

  about, 52, 70–71, 84; shepherd's pie substitute tip, 223

  Beef & Vegetable Stew, 214–*215*

  Beef Burrito Bowls, 174–175

  Kale Caesar Salad tip, 237

  Keto Spaghetti & Meatballs, *196*–197

Heirloom Tomato Lasagna, 238–*239*

hemoglobin A1C, 27, 28, 64

hemp seeds, 85, 256, 266, *278*–279

Herbed Seed Crackers, 256

herring, 70, 85

high blood pressure, 41, 53

high-fat, high-protein, low-carb diets, 43–44

high-fructose corn syrup (HFCS), 32–33, 40, 44, 55–56

Home-Style Chicken & "Rice," *232*–233

hormones. *See also* insulin; insulin resistance
    hunger and, 75–76
    incretins, 34–35, 43
    sugar and, 31–35, 44–45, 64–65
    weight set points and, 30, 71

hunger, 22–23, 32, 75–76

hunter-gatherer diet, 44

hydration, 74, 76

hydrogenation process, 37

I

incretins, 34–35, 43

infertility, 67

instant oatmeal, 35–36

insulin
    about, 20–21, 26
    athletes and, 21–22
    bear hibernation example, 23–24
    diabetes pandemic, 28, 38, 53, 54, 55, 57
    grazing (snacking) and, 33
    as growth factor, 54
    hunger and, 22–23
    insulin resistance vs. high blood sugar, 24–25

keto flu and, 73–74
measuring levels of, 25
oral insulin tolerance test (OITT), 27
overdrive, 22
pre-prediabetes, 12, 19–20, 24
regulation of, 34–35
weight set points and, 30

insulin resistance
    about, 12, 41, 55–57
    aging and, 42, 71
    atherogenic lipid profile and, 50
    blood sugar levels *vs.*, 24–25
    brain health and, 53–54
    cancer and, 54
    cholesterol and, 50–51
    cravings due to, 5–6
    fat accumulation and, 56–57
    fructose and, 40–41
    genetic influence, 56
    high blood pressure and, 41, 53
    infertility and, 67
    recommendations for, 42–43, 56
    sugar and, 34–35, 56
    in teens, 42

insulin secretion test, 12

intermittent fasting, 12, 76

Isaacson, Richard, 53–54

J

Janowitz, Warren, 51

K

kale
    about, 87
    Chicken Shepherd's Pie, *222*–223
    Kale Caesar Salad, 237
    Mexican Breakfast Bake, 160
    Portobello Shakshuka, 206–*207*
    Smoked Salmon Bowl, 142–*143*
    Spiced Turkey & Sweet Potato Bowl, 190–*191*

K cells, of small intestine, 34–35

Keto Brownies, 280–*281*

Keto Cloud Bread 2 Ways, 258–*259*

keto flu, 64, 73–75

ketones and ketosis, 14–16, 53–54, 72

Keto Spaghetti & Meatballs, *196*–197

kidneys, 41, 53, 73–74

King, David, 51

Kraft, Joseph R., 27–28

Kraft insulin secretion test, 27–28, 52, 56, 64

Kraus, Ron, 50

L

lactose intolerance, 69

lamb, 84, *224*–225

lasagna, 238–*239*

latte, 164–*165*, 167

L cells, of small intestine, 34–35

LDL cholesterol, 37, 40–41, 42, 44, 50–52

leaky gut, 67

legumes. *See* beans and legumes

Lemon-Rosemary Braised Chicken Breasts, *188*–189

lentils, 63, 89, 242–*243*

lettuce wraps, 181, 230–*231*

liquid conversion charts, 288

liver damage and failure, 39, 40–41, 53, 54–56, 89

liver enzyme tests, 64

Loja women, 44–45, 54

low-carb (keto) flu, 64, 73–75

Ludwig, David, 27, 32, 35

lunch (recipe overview), 134

Lustig, Robert H., 5, 41–42

M

Maasai tribe diet, 43, 44, 72

Macadamia nuts, 85

mackerel, 70, 85

magnesium, 74, 76

Mango Quinoa, 226–*227*

maple cinnamon trail mix, 267

marathon runners, 21–22, 54–55

marinades, *212*–213

mashed potato substitute, 222–*223*, 254–*255*

mayonnaise, 80

MCT oil, 86, 166, *278–279*

meatballs, *196*–197

meat intake, 43–44, 84. *See also specific meats*

medium-chain triglycerides (MCT), 69–70

memory problems, 53–54

microgreens, 150–*151*

milk. *See also* coconut milk; dairy products
Chia Tea Latte, 164–*165*
Creamy Protein Latte, 167
Mocha Frappé, 166

Mini Taco Salads, 234–*235*

Mocha Frappé, 166

Mongolian diet, 43, 44, 72

monk fruit, 80, 81, 89

monounsaturated fats, 70

Monterey Jack cheese, *204*–205

Moroccan Lentil Stew, 242–*243*

mozzarella cheese
Cheesy Garlic Cauliflower Breadsticks, 268–269
Pepperoni & Goat Cheese Pizza, *240*–241
Prosciutto & Gouda Pizza, 210–*211*
Warm Avocado with Egg, 150–*151*

muffins, 146–*147*, 156–*157*

muscle cramping, 74

mushrooms
Beef & Vegetable Stew, 214–*215*
Heirloom Tomato Lasagna, 238–*239*
Home-Style Chicken & "Rice," *232*–233
Portobello Shakshuka, 206–*207*
Radicchio & Mushroom Gratin, 257
Stuffed Chicken Breast with Zucchini Fettuccine, 216–217

N

Nasir, Khurram, 51

Native Americans, 43, 44

net carbs, 64–65, 66

New England Journal of Medicine
on Ecuadorian diet, 44–45
on salt intake, 75

Noakes, Tim, 54–55

nonalcoholic liver disease, 41

nonhydrogenated vegetable oils, 37–38

noodles (zoodles), 81, *196*–197, 216–217

nuts. *See specific nuts, nut flours, and nut butters*

O

oatmeal, 35–36

obesity, 28, 41–42, 54

oils
excess use of, 65
keto-friendly options, 37, 39, 52, 65, 69–70, 76, 81, 82, 86, 164
MCT oil, 86, 166, *278–279*
omega-6 oils, 18, 36–39, 45, 56, 70–71

Okinawans, 44

olive oil, 39, 52, 65, 69, 82, 86

olives, 88, 145, 150, 218–*219*

omega-3 fatty acids, 33, 38–39, 69–71, 85

omega-6 vegetable oils, 18, 36–39, 45, 56, 70–71

oral glucose tolerance test (OGTT), 27–28

oral insulin tolerance test (OITT), 27–28

P

pancetta, *144*–145, *188*–189

pancreas
fat accumulation in, 41, 54, 55, 57
fructose and, 40–41
function of, 26
incretin effect and, 34
insulin resistance and, 20, 22, 25, 42

pancreatic cancer, 54

pantry essentials, 89

Parmesan cheese
Cheesy Garlic Cauliflower Breadsticks, 268–269
Garlic & Parmesan Mashed Cauliflower, 254–*255*
Heirloom Tomato Lasagna, 238–*239*
Keto Cloud Bread topping, 258–*259*

Sticky Sesame Chicken, *212*–213

strawberries, *152*–153

strokes, 41, 50–51

Stuffed Chicken Breast with Zucchini Fettuccine, 216–217

subcutaneous fat, 44–45, 56

sugar
    addiction to, 3, 5–6, 7–8, 18, 42, 90
    digestion of, 34–36, 40
    effects of excessive sugar, 39
    history of, 32
    hormones and, 31–35, 44–45, 64–65
    insulin levels and, 34–35, 56
    metabolism, in brain, 53–54
    obesity and, 30–31, 32
    in processed foods, 34
    recommendations for, 56
    structure of, 40

sugar alcohols, 64, 66

sugar snap peas, *228*–229

sunflower seeds, 256, *278*–279

Superko, Robert, 50

supersizing meals, 33, 55–56

Sweet & Salty Trail Mix, 267

sweeteners, 64, 66, 80, 81, 89

sweet potatoes, 154–*155*, 190–*191*

sweets (recipe overview), 135

T

tacos
    Fish Tacos with Creamy Avocado Sauce, 230–*231*
    Mini Taco Salads, 234–*235*
    Spicy Parmesan Crisps tip, 266

tahini, *272*–273, *278*–279

tea, 81, 164–*165*

teen obesity, 41–42

temperature conversion charts, 289

textured soy protein, *182*–183

Thai Chickpea Curry, 186–*187*

Thai Chopped Chicken Salad, 173

Thai dressing, 173

TOFI (thin on the outside and fat on the inside), 55

tomatoes, 238–*239*, 242–*243*, 262–*263*

tomato sauces, *196*–197, 206–*207*

tortilla wraps tip, 231

trail mixes, 267

trans fats, 37

triathletes, 55

triglycerides, 42, 50, 56, 64

tuna, 70, 85

turkey
    about: shepherd's pie substitute tip, 223
    Cilantro-Lime Turkey Burgers, *220*–221
    Mini Taco Salads with Cilantro-Lime Yogurt Dip, 234–*235*
    Spiced Turkey & Sweet Potato Bowl, 190–*191*
    turkey bacon, 248
    turnips, 214–*215*
    Tzatziki Sauce, *224*–225

U

U.S. Food and Drug Administration, 37

V

vegetable oils, 18, 36–39, 45, 56, 70–71

vegetables. *See also specific vegetables and recipes*
    about, 72–73, 87, 90; dips for, 236
    Beef & Vegetable Stew, 214–215
    Chockfull of Veggie Chili, *182*–183
    Sesame-Glazed Beef & Veggie Bowl, *228*–229

veggie crumbles, *182*–183

visceral fat, 19, 41, 42, 55

VLDL (very-low-density lipoprotein), 40, 41, 56

Volek, Jeff, 14, 54, 55

W

waffles, *158*–159

walnuts
    about, 70, 85
    Grab-and-Go Nut & Berry Yogurt Bark, *152*–153
    Zucchini Feta Salad tip, 251

Warm Avocado with Egg, 150–*151*

Warm Raspberry Crisp, *274*–275

watercress, 257

weigh-in (daily), 48

weight set points, 30, 71

Weinberg, Sylvan L., 48

Westman, Eric C., 36

whey protein, 72, 80, 85

white beans, 208–209, 214–*215*

white mushrooms, 257

wraps, 181, 218–*219*

Y

yellow squash, 216–217, 238–*239*

yogurt

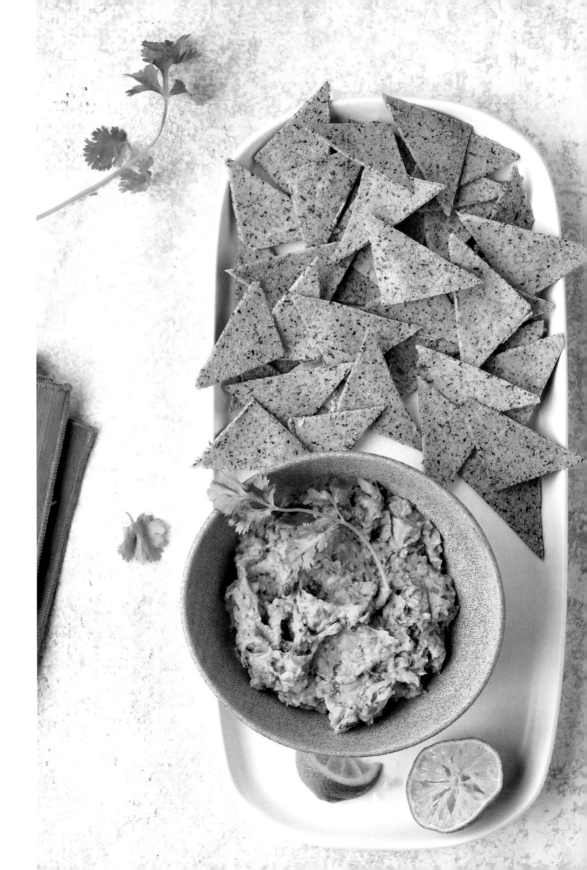

ACKNOWLEDGMENTS

First, my special thanks to the two outstanding editors who worked tirelessly and expertly with me to produce this book, Tami Booth Corwin and my wife, Sari.

From the original development of the South Beach Diet and the Coronary Calcium Score (aka Agatston Score), to the present, I have enjoyed the benefit of a remarkable continuing education. This has come from colleagues, many of whom have become friends or acquaintances; others I have not yet had the pleasure to meet but have heard their lectures and read their books and articles.

It was from one such colleague, Dr. Robert Lustig, a pediatric endocrinologist from the University of California, San Francisco, whose book, *The Hacking of the American Mind*, caused me to recognize my addiction to sugar and the critical role of sugar addiction in the obesity and diabetes epidemic. He also did much to teach me and many others about the singular metabolic role of fructose-laden sugars in our health care crisis.

Another colleague, Dr. David Ludwig, a Harvard pediatric endocrinologist and a leader in low-carbohydrate research since its early days, continues to break new ground. His recent contributions have taught us that low-carb diets decrease insulin blood levels and increase our metabolic rates, allowing for faster weight loss.

Dr. Jason Fung, a Toronto nephrologist, has been the thought leader in the area of intermittent fasting as an adjunct to low-carb dieting. We have found intermittent fasting to be an important option in helping many of our patients find success on the Keto-Friendly South Beach Diet.

The Virta Health group, led by Drs. Sarah Hallberg, Stephen D. Phinney, and Jeff S. Volek, has demonstrated for the first time in a clinical trial that diabetes can be reversed by a well-formulated keto low-carb diet when patients are remotely monitored and coached. They are great researchers and superb teachers.

Dr. Robert Superko and his RN wife, Brenda, are longtime mentors and friends. They introduced me and physicians all over the country to the importance of LDL size 25 years ago and were way ahead of their time. We now know that small LDL particles are an unfortunate result of too much sugar in our diet and are making us sick. Thank you Superkos!

Another mentor, mentee, and close friend, Dr. Khurram Nasir, has been a leader in demonstrating how the coronary calcium score can be used in everyday clinical practice to save lives and health care dollars.

Ivor Cummins, a biomechanical engineer, is the chief program officer for Irish Heart Disease Awareness, a group that promotes the use of coronary artery calcium scanning to save lives. Ivor has led the way in teaching that early detection of insulin resistance combined with early detection of coronary atherosclerosis can prevent heart attacks and diabetes. His efforts are saving lives. Our message in this book is very much along the same lines.

The amazing clinical team I work with daily has provided inspiration and support during our collective journey in the development of our keto-friendly diet program. They include my physician colleagues, Drs. Judi Woolger, Cindy Shaffer, and Jim Trice; our outstanding nutritionists Ellen Janunzzi and Shira Gluck; and our clinical RN and invaluable coordinator Rebecca Lormand.

I would also like to thank Courtney McCormick of Tivity Health for her considerable help and expertise. And a special thank you to Robin Shallow, also of Tivity Health, who knew I was excited about the latest science and pushed this project forward.

Finally, I would like to thank Mary Norris and Sheridan McCarthy at Hay House, for their editorial review under the leadership of Anne Barthel and Patty Gift.

ABOUT THE AUTHOR

Arthur Agatston, M.D., is an internationally recognized pioneer in cardiac disease prevention. Dr. Agatston worked with Dr. Warren Janowitz to develop the Agatston Score (also called the Calcium Score), a method of screening for coronary calcium as an indicator of atherosclerosis that is used at medical centers throughout the world and considered by most experts to be the best single predictor of a future heart attack.

Dr. Agatston and colleagues initiated the "Healthy Options in Public Schools" study, which demonstrated that by providing healthy school lunches, combined with an innovative education program in pre-K through grade 6, you can encourage healthy weights and improve blood pressures and standardized test scores in children. This project continues through the "Agatston Urban Nutrition Initiative" at the University of Pennsylvania.

Dr. Agatston is an associate professor of medicine at the University of Miami Miller School of Medicine and a clinical professor of medicine at Florida International University Herbert Wertheim College of Medicine. He is a member of the American College of Cardiology Nutrition Committee. He is the medical director of The Agatston Center for Private Medicine in Miami Beach, where his cardiology practice is focused on preventing heart attacks in high-risk patients. This is also the focus of his continuing research endeavors.

Known as the author of the internationally best-selling book *The South Beach Diet*, his first nonacademic work, Dr. Agatston created his balanced approach to healthy eating to help his patients improve their blood chemistries, lose weight, and prevent diabetes and heart disease. Today, the South Beach Diet remains the trusted choice of millions and there are more than 23 million copies of *The South Beach Diet* and its companion books in print worldwide. Dr. Agatston's most recent book, *The South Beach Diet Gluten Solution,* was published in 2013.

Dr. Agatston has published more than 200 scientific articles and abstracts in medical journals and is a frequent lecturer across the U.S. and around the world on diet, cardiac imaging, and the prevention of heart disease. In recognition of his contributions to cardiac prevention, the Society of Cardiovascular Computed Tomography (SCCT) created the prestigious Arthur S. Agatston Cardiovascular Disease Prevention Award in 2011, which is given annually to pioneers in cardiac prevention. He was named as one of the "Time 100" most influential people of 2004. Among his many television appearances, Dr. Agatston was featured along with President Bill Clinton on Sanjay Gupta's 2011 CNN special, "The Last Heart Attack."

We hope you enjoyed this Hay House book. If you'd like to receive our online catalog featuring additional information on Hay House books and products, or if you'd like to find out more about the Hay Foundation, please contact:

Hay House, Inc., P.O. Box 5100, Carlsbad, CA 92018-5100
(760) 431-7695 or (800) 654-5126
(760) 431-6948 (fax) or (800) 650-5115 (fax)
www.hayhouse.com® • www.hayfoundation.org

———

Published in Australia by: Hay House Australia Pty. Ltd.,
18/36 Ralph St., Alexandria NSW 2015
Phone: 612-9669-4299 • *Fax:* 612-9669-4144
www.hayhouse.com.au

Published in the United Kingdom by: Hay House UK, Ltd.,
The Sixth Floor, Watson House, 54 Baker Street, London W1U 7BU
Phone: +44 (0)20 3927 7290 • *Fax:* +44 (0)20 3927 7291
www.hayhouse.co.uk

Published in India by: Hay House Publishers India,
Muskaan Complex, Plot No. 3, B-2, Vasant Kunj, New Delhi 110 070
Phone: 91-11-4176-1620 • *Fax:* 91-11-4176-1630
www.hayhouse.co.in

———

Access New Knowledge.
Anytime. Anywhere.

Learn and evolve at your own pace
with the world's leading experts.

www.hayhouseU.com

ALSO BY
ARTHUR AGATSTON

The South Beach Diet

The South Beach Diet Cookbook

The South Beach Diet Heart Health Revolution

The South Beach Diet Quick & Easy Cookbook

The South Beach Diet Wake-Up Call

The South Beach Diet Supercharged

The South Beach Diet Gluten Solution